Mediterranean quarantines, 1750–1914

MANCHESTER 1824

Manchester University Press

SOCIAL HISTORIES OF MEDICINE

Series editors: David Cantor and Keir Waddington

Social Histories of Medicine is concerned with all aspects of health, illness and medicine, from prehistory to the present, in every part of the world. The series covers the circumstances that promote health or illness, the ways in which people experience and explain such conditions, and what, practically, they do about them. Practitioners of all approaches to health and healing come within its scope, as do their ideas, beliefs, and practices, and the social, economic and cultural contexts in which they operate. Methodologically, the series welcomes relevant studies in social, economic, cultural, and intellectual history, as well as approaches derived from other disciplines in the arts, sciences, social sciences and humanities. The series is a collaboration between Manchester University Press and the Society for the Social History of Medicine.

Previously published

The metamorphosis of autism: A history of child development in Britain *Bonnie Evans*

Payment and philanthropy in British healthcare, 1918–48 *George Campbell Gosling*

The politics of vaccination: A global history *Edited by Christine Holmberg, Stuart Blume and Paul Greenough*

Leprosy and colonialism: Suriname under Dutch rule, 1750–1950 *Stephen Snelders*

Medical misadventure in an age of professionalization, 1780–1890 *Alannah Tomkins*

Conserving health in early modern culture: Bodies and environments in Italy and England *Edited by Sandra Cavallo and Tessa Storey*

Migrant architects of the NHS: South Asian doctors and the making of British general practice (1940s–1980s) *Julian M. Simpson*

Mediterranean Quarantines, 1750–1914

Space, identity and power

John Chircop and Francisco Javier Martínez

Manchester University Press

Published by Manchester University Press
Altrincham Street, Manchester M1 7JA

www.manchesteruniversitypress.co.uk

British Library Cataloguing-in-Publication Data
A catalogue record for this book is available from the British Library

ISBN 978 1 5261 1554 6 hardback

ISBN 978 1 5261 2736 5 open access

First published 2018

Typeset
by Toppan Best-set Premedia Limited
Printed in Great Britain
by Lightning Source

Contents

List of figures

List of tables

Notes on contributors

Laurinda Abreu is Professor of History at the University of Évora, Portugal. Her specialist field is the history of poor relief and health in the Early Modern period. She is Director of the Erasmus Mundus PhD – Phoenix JDP on Dynamics of Health and Welfare. She was the coordinator (2001–09) of the Phoenix TN – European Thematic Network on Health and Social Welfare Policy. She was President (2011–13) of the European Association for the History of Medicine and Health. Her recent publications include: *The Political and Social Dynamics of Poverty, Poor Relief and Health Care in Early-Modern Portugal* (London and New York, Routledge, 2016) and a co-edited book *Hospital Life: Theory and Practice from the Medieval to the Modern* (with S. Sheard, Oxford, Peter Lang, 2013).

Jon Arrizabalaga is Research Professor in History of Science at the Spanish National Research Council (CSIC), Institución Milà i Fontanals (IMF), Barcelona, Spain. His research is mostly focused on medicine, health and disease in Pre-modern Europe; and on biomedical technologies and social movements in the modern world, with particular attention to humanitarian action and war medicine in modern Spain. His most recent publications include 'War, empire, science, progress, humanitarianism. Debate and practice within the international Red Cross movement from 1863 to the interwar period' (*Asclepio*, 2014, 66/1) and the volumes *Nicasio Landa. 'Muertos y heridos', y otros textos* (edited with Guillermo Sánchez, Pamplona, Pamiela, 2016) and *'It All Depends on the Dose'.*

Poisons and Medicines in European History (edited with Ole P. Grell and Andrew Cunningham, London, Routledge, 2017).

Dominique Bon is responsible for the Regional Fund at the Library of Monaco and a PhD student in Anthropology at the University of Nice Sophia Antipolis (LAPCOS – Laboratoire d'Anthropologie et de Psychologie cognitives et sociales). His anthropological research on the notion of contagion is carried out within the framework of an epidemiology of representations. His historical research focuses on sea and land health policies in the Province of Nice, the Sardinian States and the Principality of Monaco in the nineteenth century.

Quim Bonastra is Professor of Human Geography at the University of Lleida where he teaches at the faculty of Education, Psychology and Social Work. He is a member of the Department of Geography and Sociology. He holds a doctorate from the University of Barcelona. Currently his main research interests are in the areas of the geography and history of spaces of control at various scales ranging from the architectural to the territorial, and transdisciplinary education around and through artistic practices. He is a member of the Espai Híbrid collective (www.espaihibrid.udl.cat) and of the editorial team of *Scripta Nova*, a journal of geography and social sciences (http://revistes.ub.edu/index.php/ScriptaNova/index).

John Chircop is Associate Professor in Comparative Social and Economic History with the Department of History and Chairperson of the Mediterranean Institute, the University of Malta. He is also a co-founder of the Quarantine Studies Network. His research focuses on public health, medicine, poor relief and vulnerability in the British Mediterranean colonies (Gibraltar, Ionian Islands, Malta and Cyprus) from 1800 to the 1930s. Besides his numerous research papers in academic journals and chapters in books, his recent publications include: *Vulnerability: Social Inequality and Health* (edited with P. Bourdelais, Lisbon, Edições Colibri, 2010) and *Colonial Encounters: Maltese Experiences of British Rule 1800–1970s* (Malta, Horizons, 2015).

Malika Ezzahidi is Professor of History in the Faculty of Arts and Human Sciences, Hassan II University of Casablanca. She holds a doctorate from the Mohammed V University of Rabat. She is an active member of the doctorate programme 'History of the City in the

Mediterranean', as well as of the Laboratory of History and Translation in the same faculty. Her publications include *'Al Bâder Assafîr ...' Journey to Malta and Naples (1781–1782)* (Beirut, Arab Institute for Studies and Publishing, 2013), 'Le rachat des Captifs musulmans à Malte en 1782 ...' (*Cahiers de la Méditerranée*, 87, December 2013) and *Diplomatic Personality in the Modern Era. Ibn Othman Al Maknassî as a Model* (Rabat, CCME, 2016).

Juan Carlos García-Reyes is a research manager at Instituto de Salud Carlos III (Madrid, Spain). He was a research fellow JAE-CSIC at the Institution Milà i Fontanals (CSIC, Barcelona, 2008–13). After taking his MA in the History of Science at the Universitat Autònoma de Barcelona (2009), he is now working on a PhD thesis on the origins and early history of the Spanish Red Cross.

Angelos Hatzakis is Professor of Epidemiology and Preventive Medicine, in the Medical School of the National & Kapodistrian University of Athens, Greece. He is founder of the National Retrovirus Reference Center, Athens, Greece, and former President of the Hellenic Center for Disease Control and Prevention. He is also founder and Co-Chair of the 'Hepatitis B & C Public Policy Association', Luxembourg. He participates in many executive committees in both the private and public sectors. His research interests cover epidemiology, virology, preventive medicine and public health of infectious diseases – especially HIV/AIDS, hepatitis and other oncogenic viruses – with more than 280 international scientific publications and more than 13,000 citations.

Francisco Javier Martínez is FCT Investigator Researcher at the CIDEHUS of the University of Évora, Portugal. His research focuses on the history of medicine, public health and humanitarian relief in contemporary Morocco, especially in relation to Spanish and French colonial interventions. He has also investigated Morocco's scientific modernisation in the nineteenth and twentieth centuries and the life and writings of modern Spanish travellers to the Arab-Islamic world. Recent publications include 'The Pasteur Institutes in the Maghreb during the colonial period' in the journal *Dynamis* (2016); the chapter 'Weak Nation-states and the Limits of Humanitarian Aid: The Case of Morocco's Rif War, 1921–1927' in the volume *Dilemmas of Humanitarian*

Aid in the 20th Century (Oxford, OUP, 2016) and the biography *Viajes por Marruecos de Joaquín Gatell* (Madrid, Miraguano, 2014).

Effie Poulakou-Rebelakou graduated from the National & Kapodistrian University of Athens Medical School and Greek Literature School (Department of Medieval and Neo-Hellenic Literature). Her current position is Associated Professor of the History of Medicine and Director of the Department of the History of Medicine at the National & Kapodistrian University of Athens Medical School. She is a member of Greek, European and international societies for the history of medicine and Vice-President of the International Society of the History of Medicine.

Christian Promitzer is a Research Fellow at the Institute of History, division for Southeast European History, at the University of Graz. He was head of the multiannual research project 'Infectious Diseases and Public Health in Southeast Europe' focusing mainly on the nineteenth century and on the early twentieth century up to the Balkan Wars. He is also co-editor of the volumes *(Hidden) Minorities between Central Europe and the Balkans* (Berlin-Munster, Lit Verlag, 2009), *Health, Hygiene and Eugenics in Southeastern Europe to 1945* (Budapest and New York, CEU Press, 2011) and of *Southeast European Studies in a Globalizing World* (Berlin-Munster, Lit Verlag, 2015).

Joana Maria Pujadas-Mora is team leader of the area of Historical Demography at the Centre d'Estudis Demogràfics – Universitat Autònoma de Barcelona. She received her PhD in 2009 from the Universitat de les Illes Balears. Part of her dissertation was done at the Spanish National Research Council. From 2011–16 she worked in the Department of Geography of the Universitat Autònoma de Barcelona, as scientific coordinator of the ERC Advanced Grant Project 'Five Centuries of Marriages'. Her research interests are in the field of social history and historical demography. Some of her more recent publications are as follows: 'Bridging the Gap between Historical Demography and Computing: Tools for Computer-assisted Transcription and Analysis of Demographic Sources' (co-authored with A. Fornés, J. Lladós and A. Cabré, *The Future of Historical Demography*, Leuven, Acco, 2016), 'El cólera como conflicto y factor de legitimación, Palma 1865' [Cholera as a factor of conflict and legitimization, Palma, 1865] (with P. Salas,

Ayer, 2016) and 'Reconstructing Lifespans Using Historical Marriage Records of Catalonia from the 16th and 17th Centuries' (with F. Villavicencio and J.P. Jordà in *Population Reconstruction*, Switzerland, Springer, 2015).

Lisa Rosner is Distinguished Professor of Historical Studies at Stockton University, Galloway, New Jersey, USA. She received an AB from Princeton University and a PhD from Johns Hopkins University. Recent publications include *The Anatomy Murders* (Pennsylvania, University of Pennsylvania Press, 2009) and *Vaccination and Its Critics* (California, ABC-Clio, 2017). She is the recipient of grants and fellowships from the National Endowment for the Humanities, the American Philosophical Society and the Chemical Heritage Foundation.

Pere Salas-Vives is Associate Professor in Modern History in the History Department of the University of the Balearic Islands, where he teaches European Modern History (nineteenth century), World History (twentieth century), and European Population History (eighteenth–twentieth centuries). His main research concerns are on the study of local power, public health and local administration from a historical view. Among his publications are: 'La gestión de la salud pública en tiempo de epidemias: cordones y cuarentenas, medidas obsoletas?' [The Management of Public Health in Times of Epidemics: Cordons and Quarantines, Obsolete Measures?] in E. Perdiguero Gil and J.M. Vidal Hernández, *La ciudadela de los fantasmas. Lazaretos y protección sanitaria en el mundo moderno* (Menorca, Istitut Menorqui d'Estudios, 2010); 'Libertad y/o derecho a la vida. El resguardo sanitario durante el primer liberalismo (Mallorca, siglo XIX)' [Freedom and/or right to live. The sanitary defence during the first Liberalism (Mallorca, XIX century)], published in *Historia Social* (2010) and 'El delito de ser miserable. Seguridad pública e higiene en Palma 1852–1868' [The Crime of Being Poor. Public Safety and Hygiene in Palma 1852–1868], in the XIII Congreso de la Asociación de Historia Contemporánea: *La Historia, lost in translation?*, Universidad de Castilla la Mancha (Ediciones Universidad de Castilla la Mancha, 2016).

Eleni Thalassinou graduated from the School of Nursing, at the National & Kapodistrian University of Athens. She has a Master's Degree in Public Health from the School of Nursing of the National &

Kapodistrian University of Athens and a PhD from the Medical School of the same institution. Her PhD was entitled 'Plague an Acute Infectious Disease: Its Epidemiology through History'. She worked for the Hellenic Center for Disease Control and Prevention from 2003 until 2005 and for the National Organization Against Drugs from 2005 to date. She also worked as a Professor's Assistant in the Department of Nursing of the Technological Educational Institute of Western Greece from 2005 until 2008. Her academic interests include epidemiology, infectious diseases and the history of medicine.

Costas Tsiamis is cytologist and researcher at the Department of Microbiology, Medical School, National & Kapodistrian University of Athens, Greece. He has a PhD in Epidemiology (Department of Hygiene, Epidemiology and Medical Statistics, Medical School, National & Kapodistrian University of Athens). He teaches Historical Epidemiology at the Postgraduate Program of Historical Demography (Department of History, Ionian University, Corfu–Greece) and Humanitarian Medicine at the Postgraduate Program of International Medicine – Health Crisis Management (Athens Medical School). The main topics of his medico-historical studies are the history of epidemics and the history of public health during the nineteenth century and the interwar period.

Introduction
Mediterranean quarantine disclosed: space, identity and power

John Chircop and Francisco Javier Martínez

Histories and memories of quarantine – the well-known collective practice of defence against epidemic disease that acquired global reach in modern times – still lead back to the Mediterranean, the region which gave birth to this institution in fourteenth-century Italian city-states and embedded its evolution up until our present days. Sometimes it is the word itself, derived from the Venetian dialect *quaranta giorni* (forty days) and appropriated elsewhere around the Mare Nostrum, that still conveys effectively the medieval fear of that deadliest of pestilences, the Black Death, and the confusing horror of dying in enforced reclusion in small, beautiful islands surrounded by blue waters. Modern writers hailing from Mediterranean countries have exploited with worldwide success this memory potential in masterful works where quarantine is either literally or metaphorically used, from Albert Camus' *La peste* to Afnan el-Qasem's *Quarantaine à Tunis*, from José Saramago's *Ensaio sobre a cegueira* to Jean-Marie Gustave Le Clézio's *Quarantaine*. Other times, however, what continues to strike people is rather the material evidence that the *al-Bahr al-Abyad Mutawassiṭ* – the White Middle Sea of the Arabs – holds the most dense and impressive collection of old lazarettos in the world. In dozens of port towns on both sides of the sea, from Mahón to Istanbul, Marseilles to Ghar El Melh, Beirut to Venice, Piraeus to Algiers, Malta to Corfu, Lisbon to Essaouira (the latter two Atlantic ports, though with strong commercial and sanitary links with the Mediterranean), it is still possible to see the remains of those institutions, in some cases regretfully forgotten, left to deteriorate or ruined, in other cases restored as heritage museums and conference centres, or turned into luxury hotels and stylish restaurants.

As if following this mutation of Mediterranean lazarettos, the last decades have also seen the historiographical picture of modern quarantine deeply transformed thanks to the application of new, elaborate theoretical insights and cutting-edge research and approaches from a wide spectrum of disciplines. Traditionally, there existed an abundance of studies on the preventive strategies deployed in various localities against the recurrent epidemics of plague, cholera and yellow fever – with attention being paid to specific lazarettos and sanitary cordons, or else to specific sanitary administrations and policies – and on the long-lasting scientific debate of contagionism versus anticontagionism. This classical approach, epitomised by the works of Erwin Ackercknecht, Carlo Cipolla, Daniel Panzac or Gunther E. Rothenberg, is still alive and well today.[1] However, current historiography follows different lines of research. For example, studies on modern quarantine have been put at the centre of works on international health diplomacy and public health bodies preceding the World Health Organization, as well as on the European colonial expansion and the sanitary regulation of the pilgrimage to Mecca.[2] On the other hand, Foucaultian theoretical interpretations and approaches have led to redefinitions of lazarettos as paradigmatic 'disciplinary' and 'confinement' institutions, and have in general triggered sophisticated investigations on the medical 'bio-political technologies' deployed in those sanitation epicentres over the 'bodies' of quarantined individuals.[3] Finally, scholarly works from a variety of disciplines comprising archaeology and cultural studies have explored the multiple uses of quarantine in the construction of individual and collective identities, as well as in the creation of memories of migration and cross-border travel.[4]

As a consequence of the fertilisation from these multiple theoretical standpoints, quarantine history has been expanded into 'quarantine studies', an ever more fertile global and interdisciplinary field of inquiry. Surprisingly, major international scholarship on this emergent field in the last two decades has tended to neglect the Mediterranean in various respects. The impressive account of epidemic prevention practices and debates in nineteenth- and early twentieth-century Europe by Peter Baldwin in his book *Contagion and the State in Europe, 1830–1930* (1999), barely touches on developments in southern European and

Mediterranean countries. Mark Harrison's sophisticated account – *Contagion: How Commerce has Spread Disease* (2013) – of the relationships between quarantine and public health on the one hand and global trade and pandemics on the other hand gives the Mediterranean a central place, but largely disregards local Mediterranean historiography and case studies in favour of British ones. Alison Bashford's recently edited volume *Quarantine. Local and Global Histories* (2016) seeks to connect the histories of quarantine in the Old and New Worlds, though it actually does so by focusing on Great Britain and its various former colonial outposts (Hong Kong, Australia, the United States, New Zealand, Aden). We think these works are major landmarks in the development of the new field of quarantine studies, ones which the contributors to the present volume have used profusely as bibliographic references and for comparative purposes. However, they also reflect certain persistent biases found in international historiography about quarantine in general and Mediterranean quarantine in particular.

The present volume seeks to enrich quarantine studies by bringing local Mediterranean historiography to an Anglophone audience. For this purpose, it provides a selection of case studies presented during the first scientific meeting of the Quarantine Studies Network held at the University of Malta between 7 and 8 November 2014. We think that at this stage in research on the history of quarantine, it is important to have a new Mediterranean-focused set of essays, and especially a selection that shows clearly the similarities and differences around and across this sea, on the southern and northern shores, in Arabic, Spanish, Portuguese, Greek, Italian and French-speaking domains. Of course, the British had close connections with the Mediterranean too – more especially during the period under study (1750–1914) – and for that reason this volume includes British contributions and case studies. These join, however, a plurilingual and multinational ensemble which – though far from being comprehensive because it lacks case studies from the Italian peninsula, Egypt or the Ottoman Empire – includes discussions on quarantine in many geographical locations across the Mediterranean, from the Iberian to the Balkan Peninsula, from southern France to Morocco, from Mallorca to Malta and Corfu. The circum-Mediterranean geographical spread of this book illuminates the similarities, the differences and the overlapping of quarantine institutions and practices throughout the region, showing for instance how Christian and Islamic populations perceived, and their governments dealt with, infectious disease from plague to yellow fever and cholera. This volume is, in sum, also interested in 'joining the Anglosphere conversation'[5] and thus engaging in the global English-speaking community, offering a range of terms, sources, bibliography, interpretative tools and views produced and elaborated in the Mediterranean countries.

In this sense, the Mediterranean foundation of this collection of chapters contributes to current efforts to write a global history of quarantine. Instead of enlarging the geographical scope to draw connections with the Atlantic, the Indian and Pacific Oceans, we have actually attempted to 'disclose' the global trends underlying local Mediterranean processes to 'provincialise' Mediterranean quarantine.[6] This was actually one of the main reasons behind the selection of the long nineteenth century as our period of analysis. During this timeframe, the Mare Nostrum became much more exposed to the spread of yellow fever from the Americas and of cholera and plague from Africa and Asia as a result of multiple processes that led to an increasing global interconnectivity spurred by European colonial expansion, ever-faster land and sea transport and intensified trade exchanges. All these processes were present in the Mediterranean, though, paradoxically, they often contributed to create or deepen rivalries, divisions, conflicts and processes of domination and subordination between its northern and southern, its eastern and western coasts. Modern quarantine was, in this sense, an expression of a persistent fracture which continues to the present day. For centuries, zones, countries and whole areas in the Middle Sea implemented quarantine against each other, and when these transversal restrictions were eased it was often as a result of conquest or colonisation and therefore at the expense of the collective health of local populations. Fast forwarding to the present, old sanitary quarantines are being replaced by new, equivalent, cross-border arrangements of sanitary controls, checkpoints and detention centres for the containment, inspection – through modern biometric screening, medical and genetic techniques – selection and transfer/redirection of incoming flows of migrants and refugees. The European Union, for instance, seems to be engaged in a process of defining and demarking its southern political and sanitary borders through the construction of a 'new quarantine system for the Mediterranean' for migrants attempting to cross from the southern and eastern littorals to European countries.[7]

In the end, all these long-running tensions have contributed to the displacement of the Mare Nostrum as the perceived centre of world history – including quarantine history. It is by no means the intention of this volume to reclaim nostalgically the Mediterranean as central to the history and historiography of quarantine. Instead, we aim to use it to illuminate how a global practice was played out in local, provincial settings, what we call 'provincialisation', and to move beyond the period from the 1400s to 1700s, which still dominates the literature on the Mediterranean.[8] To disclose the global trends behind modern quarantine in this region, contributors to this volume have more or less explicitly used three fundamental categories of analysis – space, identity and power – which, although marking separate sections of the book, are actually present and indivisibly intertwined in all chapters. Before explaining in more detail the various problematics of research that can be derived from each, and discussing those that have been actually dealt with by the authors in their chapters, we would just like to make a preliminary comment. If global history, seen as different from a 'history of the world', puts most emphasis on the entanglement and interconnection of phenomena rather than on their totality across geography and time,[9] then these categories should contribute to show the inherent instability – the historicity – of the geographic, cultural/religious and political boundaries defining modern Mediterranean quarantine.

The set of chapters making up the first section of this volume focus principally on space to investigate how quarantine articulated territorial organisation, demarcated land and maritime boundaries and frontiers, substantiated national governance and economic infrastructure, and consolidated the expansionist imperial ventures of the European Mediterranean nation-states over their Islamic neighbours. Thus, Chapter 1 by Quim Bonastra investigates the modes by which lazarettos – and perhaps less significantly sanitary cordons – coevolved with the Spanish state's modern transport–communication and economic–industrial infrastructures throughout the nineteenth century. It also examines how these quarantine institutions functioned as sanitary gateways or entry checkpoints at borders, physically marking and consolidating while protecting the national territorial space. Bonastra's chapter traces the ideas underpinning the configuration and development of this quarantine network on Spanish national territory, which occurred unevenly – with the most evolved parts depending on certain strategic ports and on links with the railway transport infrastructure that was still under construction. Besides their integration in the national infrastructural grids, as the Spanish case illustrates, lazarettos also continued to develop as hubs of regional networks, connecting coastal ports to islands, islands to islands, and linking wider still with the empire and the global economic system.

The next two chapters in the first section of this book take a somewhat similar approach, exploring the development of two lazarettos and the part they played in nation- and empire-building processes, territorial demarcations and expansion. In Chapter 2, Dominique Bon investigates the lazaretto based in the port of Nice, and finds that in contrast to other similar institutions in southern Europe examined in this volume, this quarantine establishment progressively lost its importance as a tool of public health during the first half of the nineteenth century. This occurred in parallel with, and actually reflected, the geo-political shifts of the town and its neighbouring territory, then located on the 'Italian' side on the French–Sardinian border. Bon traces the gradual transformations that took place in the political, economic and sanitary interests of the port authorities, which resulted in the progressive relaxation of quarantine for arrivals from French ports, in contrast to more stringent measures for ships arriving from the Italian peninsula, and which in turn revealed and intensified an alignment with French liberal politics and free-trade commerce. The lazaretto of Nice did not shield the town against French annexationism, but rather paved the way for it.

Chapter 3 authored by Francisco Javier Martínez deals with another quarantine institution: the lazaretto of Mogador Island in Morocco. Specifically, he explores the site's centrality to the Spanish imperialist project of 'regeneration' of its southern neighbour. In contrast with the 'civilising mission' schemes deployed by the leading European imperial powers at the end of the nineteenth century, regeneration did not seek to construct a colonial Morocco but a so-called 'African Spain' complementing 'peninsular Spain'. This project was to be achieved through the support and direction of ongoing Moroccan initiatives of modernisation, as well as through the training of an elite of 'Moors' who were to collaborate with Spanish experts sent to the country, largely based in Tangier. Within this general context, the Mogador Island lazaretto became a key site of regeneration projects. From a sanitary and political point of view, it was meant to define a Spanish–Moroccan space by marking a new border and also to protect 'Moor' pilgrims against both the ideological and health-related risks associated with the Mecca pilgrimage. Martínez argues that this lazaretto's perceived ability to perform both functions derived partly from its symbolic location in front of the town of Essaouira (Mogador for Europeans). The history of this European-style city built anew in the mid eighteenth century was being reinterpreted to highlight the role played by Spain and therefore to present it as a direct precedent of the Spanish–Moroccan modernisation plans that were then being launched in Tangier.

The chapters in the second section of this book deal with the role of quarantine in the construction of multiple and diverse identities in the Mediterranean, and how they are intricately intertwined with issues of space and territoriality. In general, they consider it as an important instrument or 'technology' in the Foucauldian sense for building and defining collective identities of various kinds. More precisely, they explore how being subject to quarantine as a traveller, or having to express an opinion about it as a doctor or government official, had consequences for one's own cultural or professional identity. Thus, two chapters by Malika Ezzahidi and Christian Promitzer illuminate the experiences of individuals and collectives from countries that either were Islamic or hosted significant Muslim populations. Ezzahidi in Chapter 4 examines the writings of the renowned late eighteenth-century Moroccan ambassador Ibn Uthmân Al-Meknassî, who was the first known traveller from his country to leave an account of European quarantine as experienced during his two diplomatic missions in Spain's Ceuta (1779) and Malta's Valletta (1782). Ezzahidi shows that quarantine, on the one hand, acted as a marker of otherness by which Ibn Uthmân was identified as a Muslim – though this was not a uniform process, owing to the fact that significant differences existed in the degree of alterity experienced in Spain and Malta, and indeed other parts of the Mediterranean. The subjective opinion on quarantine, on the other hand, was also one of the means through which Ibn Uthmân situated himself within *makhzen* (Moroccan Government) elites at a time when a division between those who declared themselves in favour of European-style modernisation and those who advocated a rejection of European novelties was already visible.

Chapter 6 by Christian Promitzer provides another, more contemporary and less individualised, example of the construction of the Muslim 'other' through quarantine regulation of the Mecca pilgrimage, the *Hajj*. Promitzer investigates the under-researched case of the

Muslim pilgrimage from the Balkans during the nineteenth century. Pilgrims from Bosnia-Herzegovina (a dependency of Austria-Hungary since 1878), and Bulgaria (a tributary state to the Ottoman Empire until 1908), were subject to different quarantine policies on their return from Mecca. The author shows that while the former underwent more relaxed procedures as Austria sought to win Bosnian Muslims over to its recently established rule, the latter had to undergo strict quarantine as part of an effort by the Bulgarian authorities to consolidate their still problematic national identity against the Muslim minorities that were a reminder of their long-time oppression by the Ottomans. This, however, was not the only identity-building process going on, as sanitary measures were not always adhered to without question. Muslim pilgrims perceived the procedures of disinfection and/or fumigation of their bodies as degrading, and came to voice a heightened sensitivity towards the discrimination and stigmatisation inherent in these lengthy and stringent practices. Many came to show open discontent and even resistance to quarantine, which they identified as a Western institution.

Quarantine was also a symbolic site where the professional identity of doctors and hygienists was constructed, measured and/or altered, as the other two chapters in this section argue. Both of them address a question embedded in the larger arguments about disease aetiology and preventive strategies for cholera and other epidemics which came to dominate the medical profession during the nineteenth century, usually depicted as a confrontation between contagionism and anticontagionism (miasmatism). The authors reflect on how opinions about quarantine acted as professional boundary markers for medical bodies and individual doctors within them. A first approach is made by Lisa Rosner in Chapter 5, focusing on a particular group of British doctors, those practising with the Royal Navy. She argues that in the early nineteenth century, these physicians usually acquired their first experience of quarantine in the Mediterranean. It was an established practice for navy doctors to spend the first years of their professional trajectory in the two key British possessions in the region: Gibraltar and Malta. There, they learned to regard quarantine as a useless measure – in conformity with dominant British anticontagionism – despite the fact that it was systematically applied. Sustaining an opposite view was often incompatible with pursuing a career within the navy. At the same time, quarantine was also being used by the British medical press as a sort of 'crash-test' to define what 'professionalism' should mean in the medical corps. The press highlighted the contradiction which existed between the theoretical medical views prevalent in Britain and the routine practices of navy doctors on site in the Mediterranean outposts, and exposed this as an example of the lack of professionalism.

Jon Arrizabalaga and Juan Carlos García-Reyes explore another aspect of identity in Chapter 7, where they show how quarantine was used by the Spanish army doctor Nicasio Landa as an opportunity to elaborate not just his scientific discourse, but also his political and humanitarian views. For Arrizabalaga and García-Reyes, the classical thesis of Erwin Ackercknecht about the clear-cut dichotomy between contagionism and miasmatism in nineteenth-century Europe does not hold. On the contrary, following the work of medical historians Peter Baldwin and Chistopher Hamlin, they argue that the reality in European countries was often characterised by a plurality of intermediate positions between the two extremes. It is here, they argue, that Nicaso Landa positioned his views. The commission for the Spanish Army Health Service which he performed in the Canary Islands on the occasion of a major outbreak of yellow fever in 1862–63, served Landa as an opportunity to publicly present his views on quarantine to his chiefs in the army through administrative reports and to civil doctors during the Spanish Medical Congress held in Madrid in 1864. Landa came out as an opponent of quarantine for both scientific and humanitarian reasons, due to the additional sufferings infected patients were obliged to endure while in isolation. However, he also admitted that in practice it was necessary to adopt a pragmatic approach that did not discard quarantine as a tool to prevent the damage to public health which could result from the uncompromising confrontation of medical doctrines, especially harsh in the case of the Spanish medical community.

The third and last section of the volume explores an unavoidable issue in any serious discussion on the history of quarantine: power. The four chapters here investigate the embeddedness of quarantine within power structures. In particular they examine the use of the lazaretto and the *cordon sanitaire* as instruments of state building and colonial overseas expansion, and also as sites of contestation by local communities or colonised societies, which came to associate this institution with undesired foreign imperialist intervention. Chapter 8 by John Chircop shows how the system of maritime quarantine, which the great European powers helped to construct and operate in the Mediterranean, sustained their imperial presence and helped to expand their colonial frontiers. In this manner, they further solidified and extended their political hegemony and control over North Africa and the Levant – areas which mostly formed part of the disintegrating Ottoman Empire depicted and treated as 'the Sick Man of Europe'. In other words, during the modern imperialist era, quarantine politics came to be indivisibly entangled with the European powers' colonial partition of this part of the world. This thesis is a mainstay of the present volume, emphasised in most of the contributions, and is further explored in John Chircop's account of the contradictions in British attitudes towards quarantine. He shows, on the one hand, that Britain often took the most vociferous antiquarantinist position at gatherings such as the International Sanitary Conferences, where they argued that quarantines were inherently incompatible with free trade and liberalism, a position they supported using environmentalist or miasmatic medical theories. On the other hand, he argues, paradoxically the British also adopted a strict quarantinist position in their Mediterranean colonies. There, powerful shipping interests and colonial lobbying, the resistance of local collaborative and oppositional elites, and the popularity of quarantine measures with the native colonial populations were all factors leading British authorities to maintain draconian isolation measures. Thus, this chapter demonstrates the extent to which quarantines in these colonial ports were transformed into sites of power brokerage and negotiation between colonial masters and sections of the colonised people, and between various economic and political interests.

In Chapter 9, Laurinda Abreu explores the historical endeavours of the Portuguese crown to construct a modern nation-state and organise a functioning mode of governance with the use of public health institutions – specifically through quarantine. It is shown how, from the sixteenth century, the king considered sanitation and plague control to be one of his principal responsibilities, justifying his direct intervention during outbreaks of epidemics and affirming his duty to mitigate collective calamities. For Abreu, this historical precedent was behind the use of quarantine during the second half of the eighteenth century to strengthen the centralisation of the Portuguese state. Abreu examines three particular examples of that process. On the one hand, she studies how the quarantine measures decreed by the Marquis of Pombal, Portugal's first minister between 1750 and 1777, for preventing an unlikely importation of plague from Algeria, actually served to reinforce his political power. On the other hand, she analyses how the establishment of a sanitary cordon on the frontier with Spain in 1800 for fear of importation of yellow fever from Cádiz was actually an instrument for the mobilisation and organisation of military forces against an eventual Spanish invasion. By contrast, another sanitary cordon set up in 1804 in the same frontier would have a primary sanitary goal and would follow modern procedures.

The third chapter in this section, by Costas Tsiamis, Eleni Thalassinou, Effie Poulakou-Rebelakou and Angelos Hatzakis (Chapter 10), deals specifically with the quarantine measures that operated in the British protectorate of the Ionian Islands (1815–64). More precisely, this team of researchers shows how, in reality, Great Britain – the anti-contagionist nation par excellence in principle – strengthened rather than abandoned the strict quarantine measures in the Ionian Islands during that period. Actually, Britain reinforced quarantine throughout its network of Mediterranean possessions (Gibraltar, Malta, Corfu/Ionian Islands) as a forefront yet distant barrier against the spread of cholera, plague and other contagious diseases, but also as a means to regulate regional shipping and trade as well as to facilitate its own shipping passing through a densely quarantined Mediterranean. Strict quarantine in the remaining British possessions, as in the other regional ports, became even more pronounced with the opening of the direct maritime route to India through the Suez Canal from 1869. By this time, there had been a reversion to quarantine in Britain itself in parallel with the stricter quarantine measures adopted in the southern European ports – a general process which Peter Baldwin has termed 'neoquarantinism' and which has also been called 'the English system' (for the British case) by various authors including Krista Maglen.[10]

Examples of the correlation of quarantine institutions with state power and modes of governance over national territories are found in all sections of this volume, and is further examined in the last Chapter 11 by Joana Maria Pujades-Mora and Pere Salas-Vives on the connections between quarantine and the structures of power of the liberal state in Spain. Their study shows that the setting up and the actual configuration of sanitary cordons during the nineteenth-century epidemics in Mallorca were, to various extents and in different measures, shaped by the problematic relation between the central, provincial and municipal health administrations. Enacted by the state and guarded by the army, sanitary cordons were usually repressive, shaped by national frontier politics. Yet, in the case of Mallorca, *cordons sanitaires* were also an expression of how local communities, assisted by their local medics, continued to believe in the strength of the 'inland isolation [by cordons] which had a long historical tradition' as protection against the spread of contagion. This popular pro-quarantinist mentality was still encountered as late as 1880, as manifested in the local people's protests against the central government's attempts to relax quarantine, and specifically against the prohibition of cordons following the Health Law of 1855. Similar pro-quarantine philosophies remained very strongly rooted in the population and the local medical bodies, not only in Mallorca, but in most other parts of southern Europe and the islands.

In conclusion, by making the complex interfaces of space, power and identity apparent, all chapters in this volume have sought to contribute to the 'disclosure' of the heterogeneous practices of Mediterranean quarantine that were sources of significant political and cultural transformation, and the 'provincialisation' of the history of modern quarantine in the Mediterranean to show how global practices were expressed in local, provincial settings. In this way, they have sought to contribute to the writing of an interdisciplinary and global history of quarantine. These chapters do not pretend to be the last word on quarantine in the Mediterranean or elsewhere. Rather, they seek to open the field to further historical work, and illuminate what the past has to say about current efforts to find solutions for ongoing problems of cross-border migration within this region. These problems have brought back to the fore, albeit in new ways, some of the old realities and debates that always made of quarantine much more than a purely sanitary issue.

Notes

1 See, for instance, the works of Oleg Shepin and Waldemar Yermakov, *International Quarantine*, Madison, International Universities Press, 1991; Christopher Hamlin, 'Predisposing causes and public health in early nineteenth-century medical thought', *Social History of Medicine* 5, 1, 1992, 43–70; Mohammed A. El-Bezzaz, *The International Sanitary Council of Morocco, 1792–1929* [in Arabic], Rabat, University Mohammed V, 2000; Krista Maglen, '"The first line of defence": British quarantine and the port sanitary authorities in the nineteenth century', *Social History of Medicine* 15, 3, 2002, 413–428; Pierre-Louis Laget, 'Les lazarets et l'émergence de

nouvelles maladies pestilentielles au XIXe et au début du XXe siècle', *In situ. Revue des Patrimoines* 2, 2002, 1–16; María José Betancor, *Epidemias y pleito insular. La fiebre amarilla en Las Palmas de Gran Canaria en el periodo isabelino*, Madrid, CSIC, 2002; Peter Baldwin, *Contagion and the State in Europe 1830–1930*, Cambridge, Cambridge University Press, 2005; John Booker, *Maritime Quarantine: the British Experience, c. 1650–1900*, London, Ashgate, 2007; Birsen Bulmuş, *Plagues, Quarantines and Geopolitics in the Ottoman Empire*, Edinburgh, Edinburgh University Press, 2012.

2 Jean-David Mizrahi, 'Politique sanitaire et impérialisme à l'heure de la révolution pastorienne: le Conseil sanitaire de Constantinople, 1839–1923', in Jacques Tobie and Walid Arbid (eds) *Méditerranée, Moyen-Orient, deux siècles de relations internationales: Recherches en hommage à Jacques Thobie*, Paris, L'Harmattan, 2003, 221–242; Alison Bashford, *Imperial Hygiene: A Critical History of Colonialism, Nationalism and Public Health*, London, Palgrave-MacMillan, 2004; Valeska Huber, 'The unification of the world by disease? The International Sanitary Conferences on cholera (1851–1894)', *The Historical Journal* 49, 2, 2006, 453–476; Mark Harrison, 'Disease, diplomacy and international commerce: the origins of international sanitary regulation in the nineteenth century', *Journal of Global History* 1, 2, 2006, 197–217; Sylvia Chiffoleau, 'Entre initiation au jeu international, pouvoir colonial et mémoire nationale: le Conseil Sanitaire d'Alexandrie, 1865–1938', *Egypte-Monde Arabe* 4, 2007, 55–74; Michael Christopher Low, 'Empire and the Hajj: pilgrims, plagues, and pan-Islam under British surveillance, 1865–1908', *International Journal of Middle East Studies* 40, 2, 2008, 269–290; Saurabh Mishra, *Pilgrimage, Politics and Pestilence. The Haj from the Indian Subcontinent, 1860–1920*, New Delhi, Oxford University Press, 2011; Mark Harrison, *Contagion. How Commerce has Spread Disease*, New Haven, Yale University Press, 2012; Luc Chantre, 'Le pèlerinage à La Mecque à l'époque coloniale (v.1866–1940). France, Grande-Bretagne, Italie', unpublished PhD thesis, University of Poitiers, 2012; Sylvia Chiffoleau, *Genèse de la santé publique internationale. De la peste d'Orient à l'OMS*, Rennes, Presses universitaires de Rennes/Ifpo, 2012; Allison Bashford, *Quarantines. Local and Global Histories*, Basingstoke, Palgrave, 2016; Francisco Javier Martínez, 'International or French? The early international sanitary conferences and France's struggle for hegemony in the mid-19th century Mediterranean', *French History* 30, 1, 2016, 77–98.

3 Stuart Eden, 'Plague, panopticon, police', *Surveillance and Society* 1, 3, 2003, 240–253; Quim Bonastra, 'Ciencia, sociedad y planificación territorial en la institución del Lazareto', unpublished PhD thesis, University of Barcelona, 2006; Alan McKinlay, 'Foucault, plague, Defoe', *Culture and Organization* 15, 2, 2009, 167–184; Quim Bonastra, 'Recintos sanitarios y

espacios de control. Un estudio morfológico de la arquitectura cuarentenaria', *Dynamis* 30, 2010, 17–40; Enrique Perdiguero and Josep M. Vidal Hernández (eds), *La ciudadela de los fantasmas. Lazaretos y protección sanitaria en el mundo moderno*, Mahón, Institut d'Estudis Menorquins, 2010.

4 Quim Bonastra, 'Los orígenes del lazareto pabellonario: la arquitectura cuarentenaria en el cambio del setecientos al ochocientos', *Asclepio* 60, 1, 2008, 237–266; Biswamoy Pati and Mark Harrison (eds), *The Social History of Health and Medicine in Colonial India*, London and New York, Routledge, 2008; Paola Schiappacase, 'Archaeology of Isolation: The 19th Century Lazareto de Isla de Cabras, Puerto Rico', unpublished PhD thesis, University of Syracuse, 2011; Anne-Marie Moulin, *Islam et révolutions médicales. Le labyrinthe du corps*, Paris, IRD-Khartala, 2013; Michael C. Lemay, *Doctors at the Borders: Immigration and the Rise of Public Health*, Santa Barbara, Praeger, 2015; Peter Hobbins, Ursula K. Frederick and Anne Clarke, *Stories from the Sandstone: Quarantine Inscriptions from Australia's Immigrant Past*, Crows Nest, Arbon Publishing, 2016.

5 Peter Baldwin, 'Smug Britannia: The dominance of (the) English in current history writing and its pathologies', *Contemporary European History* 20, 3, 2011, 351–366.

6 We take the concept from Dipesh Chakrabarty, *Provincializing Europe. Postcolonial Thought and Historical Difference*, Princeton, Princeton University Press, 2007.

7 www.theguardian.com/world/2015/jun/23/eu-to-create-new-quarantine-system-for-mediterranean-migrants (accessed 26 September 2016).

8 Some recent works on Medieval and Early-Modern Mediterranean quarantine include, for example, Nelli-Elena Vanzan Marchini, *Venezia e i lazzaretti mediterranei*, Venezia, Edizioni della Laguna, 2004; Salvatore Speziale, 'Le domaine sanitaire tunisien aux temps d'Hammoudah Pacha (1782–1814)', *Revue d'Histoire Maghrebine* 32, 117, 2005, 123–135; Birsen Bulmuş, 'Plague in the Ottoman Empire, 1300–1838', unpublished PhD thesis, Georgetown University, 2008; Blazina Tomic and Vesna Blazina, *Expelling the Plague. The Health Office and the Implementation of Quarantine in Dubrovnik, 1377–1533*, Montreal-Kingston, McGill-Queen's University Press, 2015; Jane L. Stevens Crawshaw (ed.), *Plague Hospitals: Public Health for the City in Early Modern Venice*, London and New York, Routledge, 2016.

9 Bruce Mazlish, 'Comparing global history to world history', *The Journal of Interdisciplinary History* 28, 3 (1998), 385–395; Diego Olstein, *Thinking History Globally*, Basingstoke, Palgrave MacMillan, 2015.

10 Krista Maglen, *The English System: Quarantine, Immigration and the Making of a Port Sanitary Zone*, Manchester and New York, Palgrave MacMillan, 2014.

I

Space

1

Quarantine and territory in Spain during the second half of the nineteenth century

Quim Bonastra

Introduction

In this chapter, I seek to examine the evolution of the quarantine network in Spain during the second half of the nineteenth century, and to highlight the ideas underlying its configuration and evolution. This network evolved in tandem with the development of the transport–communication and economic–industrial infrastructures, and served as a gateway or checkpoint, physically marking borders and consolidating and protecting the national territory. Thus, the expansion and articulation of this network happened unevenly, generally in strategic ports or where the railway transport infrastructure was most developed. I also suggest that the gradual relaxation of quarantine in liberal Spain was periodically called into question by economic and political policies that defined the relation between the coastal and inland regions of the country. This, then, is a story of how – from the *Ley de Sanidad* (Health Law) of 1855 to the *Reglamento de Sanidad Exterior* (Border Sanitary Regulations) of 1899 – quarantine was about much more than attempts to protect against epidemics, but was also implicated in efforts to configure Spanish territory and the foreign trade policies of the Spanish liberal state.

In approaching this subject, I see quarantine as a form of spatial practice that is translated into socially constructed territorial production, which involves *maillage*, *noeud* and *réseau*, that is, the demarcation and division of areas, the establishment of nodes and network design. Such territorial systems, hierarchically organised, allow – among other things – the integration and cohesion of space and constitute the mantle under which power relations are developed. In addition, as the geographer Claude Rafesttin argues, territorial systems are simultaneously a means and an end. As a means, they denote a territory, a territorial organisation, but as an end they imply an organisational ideology.[1] Thus, quarantine networks, formed within the territorial confines of states to protect them from epidemics, are a vantage point from where to analyse underlying ideas in the configuration and planning of territorial systems. Their frontier location, either in the states' maritime or land borders, made them interdepend on other networks, such as those of ports, customs, railways or roads, and therefore capable of influencing their configuration and evolution. We should bear in mind that territorial networks are, by definition, in constant growth. As Raffestin again points out, they depend on the actors who manage and control different points within the network, or on the actors' position in relation to the flows circulating within each network.[2]

Major national and international debates

The concept of territory in liberal Spain

During the nineteenth century, Spain underwent a double process involving the loss of its overseas empire and the birth of the metropolitan nation-state. In this context, the new liberal state arising from the gradual collapse of the Old Regime delineated a territorial model in which, according to Françesc Nadal, both the interests and the internal logic found at its base were represented.[3] The new Spanish liberal state championed a unitary, centralised and legalistic model of territorial administration based on egalitarian, uniform and rational criteria. However, as Nadal and other authors have shown, the introduction of the liberal territorial system was hindered by various factors: a defective articulation of the national market, the failure of the industrial revolution in vast areas of the Iberian Peninsula and the inefficiency of the central administration, which was awkward and oversized.[4] During the 1830s, a provincial division was established throughout Spain, which abolished the old historic regions and undermined regional identities, albeit in different ways and to different extents across the nation. Certainly, the provincial division addressed key territorial needs of the country, such as rationalising and standardising its administrative map. However, from about mid century, the debate over the country's territorial organisation began to revolve around the need to reframe the territory again in regions. This was due to a widely shared demand for decentralisation that was presented under different political guises, either as regionalisation of the state's peripheral administration, as administrative autonomism or as federalism.

On the other hand, one of the key novelties brought about by liberal regimes in Europe with regard to the earlier conception of territory introduced during the Enlightenment – although the idea had been used even before then[5] – concerned the specificity and specialisation of the different areas and urban spaces of each country, and the understanding of their different needs, which in turn had to be subordinated to a general programme.[6] During the nineteenth century, this conception ultimately came to mean the specialisation of the regions in those fields (agriculture, industry, mining, commerce, etc.) in which they possessed a greater comparative advantage or a lesser disadvantage in relation to other regions. This 'productive specialisation' would eventually benefit each of the regions involved in the subsequent exchange of their products. Spain joined this general tendency, though it would be affected by the same structural constraints outlined above.

The creation of an international consensus regarding maritime sanitary protection and its impact in Spain

The nineteenth century saw the establishment of the quarantine system on a truly global scale, beyond the few European countries that had previously adopted this sanitary institution. This expansion saw in parallel the search for an international consensus in order to standardise the application of quarantine regulations,[7] owing to the fact that the system was being developed in different ways by a great number of countries, with the ensuing diversity in regulations and severity of their enforcement.[8] The consensus was also meant to stop the use of quarantine as a diplomatic and commercial weapon in the relations between states. In this context, during the period from the 1830s to 1850s, national quarantine reforms, the first International Sanitary Conferences and the introduction of the 'English System' for the prevention of epidemics (which will be described below) all assisted in the relaxation and standardisation of quarantine regulations on an international level.

Quarantine reform resulted from a combination of technological advances arising from the application of steam to maritime transportation, and novel scientific ideas about the aetiology and incubation periods of the main infectious diseases (cholera, plague, yellow fever). Progress, represented at this time by steam-powered navigation, was hampered by the lengthy quarantine procedures imposed on vessels across the Mediterranean. In 1841, England decided to reduce the period of quarantine to fourteen days, to be counted from the moment the ship departed.[9] In practice, this meant that on the British coast quarantine against plague disappeared in the case of ships on which no deaths had occurred during the voyage. Austria and some Slavic countries followed the British example. In France, however, the response was more complicated, notably in Marseille where the *Intendance sanitaire* (sanitary board) was mostly composed of supporters of contagionism.[10] The intense debate that followed resulted in the creation of an inquiry committee on plague in the *Académie Royale de Médecine,* headed by Clovis-René Prus (1793–1850), which reported in 1846, proposing a modified quarantine regime in which the length of quarantines for vessels arriving to French ports from the Ottoman Empire and North Africa should be substantially reduced.[11] The regime proposed by the Prus committee was adopted after eight months of deliberation at the *Académie* and was translated into the Royal Decree of 18 April 1847 that replaced the old ordinance of 7 August 1822, whose stringent regulations had been agreed in the context of the yellow fever epidemic prevailing in Spain at that time. This decision marked the beginning of quarantine reform in France, according to the Spanish hygienist and member of Spain's *Consejo de Sanidad del Reino* (Royal Health Council) Pedro Felipe Monlau (1808–71).[12]

The first International Sanitary Conference (ISC) held in Paris in 1851 sought initially to establish uniform quarantine measures for all the Mediterranean ports, but in practice came to be concerned mainly with fixing the minimum duration of quarantine. The conference debates were cut short by the different points of view expressed by the delegates, either on scientific issues, or regarding the political and commercial goals of the different states.[13] The second ISC took place in 1859, again in Paris, and its main purpose was to revise the text of the failed convention prepared eight years earlier, which had only been ratified by France and Sardinia. It was purely diplomatic in nature,[14] with the main debate revolving around the tensions between free trade and 'sanitary protection'. In this case, and for the same reasons, it was again impossible to reach an agreement. In 1866, the third ISC, held in Constantinople, had cholera as the main subject of discussion. The conference had two main goals. First, to agree on the theoretical guidelines for sanitary protection in view of the latest scientific knowledge about the causes, transmission and propagation of cholera. Second, to create structures for the control of cholera epidemics on an international scale, which would be mainly deployed in Eastern countries to prevent the disease from reaching Europe.[15] There was also a proposal to impose quarantine measures on some Asian and African countries in order to prevent the introduction of cholera into Europe by land or by sea, thus creating a first wall of defence and a 'cholera-free' European space.[16]

In general, France and the majority of Southern European countries took a pro-quarantine *status quo* position, while Great Britain voted against almost all measures tending to maintain quarantine and regulate commercial traffic. Britain had in fact practically abolished quarantine in its metropolitan territory, implementing it rarely or only lightly during the late 1840s and early 1850s while Edwin Chadwick (1800–90) still presided over the General Board of Health. In the 1870s, after a short period in which there was a reversion to quarantine in Britain,[17] the so-called English system definitely replaced quarantines. Customary information about the vessel's country of origin and its sanitary status, the ports of call and other information were thereby substituted for a medical inspection of the whole vessel and crew coming into English ports. Thus, passengers were considered suspect only if they showed symptoms of an infectious disease. This was a much stricter understanding of the term than that of the classic quarantine system in which, as mentioned above, the place of origin and its sanitary condition were the main factors taken into consideration.[18] With this new system, the detention of a ship would only last the time necessary to locate and isolate the sick or suspect individuals, and to carry out the disinfections deemed pertinent.

The fourth ISC, held in Vienna in 1874, represented a revision of the conclusions of the previous conference.[19] Although no agreement was reached for an international sanitary convention on quarantine against cholera epidemics, or for the complete suppression of quarantines, it was recommended that both the quarantine system and the English system should coexist at the international level.[20] The following sanitary conference, held in Rome in 1885, highlighted, among other subjects, the deployment of a systematic quarantine policy in the Near and Middle East.[21] For half a century, in general, the International Sanitary Conferences had attempted to establish a peripheral sanitary network in some key dependencies of the Ottoman Empire that eventually fell under colonial control (Egypt, Tunisia, Yemen), while within Europe an effort was made to relax the quarantine system and even replace it with the English system or, to use Peter Baldwin's term, 'neoquarantinism' – as Dominique Bon, Christian Promitzer and other authors show in this volume. The latter would be finally adopted as the basis for international pre-emptive action after the conferences of Venice (1892)[22] and Dresden (1893).[23]

With regard to the case of Spain, the International Sanitary Conferences had hardly any practical repercussions on its maritime sanitary policy beyond the adoption of the quarantine reform enacted at the first conference, which became embedded in the text of the Health Law of 1855. Spain maintained strict quarantine regulations until the end of the century. Only in the last decade did the Spanish delegate at the Dresden conference, Dr Alejandro San Martín, accept, in his report of the meeting, the possibility of switching to a mixed system in some ports by adding elements of the English system to the existing quarantine structure. However, this would be done only in case the Spanish Government was put under diplomatic pressure to relax its strict maritime sanitary procedures.[24]

Another important element in the international debate on quarantines was the foreign trade policies which the different governments adopted for their own economic interests. The economic theory of *laissez faire*, formulated in the second half of the eighteenth century, set the stage for the debate between the two types of commercial policies that competed against each other on the international scene throughout the nineteenth century: protectionism versus free trade. This economic debate would become intrinsically linked to the design and implementation of quarantine policies, which tended to slow the traffic of goods. England was the standard bearer and promoter of free-trade ideas, as the abolition of its protectionist Corn Laws in 1846 clearly demonstrated.[25]

When it comes to Spain, it is possible to distinguish two fairly clear stages in the establishment of free trade. The first was characterised by a strong protectionist tendency inherited from the previous century and which remained in force until approximately 1840, despite the liberal tendency of the Cádiz Cortes of 1810–14. The second stage began with the advent of the new customs duties in 1841 and 1849, which embodied some of the liberalising policies being introduced at the time in other European countries.[26] With the rise of liberalism in Spain during this decade, Spanish free-trade supporters launched a propaganda campaign to exalt the virtues of their cause,[27] which set the stage for Laureano Figuerola (1816–1903), then Minister for Finance, to introduce a bill into Parliament to eliminate restrictions on imports and exports and do away with the 'flag tax' for foreign vessels loading and unloading goods which imposed duties twice as high as those levied on Spanish vessels: Parliament passed this 'free-trade tariff'. After 1890, and following international economic trends, Spain re-embraced protectionism, forced by the economic crisis, the rise of nationalism and imperialism and the mounting pressure of working-class demands,[28] although it could be said that protectionism had never been entirely abandoned.[29]

Sanitary protection and the articulation of coastal territory in liberal Spain

The construction of the liberal state in Spain from the 1830s brought about a period of important transformations in the sanitary domain. Not only was the scope of public health defined, but a 'framework of action for the different administrations of the state' was also drawn up.[30] This modernising process was undertaken against the background of a constantly changing political climate that acted sometimes as deterrent, sometimes as catalyst, for sanitary reform. In 1855, with the Progressive party in power after the revolutionary uprising of the previous year, and cholera threatening rapid expansion throughout the peninsula, the first major sanitary regulation in our period of study was passed: the *Ley de Sanidad* (Health Law) of 1855. Inspired by the English Public Health Act of 1848, this law provided Spain with a health system designed along the lines of liberal thought on the subject.[31] On the one hand, it ratified the structure laid down in the previous *Real Decreto Orgánico de Sanidad* (Royal Sanitary Decree) of 1847 and, on the other hand, it regulated how the health system should be administered, especially in the maritime health service. This meant in theory that the law created the first comprehensive organisation of sanitary protection in Spanish maritime health; in practice, the organisation took longer to begin to realise its comprehensive ambitions. The subordinate decree that was to determine the actual location of the various facilities of the quarantine network would not be passed until 1860, and the budget needed for their development would come only in 1867. Moreover, the general rules governing the system created by the Health Law would not be ready until 1887. For all these reasons, the maritime sanitary service operated poorly, and infringement of regulations was the norm almost until the turn of the century.[32]

As I have shown elsewhere,[33] the Spanish maritime sanitary network was fragmented and 'cumulative' (i.e. asystematic or largely unplanned) before 1855,[34] although it is also true that there were several attempts, projects and proposals to provide the state with a planned, uniform and hierarchical protection system. One of the main novelties of the new sanitary protection network resulting from the law of 1855 consisted in the *Direcciones Especiales de Sanidad* (Port Sanitary Inspections – DES) replacing lazarettos as the cornerstone of the system. The pre-eminence of the DES meant that the main lazarettos had to be located in second-tier ports that were less important for trade within the Spanish port network. Meanwhile, the DES, placed under the command of a port sanitary inspector, were to be set up in the most important ports authorised for trade, and divided into three categories depending on the port's commercial and sanitary relevance. Quarantines would be carried out in the so-called 'foul' or 'observation' lazarettos. Save for exceptional cases, vessels with a 'foul bill of health', due to plague or yellow fever, would undergo their quarantine in the former, and those with Asiatic cholera would do so in the latter. It is quite significant that the relaxation of quarantine for ships with cholera – which in the draft bill were still meant to be confined in foul lazarettos as those infected by plague and yellow fever – reflected the liberal positions promoted in the ISC of 1851 and came from an amendment to the legislative text proposed by Laureano Figuerola, the liberal Catalan politician who would later, as Minister for Finance, sanction the tariff that would start free trade in Spain. As we have pointed out, the legislative text did not specify in which coastal localities DES or lazarettos should be placed. The law left it up to the government to arrange things, and it wasn't until the *Reglas generales para el servicio de Sanidad* (General Rules of the Sanitary

Service) were passed by the Royal Decree of 6 June 1860 (Figure 1.1) that the configuration of the network was finalised as follows:

Port Sanitary Inspections (DES):

> 1st class: Alicante, Barcelona, Cádiz, Málaga, Santander and Valencia.
> 2nd class: Almería, Bilbao, Cartagena, Coruña, Las Palmas (Canarias), Mahón, Palma (Mallorca), Sanlúcar de Barrameda, Santa Cruz de Tenerife (Canarias), Tarragona, Torrevieja (Alicante) and Vigo.
> 3rd class: San Sebastián, Sevilla, Carril, Palamós, Rivadeo, Huelva.

Quarantine stations:

> Foul lazarettos: Mahón, San Simón (Vigo).
> Lazarettos of observation: Alicante, Barcelona, Cádiz, Málaga, Santander and Valencia.

If we compare the sanitary network with other infrastructural networks deployed in the Spanish coastal system, we can observe, with some exceptions, a series of overlaps between their most important nodes. For example, the localities where a first-class DES was to be set up usually happened to be 'ports of general interest' for the Ministry of Public Works.[35] When comparing both networks we can see that, except for Alicante, the other five ports assigned a first-class DES were among those of 'general interest', either for trade or for the berthing/shelter of vessels. Thus, the sanitary network gave preference (by placing a first-class DES) to those ports that in most circumstances acted as indispensable stops for merchandise and passengers before these were re-routed to other ports of the peninsula, with all the benefits that this entailed. With regard to commercial imports, one can observe again a visible coincidence between those ports where first-class DES were to be established and those considered of 'general interest'. Barcelona led the way, receiving twice as much import trade as Cádiz, which came second. These two were followed in order by Málaga, Alicante, Santander, Cartagena, Sevilla, Bilbao and Valencia.[36]

On the other hand, the list of ports with first-class Maritime Customs included all the localities with first-class DES, the two with foul lazarettos and a series of ports with some relevance for local trade, the general idea being once again 'to articulate a trade policy to foster the development of the Spanish economy'.[37] Furthermore, each DES matched an

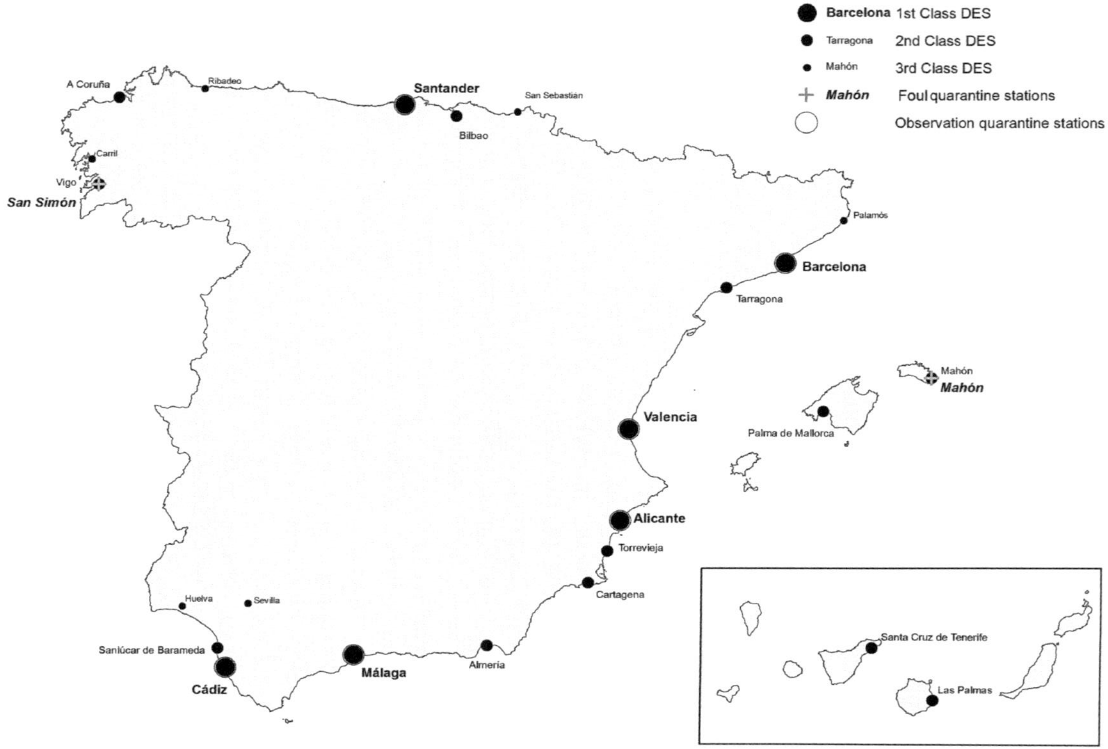

Figure 1.1 Map of the maritime sanitary network proposed in the Health Law of 1855 and the Royal Decree of 6 June 1860.

important node within the urban network as it was then configured, that is, the major cities in the Spanish coastal system. These had an important degree of functional diversification, meaning that they were administrative, economic and military centres.[38] This made them also the terminal stations of the 'general interest' railway lines established by the 1855 Railway Law. By contrast, when it came to the territorial network of the Navy, one observes a strategy of complementarity, a plan to distribute functions among the different ports. In this case, the territorial network of the Navy, well defined since the late eighteenth century, departed ostensibly from all the other networks, which were ultimately related to trade, including the sanitary network. Ports with a first-class DES were thus exempt from Navy-related matters, the great exception to all this being the port of Cádiz, where civil and military functions had traditionally overlapped.

In general, we are dealing with a scheme in which, save for a few exceptions, it is evident – at least on paper – that the authorities possessed an idea of how Spain's coastal territory ought to be articulated. The different networks imbricated in the coastal system overlapped in their most important nodes, except where complementary functions were sought between different ports, as we have seen was the case for the territorial network of the Navy. This was not incompatible with the existence of far fewer overlaps in secondary nodal points. In any case, the political and economic misfortunes suffered by Spain throughout the century – the French invasion of 1808, the loss of the American continental colonies and three civil wars, among other things – and the chronic malfunction of the government prevented in practice a satisfactory territorial cohesion that would help articulate a national market, extend industrialisation all over the peninsula and, ultimately, contribute to the development of the most depressed regions.

The 1866 amendments to the Health Law

In 1866, the concerns of several local health boards about the new major epidemic of Asiatic cholera ravaging Europe led to major changes in the Health Law of 1855, now deemed to be too much influenced by anticontagionist ideas.[39] After the publication of the amendments in the *Gaceta de Madrid* (the central government's bulletin) on 24 May 1866, the machinery in charge of creating the new quarantine network was promptly set in motion. Just weeks after the legislative sanction, the Home Office issued a series of regulations and interim provisions. The quarantine network was configured in less than a year, at least at the legislative level (the actual consequences that such provisions entailed for the design and erection of infrastructure deserve a separate study). On 8 June 1866, the government issued a Royal Order establishing a provisional network – while the necessary studies to create the permanent system were carried out – following the lines of article 27 of that decree. Foul lazarettos, which would double as observation stations during this interim period, would be located in the Balearic Islands (Palma and Mahón) and in Galicia (Vigo and Tambo). The ports of Santander, Cádiz and Cartagena would serve as lazarettos of observation too. On 25 January 1867, a Royal Order arranged the creation of another lazaretto of observation at the port of Barcelona, and a final one would be established at Santa Cruz de Tenerife, in the Canary Islands, through a Royal Order of 5 April of the same year.

The Port Sanitary Inspections proposed in the Health Law of 1855 were finally established in 1867.[40] It seems that, apart from an interest in ensuring the proper functioning of the Spanish quarantine system, another influential factor in this decision was the fact that income derived from sanitary taxes during the three preceding years had far exceeded the personnel salaries and current expenses.[41] It was argued that 'while our ports are not diminished in standing, every day more national and foreign vessels sail our seas, coming to facilitate mercantile and commercial transactions, and providing true and desirable development to the nation's public wealth.'[42] These words did nothing to hide the protectionist ideas of the time which still prevailed in Spanish economic policy. The last expression of this short-lived 'regulative fever' would be, first, a Royal Decree issued on 24 April 1867 establishing, after the sanction of the Royal Sanitary Council, the ports that were to act as 'foul' lazarettos and those that were to function as 'observation' quarantine stations. On 26 April, another decree was passed regulating the maritime sanitary service in a provisional fashion until a final version of the regulations would be approved. This decree included the sanitary classification of the ports. After new observation lazarettos were added by a Royal Order of 2 August of the same year, the network presented this configuration (Figure 1.2):

Port Sanitary Inspections:

1st class: Barcelona, Valencia, Alicante, Cartagena, Málaga, Cádiz and Santander.
2nd class: Tarragona, Almería, Sevilla, Vigo, Coruña and Bilbao.
3rd class: Mahón, Palma de Mallorca, Torrevieja, Águilas, Algeciras, Las Palmas, Santa Cruz de Tenerife and San Sebastián.
4th class: All other ports not authorised or included in the preceding division.

Quarantine stations:

Foul lazarettos: Mahón, San Simón (Vigo) and Tambo (Pontevedra).
Lazarettos of observation: Barcelona, Tarragona, Valencia, Alicante, Torrevieja, Cartagena, Almería, Málaga, Ceuta, Cádiz, Santa Cruz de Tenerife, La Coruña, Santander, Bilbao and San Sebastián.

The sanitary network created under the Health Law reform of 1866 brought about a great change in the planning and articulation of Spain's coastal territory. The five foul lazarettos (the fifth one was to be set up in Gando, in the Canary Islands) stipulated by the original law were reduced in practice to the three that had been in operation during the cholera epidemic of 1865. Two of them, San Simón and Tambo, were built in contiguous tidal inlets on the Galician coast, missing the opportunity to serve Spain's Atlantic coast with a more balanced territorial distribution of facilities. The San Simón lazaretto had been in operation since 1842[43] and the choice of Tambo seemed natural, as it had existing quarantine facilities dating back to the above-mentioned epidemic. This did not make the latter's choice any more rational, since a new foul lazaretto would have made more sense in one of the eastern ports of the Bay of Biscay.[44] On the other hand, the new distribution of observation lazarettos also introduced great changes. The previous allocation was based on the pre-eminence of six ports for health and trade. Four of them were on the Mediterranean coast (Barcelona, Valencia, Alicante and Málaga), one on the South Atlantic coast (Cádiz) and one in the Bay of Biscay (Santander), a reasonable distribution if we consider the importance of foreign trade at each port at the time. The creation of a quarantine station in Santander had actually been an exercise in 'territorial balance', aimed at completing a territorial network that was very hierarchical and had great internal coherence.

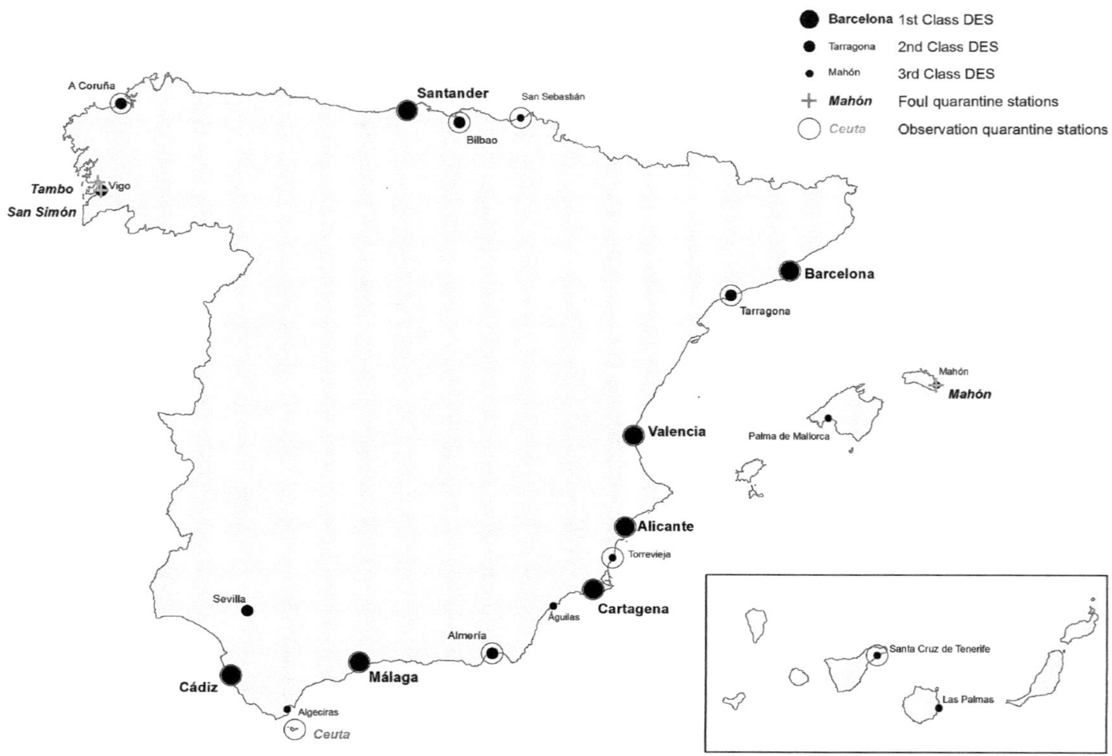

Figure 1.2 Map of the quarantine network arising from the amendments of 1866 to the Health Law.

By contrast, in 1867 a total of fifteen observation lazarettos were set up around the peninsula, both on the Mediterranean and Atlantic coasts, the North African possessions and the Canary Islands. The major novelty resided in the sharp increase in their number, a fact which apparently contradicted the spirit that had inspired the legislative reform, since re-directing the arrival of vessels with cholera on board to foul lazarettos aimed at drastically reducing the operations of observation quarantine stations. However, it must be borne in mind, as before, that income from sanitary taxes largely exceeded the cost of the service, which explains, together with eventual lobbying by local authorities, this profusion of observation quarantine stations. It is also true that this helped improve the service in some regions which, lacking commercial relevance, had previously been pushed into the background, such as those on the coast along the Bay of Biscay, which had few facilities, the North African Spanish possessions and the Canary Islands. As for the DES, the situation changed from a scenario in which the first-class DES coincided with observation lazarettos and second-class DES with foul lazarettos, to a new one in which quarantine facilities were located at any of the four existing categories of ports.

The years preceding the 1868 *Gloriosa* Revolution were marked by a return to ultra-conservative positions, great instability and a high degree of corruption in the political sphere. There was also a profound economic crisis resulting from a period of increased market, speculative and protectionist positions with a few free-trade overtones, all of it resulting from adverse circumstances in the field of tariff policies. With regard to epidemic prevention, the belief in the contagious character of cholera, the disease that most worried the public at that time, was strengthened and for this reason barriers were reinforced to prevent its entrance into the country. All these elements resulted in demands for the revision of some of the articles of the 1855 Health Law – in particular those dealing with the organisation of the quarantine system. The wording of the contested articles in the law made the contagious character of cholera appear quite mild. Claims for revisions of the law intended cholera to be treated as a disease as contagious as plague and yellow fever.

The new network's design did away with the hierarchy of ports in the previous network, even more so if we bear in mind that the latter coincided (with very few exceptions) with the port classification made by the Ministry of Development in 1852.[45] According to that classification, those ports 'through which trade of interest to a large number of provinces is carried out, which are in direct communication with the main inland production centres in the peninsula facilitating the import and acquisition of the objects they lack, and which are necessary for the prosperity and promotion of agriculture and industry' were supposed to be counted among the general interest ports. Also of general interest were those capable of providing shelter to vessels in the event of storms. Of 'local interest, first order', were those 'of interest not only to the city or province where they are located, but to other cities, territories or provinces; and which, according to their trade, can be eventually declared of general interest'.[46] In the 1855 Health Law, quarantine stations were located in ports of general interest, whereas in the network established in 1866–67, they were set up both in ports of general and local interest. From the administrative point of view, this presented a problem as not all of them enjoyed the same rights in the eyes of the Ministry of Public Works. This Ministry only took charge of the full cost of building, operation and cleaning expenses at ports of general interest. In the case of ports of local interest, the responsibility for such expenses was shared with the local administrations.[47] This situation meant that two ports belonging to the same category from the sanitary point of view could be considered differently by the Ministry.

When we contextualise the network emerging from the legislative reform of 1866 and the subsequent regulations in the territorial system, it is clear that the idea of a general programme is lost. As I have already argued – when comparing the quarantine network with other networks – there was no longer any an overlap or hierarchical complementarity in the key nodal points between the system's networks. This resulted, for example, in a lack of correspondence between the network of main ports of the Ministry of Public Works, the territorial network of the Navy and the sanitary network, or even within the sanitary network itself where there existed a mismatch between the lazarettos and the Port Sanitary Inspections. There was, however, a correspondence – by no means absolute – between the observation lazarettos, the main foreign trade ports and the railway network. In general, we are dealing with a network designed at a moment of profound economic crisis; therefore, the rationale behind the multiplication of observation quarantine stations must be interpreted as a means to favour the flow of goods through a greater number of ports (and therefore to increase and diffuse the sources of income), regardless of the general programme existing in the previous territorial system.

The Border Sanitary Regulations of 1899

It would take too long to review the different changes that were introduced in the sanitary network between 1867 and 1898, and in any case this would be a diversion from the main purpose of this chapter. Thus, I will focus my analysis on one last issue: the sanitary network set up by the *Reglamento de Sanidad Exterior* (Border Sanitary Regulations) of 1899. These regulations came about at a time of deep economic, political and social crisis. The Spanish monarchy had just lost its last overseas colonies and the economic effort demanded by the wars in Cuba and the Philippines, together with the deficient development of the country's industrial production, commerce or public health, resulted in an intensification of the so-called 'regenerationist' movement, which, as Francisco Javier Martínez also argues in his contribution to this volume, aimed at rescuing Spain from the secular backwardness in which it was stuck. In light of all this, the Border Sanitary Regulations of 1899 should be seen as one of the many convergent attempts to regenerate the country[48] and take it back into the ranks of the most-developed nations.

In this context, the new conservative cabinet in power from March 1899 issued a Royal Decree on 5 October ratifying a previous one issued on 15 August which re-established the *Dirección General de Sanidad* (National Health Board), suppressed in December 1892. The new Royal Decree was aimed at reorganising the sanitary administration in Spain and improving public health. In addition, as the project for a new Health Law (*Proyecto de bases para una ley de sanidad*) had been postponed by Parliament, as had happened on many other occasions in the preceding decades, a Royal Decree was issued on 28 October approving the Border Sanitary Regulations which would later be incorporated into the *Instrucción de Sanidad* (Public Health Act) of 1904. These regulations stemmed from two major facts. On the one hand, Spain had adhered to the convention resulting from the tenth ISC held in Venice, thereby committing itself 'to put our health legislation, particularly in the Border or International Sanitary aspect, in consonance with the agreed and accepted conclusions'.[49] On the other hand, as had been characteristic of the history of epidemic prevention in Spain, the legislative change came about due to pressure from a renewed sanitary emergency: the threat posed by the third plague pandemic, which, spreading worldwide from China since 1893, had just caused a major outbreak in the Portuguese city of Porto in the summer of 1899.[50]

The great novelty of the 1899 Regulations consisted in the adoption of a mixed system that began to embrace health inspections, while maintaining the quarantine system for all passengers of ships with an infectious disease on board[51] – in agreement with the statements made by the Spanish representative at the eighth ISC in Dresden, Alejandro San Martín. Furthermore, these regulations established a new system of territorial division and a new hierarchy in the quarantine network. The Spanish coast was divided into a series of 'sanitary districts' under whose jurisdiction were placed first- and second-class 'sanitary stations' and 'local inspections' varying in number according to each district (see Table 1.1). This new territorial division was novel in its attribution of territorial boundaries to each of its divisions, be they districts or sub-districts. This fact is important if we consider two points: on the one hand, during most of the eighteenth century, as part of the early establishment of a centralising administration of quarantines, there existed a fairly decentralised configuration of the network, with a port of reference for quarantines located in each of the old 'kingdoms' (Aragón, Castilla, Granada, León, Navarra) which used to make up the State. On the other hand, we must remember that from the mid nineteenth century the idea of a need to reorganise the territory into regions had been gaining ground, a need interpreted in decentralisation terms and which matched the growing appeal of local nationalist movements in some of the abovementioned 'old kingdoms'. During this period, we also find several regionalisation projects, some of which coincided to a great extent with the plan presented in the Border Sanitary Regulations of 1899. We are referring to territorial projects such as the one included in the Federal Constitution of 1873, or the one presented by the Liberal party member Segismundo Moret in 1884.[52]

Regarding the integration of the network of quarantines with others, particularly that of the railway – as had been happening since mid century – one observes that the first-class sanitary stations were all located at the final destinations of the railway lines (Figure 1.3). In addition, many of the second-class sanitary stations (Tarragona, Alicante,

Table 1.1 The quarantine network resulting from the Border Sanitary Regulations of 1899

	1st class sanitary stations	2nd class sanitary stations	Local inspections	Provinces
Palma de Mallorca Sanitary District	Palma de Mallorca	>>	Puerto Colón Alcudia Ibiza Manacor Andraitx	Baleares
		Mahón, with the quarantine station of the same name	Ciudadela	
Barcelona Sanitary District	Barcelona	>>	Cadaqués Rosas La Escala Palafrugell Palamós	Gerona
		>>	San Feliu de Guíxols Tossa Blanes Malgrat Mataró Villanueva y la Geltrú	Barcelona
		Tarragona	Vendrell Torredembarra Salou Tortosa San Carlos de La Rápita	Tarragona

Table 1.1 The quarantine network resulting from the Border Sanitary Regulations of 1899 (continued)

	1st class sanitary stations	2nd class sanitary stations	Local inspections	Provinces
Valencia Sanitary District	Valencia	>>	Vinaroz	Castellón
			Benicarló	
			Graó de Castellón	
			Burriana	
		Gandía	Cullera	Valencia
		Alicante	Denia	Alicante
			Jávea	
			Altea	
			Torrevieja	
Cartagena Sanitary District	Cartagena	>>	Mazzarón	Murcia
			Águilas	
			San Pedro del Pinatar	
		Almería	Adra	Almería
		Garrucha	>>	
Málaga Sanitary District	Málaga	>>	Albuñol	Granada
			Motril	
			Almuñécar	
			Torrox	Málaga
			Torre del Mar	
			Fuengirola	
			Marbella	
			Estepona	

Table 1.1 The quarantine network resulting from the Border Sanitary Regulations of 1899 (continued)

	1st class sanitary stations	2nd class sanitary stations	Local inspections	Provinces
Cádiz Sanitary Districts	Cádiz	Algeciras	Puerto Mayorga	Cádiz
			Palmones	
			Tarifa	
		>>	Vejer	
			San Fernando	
			Trocadero	
			Puerto de Santa María	
			Rota	
		Ceuta	>>	
		Sevilla-Bonanza	>>	Sevilla
		Huelva	Moguer	Huelva
			Sanlúcar de Guadiana	
			Ayamonte	
			Cartaya	
			Isla Cristina	
Vigo Sanitary District	Vigo, with the quarantine station of San Simón	>>	La Guardia	Pontevedra
			Bayona	
			Marín	
		Villagarcía-Carril	>>	
La Coruña Sanitary District	Coruña, with the quarantine station of Oza	>>	Puebla del Deán	Coruña
			Riveira	
			Puente Cesures	
			Padrón	
			Noya	
			Muros	
			Corcubión	
			Camariñas	
			Puentedeume	
			Betanzos	
			Ferrol	

Table 1.1 The quarantine network resulting from the Border Sanitary Regulations of 1899 (continued)

	1st class sanitary stations	2nd class sanitary stations	Local inspections	Provinces
Gijón Sanitary District	Gijón	Avilés	Vivero	Lugo
			Puebla de San Ciprián	
			Ribadeo	
			Vega de Ribadeo	Oviedo
			Tapia	
			Navia	
			Luarca	
			San Esteban de Pravia	
		>>	Luanco	
			Villaviciosa	
			Ribadesella	
			Llanes	
Santander Sanitary District	Santander, with the quarantine station of Pedrosa	>>	San Vicente de la Barquera	Santander
			Suancés	
			Santoña	
			Castro Urdiales	
Bilbao Sanitary District	Bilbao	>>	Poveña	Vizcaya
			Bermeo	
			Lequeitio	
		San Sebastián	Deva	Guipúzcoa
			Zumaya	
		Pasages	Fuenterrabía	

Table 1.1 The quarantine network resulting from the Border Sanitary Regulations of 1899 (continued)

	1st class sanitary stations	2nd class sanitary stations	Local inspections	Provinces
Santa Cruz de Tenerife Sanitary District	Santa Cruz de Tenerife	>>	Puerto de la Cruz (Island of Tenerife) San Sebastián (Island of la Gomera) Valverde (Island of El Hierro)	Canarias
		Santa cruz de la Palma (Island of la Pala)	>>	
Las Palmas Sanitary District	Las Palmas, with the quarantine station of Gando	>>	Puerto de Cabras (Island of Fuerteventura) Reef of Lanzarote (Island of Lanzarote)	Canarias

Source: *Border Sanitary Regulations of 1899*

Almería, Algeciras, Huelva and San Sebastián) were also connected to this network. The classification of ports by the Ministry of Public Works gives us, by contrast, an idea of the problems in the functioning of the country's infrastructure. Many towns and economic interest groups lobbied the government in different ways to have certain ports promoted to the category of general interest, as this guaranteed the government took full charge for their improvement projects. As a result, several laws were passed in the second half of the century reclassifying ports. The disastrous result of the central government's

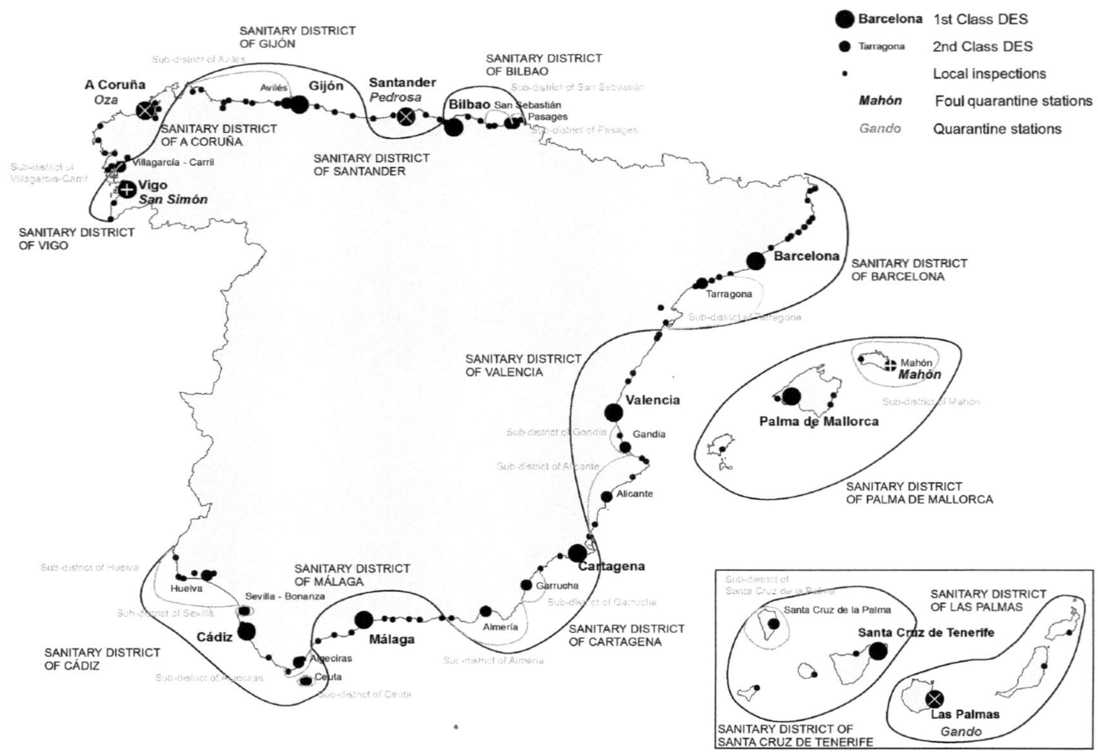

Figure 1.3 Map of the quarantine network resulting from the Border Sanitary Regulations of 1899.

yielding to local pressures and accepting most of these petitions can be summed up in the fact that, in 1903, Spain had 121 ports declared of general interest, most of which had no maritime traffic, works or services to justify such a classification. In this way, the government fell short of its goal to develop some major ports with direct funding from the state.

If we turn our attention to the urban network,[53] we realise that on the Mediterranean coast, the first-class sanitary stations coincided with the key cities in the network, except for the cases of Cartagena and Palma, which were only important cities at the provincial administration level. On the Atlantic coast, only Cádiz and Bilbao were major cities in the Spanish urban network. The rest fell into the provincial administrative category, except for Gijón, which was a major industrial city. Thanks to the adoption of the English system in the 1899 Regulations, the new sanitary law was more extensive than the previous ones, a fact reflected in its design. It is interesting to note, however, that on the whole southeastern coast of the peninsula, which carried most weight within the Spanish urban network, there were no lazarettos – a fact to which Francisco Javier Martínez refers in more detail in his Chapter 3. This area was covered by Mahón, which serviced arrivals from the Mediterranean, and Gando, which serviced arrivals from the South Atlantic. We see in this a clear strategy to free the most important trade ports from the 'threatening presence' of lazarettos. This also occurred, to a certain extent, on the northern Atlantic coast of the peninsula.

Conclusion

The Spanish quarantine network during the second half of the nineteenth century was an essential element in the hierarchical organisation of the state's coastal territory by way of the three main configurations of 1855, 1866–67 and 1899 which we have presented in this chapter. In this process, it interacted in various ways with other networks being deployed by the liberal state, mainly those of the main commercial ports and the railway network which started to be built from 1855. It also came to reflect the periodic shifts between the officially sanctioned provincial organisation of the state and alternative regional or federal models of political and geographical structuring. Finally, the quarantine network was mainly defined in this period by the Health Law of 1855 and the Border Sanitary Regulations of 1899, both of which brought forward measures aimed at the relaxation of detention procedures, especially with regard to cholera, agreed in the ISCs of 1851 in Paris and of the 1890s in Venice, Dresden and Paris.

The three configurations of 1855, 1866–67 and 1899 reveal different ideas with regard to territorial organisation, the main focus of my chapter. The first, quite rational in nature, aimed at harmonisation with other complementary networks (both on the Spanish coastal system and within the urban system), promoting a nodal overlap within the different networks of both systems. The second configuration, drafted in a climate of crisis, broke the coherence, balance and complementarity of the previous one's general programme in favour of a maximalist solution. It tried to make the most of all the business opportunities favoured by trade through a large number of ports, making it in essence a solution based on compromise. The last configuration, which can be defined as realistic, adapted to inherited circumstances and took advantage of new ones. For example, it gave up on achieving total articulation with other networks, but adapted to the novel regionalising trends of the territory, and left a great number of ports ready for trade thanks to its partial adoption of the English system.

Notes

1 Claude Raffestin, *Pour une géographie du pouvoir*, Paris, LITEC, 1980, 135–136.
2 Ibid., 141 and following.
3 Francesc Nadal, *Burgueses, burócratas y territorio, la política territorial en la España del siglo XIX*, Madrid, Instituto de Estudios de la Administración Local, 1987, 21.
4 Ibid., 21–45.
5 In late sixteenth-century Spain, Castillo de Bovadilla already talked of the possibilities which the soil and climate conditions of the peninsula offered for productive specialisation. Jerónimo Castillo de Bovadilla, *Política para Corregidores y Señores de Vasallos, en tiempo de paz, y de guerra …*, Madrid, Luís Sánchez, 1597.
6 With regard to this, see Carlos Sambricio, *Territorio y ciudad en la España de la Ilustración*, Madrid, Ministerio de Obras Públicas y Transportes, 1991, 36. On Spanish territorial policy in the late eighteenth century, see also Antonio T. Reguera, *Territorio ordenado, territorio dominado, Espacios,*

políticas y conflictos en la España de la Ilustración, León, Secretariado de Publicaciones de la Universidad de León, 1993.

7 For an overview of the early period of this consensus-building effort against quarantines, see Mark Harrison, 'Disease, diplomacy and international commerce: the origins of international sanitary regulation in the nineteenth century', *Journal of Global History* 1, 2, 2006, 197–217.

8 These used to be less stringent in those countries that were more dependent on trade, as can be seen in Richard J. Evans, 'Epidemics and Revolutions: Cholera in Nineteenth-century Europe', in Paul Slack and Terence Ranger (eds), *Epidemics and Ideas*, Cambridge, Cambridge University Press, 1992, 149–174, 168–169.

9 E.A. Heaman, 'The rise and fall of anticontagionism in France', *Canadian Bulletin of Medical History* 12, 1, 2005, 16.

10 Ibid. See also Francisco Javier Martínez, 'International or French? The early International Sanitary Conferences and France's struggle for hegemony in the mid-nineteenth century Mediterranean', *French History* 30, 1, 2016, 77–98.

11 Réné-Clovis Prus, *Rapport à l'Académie royale de médecine sur la peste et les quarantaines: fait au nom d'une commission*, Paris, Chez J.-B. Baillière, 1846.

12 Pedro Felipe Monlau, *Elementos de Higiene Pública ó arte de conservar la salud de los pueblos*, 2nd edn, Madrid, Impr. and Est. de M. Rivadeneyra, 1862, 265.

13 Oleg Schepin and Waldemar Yermakov, *International Quarantine*, Madison, International University Press, 1991, 66–70.

14 Ibid., 75.

15 See the *Annexe au Procès-verbal no 44* from the second tome of the conference proceedings: *Annex au Proces-verbal de la Conference Sanitaire Internationale ouverte a Constantinople*, Constantinople, Imprimerie Centrale, 1866, Tome II.

16 Ibid., *Procès-verbal no 30*, 17; adopted by unanimity. Ibid., *Procès-verbal no 31*, 14. Ibid., *Procès-verbal no 33*, 15; adopted by thirteen votes in favour, three against and four abstentions. Ibid., *Procès-verbal no 34*, 14, Inter alia.

17 See Peter Baldwin, *Contagion and the State in Europe, 1830–1930*, Cambridge, Cambridge University Press, 1999.

18 On the English system, see Anne Hardy, 'Cholera, quarantine and the English preventive system, 1850–1895', *Medical History* 37, 3, 1993, 250–269; and Krista Maglen, *The English System: Quarantine, Immigration and the Making of a Port Sanitary Zone*, Manchester, Manchester University Press, 2014. On the shift to the 'English system' and the change from a disciplinary power mechanism to one with a focus on security, see Quim Bonastra, 'La sanidad internacional en el siglo XIX. Entre la disciplina y

la seguridad', in I. Porras (ed.), *Transmisión del conocimiento e internacionalización de las prácticas sanitarias: una reflexión histórica*, Ciudad-Real, Sociedad Española de Historia de la Medicina, 2011, 267–271.

19 Norman Howard-Jones, *The Scientific Background of the International Sanitary Conferences 1851–1938*, Geneva, World Health Organization, 1975, 35.

20 'Ces deux systèmes, qui ont leurs mérites et leurs inconvénients propres, on été soutenus avec une égale ténacité et finalement proposés, l'un et l'autre, comme pouvant servir de base à une entente, d'une parte, entre les Etats partisans de la simple inspection médicale ou révision, et, d'autre part, entre ceux qui persistent à croire à l'utilité des quarantaines appliquées en Europe contre le choléra.' *Procès-verbaux de la Conférence sanitaire internationale, ouverte à Vienne le 1 juillet 1874*, Vienne, Impr. Impériale et Royale, 1874, 374.

21 *Protocoles et procès-verbaux de la Conférence sanitaire internationale de Rome, inaugurée le 20 mai 1885*, Rome, Imprimerie du Ministère des affaires étrangères, 1885, 341–366.

22 *Protocoles et procès-verbaux de la Conférence sanitaire internationale de Venise inaugurée le 5 janvier 1892*, Rome, Impr. Nationale de J. Bertero, 1892.

23 *Procès-verbaux de la Conférence sanitaire internationale de Dresde, 11 mars–15 avril 1893*, Dresde, Impr. B.G. Teubner, 1893.

24 Alejandro San Martín, *Conferencia sanitaria internacional de Dresde: memoria presentada por...*, Madrid, Ricardo Rojas, 1893, 29–30. See also Josep Lluís Barona and Josep Bernabeu-Mestre, *La salud y el Estado. El movimiento sanitario internacional y la administración española (1851–1945)*, Valencia, Publicacions de la Universitat de València, 2008, 47–49.

25 A new approach to the ideological and political framework behind this decision can be read in Cheryl Schonhardt-Bailey, *From Corn Laws to Free Trade. Interests, Ideas and Institutions in Historical Perspective*, Cambridge, MIT Press, 2006.

26 Ibid., 631–632.

27 Rocío Román Collado, *La escuela economista española*, Sevilla, Servicio de Publicaciones de la Universidad de Sevilla/Sevicio de Publicaciones de la Universidad de Cádiz, 2003, 189–196.

28 Juan Martín Fernández, 'La economía española y la articulación de su mercado (1890–1914): los orígenes de la vía nacionalista del capitalismo español', PhD thesis, Universidad complutense de Madrid, 2002, 124–125.

29 On this subject and the different stances taken by economic historians on it, see Antonio Tena, 'Por qué fue España un país con alta protección industrial? Evidencias desde la protección efectiva 1870–1930', *Documentos de*

Trabajo. Universidad Carlos III. Serie de Historia Económica e Instituciones, 01–72 (04), november 2002, 1–40.

30 Carmen Barona, 'Organización sanitaria y de la higiene pública en la provincia de Valencia (1854–1936)', PhD thesis, Universidad de Valencia, 2002, 39.

31 Ibid., 44 and 49.

32 Ibid., 42.

33 Bonastra, 'Recintos sanitarios y espacios de control', 453–472.

34 '(…) our (health) legislation, dating from different times and circumstances, pieced together as a puzzle if you will, without harmony or coherence (…)' (phrase taken from the introduction to the 'Draft Health Bill presented before the Courts on March 27, 1855', in *Diario de Sesiones de la Cortes Constituyentes …*, 1880–1881, Tomo IV, apéndice tercero al no. 119, 3372.

35 See *Regulations for the implementation of the orders in the Royal Decree from December 17, 1851 regarding the administration, construction service, cleaning and conservation of trade ports in the peninsula and adjacent islands*, 30 January 1852.

36 Weight of imports in each one of those ports in percent: Barcelona, 24%; Cádiz, 13.5%; Málaga, 8.6%; Alicante, 7.8%; Santander, 7.7%; Cartagena, 7%; Sevilla, 4.8%; Bilbao, 4.2%; Valencia, 3.6%. Calculations based on the *General Statistics of Foreign Trade of Spain, 1860.*

37 Juan Pro Ruiz, 'Inventario y extracción de los recursos: Reclutamiento, recaudación y estadística en la construcción del estado nacional', in Joaquín del Moral, Juan Pro and Fernando Suarez Bibao, *Estado y territorio en España, 1820–1930*, Madrid, Libros de la Catarata, 2007, 579.

38 Gaspar Fernández Cuesta, 'Crecimiento urbano y modernización en España entre 1857 y 1900', *Ería* 84–85, 2011, 5–46.

39 The debate is reviewed in depth in Quim Bonastra, 'Del programa general a la solución de compromiso. Cuarentenas y territorio en la modificación de la ley de sanidad de 1866', in Quim Bonastra and Gerard Jori (eds), *Imaginar, organizar y controlar el territorio. Una visión geográfica de la construcción del Estado-Nación*, Barcelona, Icària, 2013, 123–165.

40 Royal Order of 17 April 1867.

41 In the budget passed on 25 June 1867, total personnel expense for the maritime sanitary service was 135,000 *escudos*, expense on materials 89,000 *escudos* (section 6, subsections 11/2 and 12/2), while the income expected from taxes generated by the sanitary police amounted to 300,000 *escudos*.

42 This is the introductory text to the Royal Order signed by González Bravo. See *Colección Legislativa Española*, Primer semestre de 1867, Tomo XCVII, 1867, 676.

43 Antonio Meijide, 'Orígenes de la prevención sanitaria marítima en Galicia. El lazareto de San Simón (1838–1857)', *Medicina Galaica* 37, 38, 1987, separata, 1–12.

44 This case confirms, on an intra-state scale and with regard to the infrastructures, Baldwin's geo-epidemiological argument, according to which geographical proximity to the sources of contagion and the countries' cultural traditions carried more weight than political and economic arguments when it came to implementing epidemic-prevention strategies. The Spanish coast along the Bay of Biscay, being the furthest from the usual foci of contagion, lacked important quarantine infrastructures until the lazaretto of Pedrosa was built in Santander. We should not forget that in spite of this, during our period of analysis, that section of the Spanish coastal territory was integrated into the protection system we have described, and was subject to its regulations, which means that we should consider it part of the quarantine system (see Baldwin, *Contagion and the State in Europe*).

45 Regulations of 30 January 1852.

46 Article 4 of the above regulations.

47 Royal Decree from 17 December 1851, article 5.

48 On this subject and in relation to public health, see, for example: Esteban Rodríguez Ocaña, 'La salud pública en España en el contexto europeo, 1890–1925', *Revista de Sanidad e Higiene Pública* 68, 1994, 11–27 and Delfín García Guerra and Víctor Álvarez Antuña, 'Regeneracionismo y salud pública. El bienio de Ángel Pulido al frente de la Dirección General de Sanidad (1901–1902)', *Dynamis* 14, 1994, 23–41.

49 *Colección Legislativa Española*, tomo IV, vol. 2 from 1899, 398.

50 Ibid., 399.

51 See Chapter XI of the Regulations, entitled *Medidas sanitarias en los puertos de llegada*.

52 On these and other territorial division projects, see Jesús Burgueño, 'Geografía política de la España constitucional. La división provincial', Madrid, Centro de Estudios Constitucionales, 1996.

53 Fernández Cuesta, 'Crecimiento urbano y modernización en España', 22.

2

Cholera epidemics, local politics and nationalism in the province of Nice during the first half of the nineteenth century

Dominique Bon

Introduction

Over most of the nineteenth century, the health policy of the Kingdom of Sardinia underwent substantial change due to several factors. The threat of new 'exotic' epidemics – yellow fever and especially Asiatic cholera – cast doubts on a quarantine protection system designed, as Daniel Panzac showed for European Mediterranean countries at large, for the prevention of bubonic plague.[1] Besides, following the liberal thrust associated with the movement for Italian Unification, Sardinia undertook a series of reforms on the basis of its first constitution, the *Statuto Albertino* of 4 March 1848. As the medical historian Erwin Ackerknecht argues, political regime changes had a direct influence on the relaxation of quarantines.[2] Finally, the first ISC held in Paris in 1851, whose ensuing Convention was endorsed by Sardinia (the only country apart from France), was a breaking point in the Italian contagionist tradition. From this general standpoint, we will try to develop different levels of analysis in this chapter by discussing, on the one hand, the connections between economic interests and public health in Nice and, on the other hand, the changing relations between the province of Nice and the province of Genoa.

From the integration of the centuries-old Republic of Genoa into the Kingdom of Sardinia in 1815, Nice had suffered a triple demotion: it had become a second-class administrative jurisdiction, it had lost its free port privileges (1851–54) and the Sardinian *Real Marina* base located at nearby Villefranche was transferred to Genoa. Railway networks never connected Turin with Nice as they did with Genoa. The expansion of its maritime trade being also compromised, the whole situation ultimately resulted in a change of sovereignty: the annexation of Nice to France following Napoleon III's intervention in the Second Italian War of Independence of 1859–60. The part played by Catholic circles in garnering popular support to French annexation, partly influenced by public health measures, was significant, as we will try to show.

Quarantine during the Restoration period, 1814–48

Beginning in the fourteenth century, the province of Nice became the only maritime outlet of the Duchy of Savoy, the direct predecessor of the future Kingdom of Sardinia. From then onwards, commercial and sanitary institutions flourished, including late seventeenth-century creations such as the *Consulato del Mar,* the commercial court having jurisdiction over the nearby Freeport of Villefranche and the *Reale Senato di Nizza* – the supreme court from which the *Magistrato di Sanità* (health magistrate) emanated. But for my purposes, the most crucial institution was the establishment, at about the same time, of the Royal Harbour and the new lazaretto in the large nearby bay of Villefranche. During the Restoration period following the Napoleonic conquest in 1818, this lazaretto would be renovated while the one at Nice was abandoned in 1820[3] – although a quarantine facility persisted in its harbour until mid century. On 13 May 1818, the city of Nice asked King Vittorio Emanuele I for permission to reorganise the lazaretto of Villefranche. The motivations and arguments behind this request are important in order to understand the role played by the port in the development of the province. The lazaretto was regarded as an advantage for economic development at a time when Villefranche was declining as a free port due to competition from neighbouring countries and rising custom duties that slowed down commerce. The city of Nice insisted that the lazaretto was also an opportunity for the economy of the kingdom as a whole. It should be noted that the permission for renovation was requested by the *Magistrato di Sanità* on behalf of the local council. Thus, health and economy were not in conflict but converged with a view to co-opting the maritime traffic from the Near and Middle East and South America. With cholera still unknown at that time in Europe, the risk associated with the lazaretto seemed to be under control.[4]

The French doctor A. Brayer, a supporter of anticontagionism who had taken up practice in Constantinople from 1816,[5] experienced the rigorous measures against plague in the lazarettos of Marseille and Villefranche in 1820, which he later criticised in his book *Neuf années à Constantinople* (1836). A chapter titled 'My first quarantine in Villefranche' described the difficulties met there by ships arriving from the Black Sea: a quarantine of forty days, three purifications, a dangerous trip to the coast and an unequipped lazaretto.[6] France had not yet begun its move away from contagionism and Sardinia would remain contagionist for a long time. It is not strange, then, that Villefranche was perceived as a 'supercontagionist' lazaretto, the phrase used by Ackerknecht to describe Marseille's lazaretto. During the smallpox epidemic of 1828 in Marseille, the *Magistrato di Sanità* of Nice imposed a twenty-day quarantine for arrivals from that port and ordered the establishment of a *cordon sanitaire* along the land border with France, as had been done during the Great Plague of Marseille in 1720. Soldiers killed some people crossing the border, and although this rigorous implementation of quarantine measures enhanced the port's reputation, it also proved to be an obstacle to the development of steamship companies.[7] In 1831, responding to the first cholera epidemic that reached Europe, the Sardinian Government created a *Giunta Superiore di Sanità Pubblica* (Superior Board of Health) by Royal Patent of 28 July 1831, to coordinate all the *Magistrati di Sanità* of the kingdom, fix the duration of quarantines and recognise the contagiousness of cholera.[8] Shortly after, Pierre Richelmi (1769–1841), a Nice doctor who had enrolled in the French army during the Napoleonic Wars, published his renowned *Essai sur le cholera morbus épidémique et contagieux* (1832), in which he defended the contagiousness of the disease.

But times were changing for quarantine in Europe. After the English and the Austrians began to suppress or greatly reduce quarantine for arrivals from the Ottoman Empire and Egypt, the French followed suit. As Ackerknecht noted, 'the first changes in France occurred in 1828 and 1832. In 1835 even Marseilles, 'supercontagionist' since the plague of 1720, softened her quarantines.'[9] Relaxations were substantial. When the *Intendance Sanitaire* of Marseille revised its regulations in 1835, quarantine was reduced by a third for vessels with foul and suspect bills of health. By the Royal Orders of 11 September 1834 and 5 January 1836, Marseille and Toulon stopped being the exclusive lazarettos for the Levant in France, arrivals from that region being henceforth admitted to ports on the Atlantic coast as well.[10] In contrast to these changes, when some cases of cholera were reported in Marseille and Toulon in 1834, Nice established the usual *cordons sanitaires* along the Var River that marked the land border with France. When cholera broke out in Marseille in 1835, the Nice health administration acted again with the utmost severity. As the anecdote goes: when Sir Henry Brougham, an English Lord on his way to Nice, was forced to retrace his steps because of the rigorous implementation of cordons, he settled in a small fishing village. His accidental stop would make Cannes the new place to be for the European aristocracy.[11]

However, things turned out unexpectedly for Nice when bad weather obliged a ship bound for the lazaretto of Villefranche to be placed under quarantine in its port (without a lazaretto). Fifteen days later, sailors came into contact with the population and an epidemic was declared in the city – which spread to Cuneo, Turin, Genoa and the entire Kingdom of Sardinia. The *Magistrato di Sanità* did not yield to French pressure to resume trade, despite the fact that the economy of Nice was grinding to a standstill and the population suffering from incipient famine:[12] 'the port is abandoned, commerce is forbidden by land or sea, stagnation is complete'.[13] After the epidemic, the consul of France in the city addressed a report to the French Ministry of Foreign Affairs in which he criticised the president of the *Magistrato di Sanità* in Nice for the 'measures tainted by stubbornness which fear has made him adopt and which, I like to believe for his honour, were instilled in him from Turin. Among them, the rigor of quarantines and the absurdity of sanitary cordons must be mentioned.'[14] The consul went further in his criticism by affirming that the sanitary cordons placed along the French border were malicious because the danger of contagion for Nice actually came from Genoese immigrants.

Breaking point: sanitary consequences of the 1848 Revolution

In the context of the European revolutions of 1848, the Sardinian Government issued a set of liberal reforms that targeted many domains, including public health. By the Royal Edict of 30 October 1847, the

Magistrato di Sanità, regarded as a symbol of absolutism, was removed while a new sanitary administration composed of the *Consiglio Superiore di Sanità* (Superior Health Council located in Torino) and Provincial Health Councils (responsible for public hygiene and hospitals, chaired by an *Intendente Generale*) was established with a view to strengthening centralisation. By an edict of 22 April 1848, a reorganisation of the maritime health service further advanced this process by placing Nice under the authority of a *Consiglio Generale di Sanità Marittima* (General Maritime Health Board) located in Genoa. This board was headed by the renowned doctor Angelo Bo (1801–74), who was also professor of medicine at the Royal University of Genoa and would act as the Sardinian delegate at the first ISC.

The cholera epidemic of 1849 tested the new system. The *Consiglio Generale di Sanità Marittima* decided to impose five days of quarantine. Following the recommendation, the *Consulta di Sanità Marittima* of Nice (the city's Local Health Council) addressed a note to the *Intendente* of the Provincial Council of Health in August 1849 to inform him that all vessels arriving from France's southern coast to that port were henceforth only subject to a quarantine of observation of five days instead of the previous seven. When the French consul found out about this, he reminded the *Intendente* that quarantine measures, no matter how relaxed, were burdensome and needless. At a time when 'enlightened medicine' ranked cholera among the epidemic diseases, he argued, quarantines 'will have negative consequences for the interests of maritime commerce'. However, the case of Menton, a former commercial port of the Principality of Monaco, was raised by the authorities of Nice. Menton had broken away from Monaco in 1848 and, after declaring itself a 'free city', had created its own board of health (*Junte de Santé Maritime*) which, while waiting to see its status legitimised, decided to take instructions from Nice's *Intendente*.[15] By contrast, the Monegasque enclave, diminished by 80% of its territory, continued to follow the health policy of Marseille.[16] As a result, along the approximately 60 km of coastline from Cannes to Menton, opposing health policies were implemented in consecutive localities. Nationalist rivalry between France, Sardinia and Monaco was already complicating public health relations and cooperation.

To Nice's dismay, Sardinia would move closer to French sanitary policies during the first ISC of 1851, when it adopted an anticontagionist stance that set it apart from the rest of the states in the Italian Peninsula (Tuscany, the Kingdom of Two Sicilies and the Papal States). Dr Bo claimed that quarantine against cholera was an ineffective measure and a harassment to trade, especially when applied to land borders (Session 5, 1 August). He affirmed that 'science must develop a doctrine other than that followed in Italy on the spread of cholera' (Session 14, 4 October). The implementation of quarantine against plague and yellow fever was still an option for him, but he opposed it for cholera. In his opinion, there was no contradiction in this: 'I have made popular and contagious diseases the object of my research for almost the whole of my life and I do not renounce any of my principles' (Session 5, 14 August). Such change in policy had been thoroughly discussed in Genoa prior to the ISC. Dr Bo noted that the *Consiglio Generale di Sanità Marittima* subscribed to studies on cholera that defended an incubation period for the disease of three to four days maximum. Thus, all vessels arriving from infested places and where the voyage had lasted less than five days should be only subject to a quarantine of observation, as the period of navigation acted as a 'kind of sea quarantine' (Session 14, 4 October). An 'optional quarantine of observation' of another five days maximum could nevertheless be allowed (Session 16, 9 October). If one could still distinguish between *temps ordinaires* and *temps d'épidémie*, the termination of cholera occurred within ten days in both situations. During the ISC, Dr Bo acted as a member of the committee working on lazarettos and health administrations, while the Sardinian diplomatic representative asked to be the editor of the International Health Regulations (Session 18, 14 October).[17] This shows the close involvement of Sardinian delegates in the conference alongside Dr François Melier (1798–1866) from France, probably because the French had actually co-opted the Sardinian plan for organising a similar conference in 1850, and, therefore, counted on their support and complicity.[18] Sardinia would be the only country to ratify the sanitary convention apart from France itself.[19]

In spite of all this, when the *Accademia di Medicina* in Genoa examined the conference proceedings, it expressed reservations. First, it recalled that Italy, 'Mother of Arts and Sciences', was the inventor of quarantine measures. Hygienic progress should not turn the *leggi quarantenarie* (quarantine laws) into careless *laissez faire* policies. Abandonment of quarantine was regarded as 'a break' from previous practice.

Second, according to the Academy, if the ISC recognised quarantines, then it implicitly admitted the doctrine of contagion. Finally, land and sea measures were considered asymmetric.[20] Because plagues easily crossed land borders, the latter ceased to be perceived as barriers.[21] In spite of these objections, the International Health Regulations drafted during the ISC would be approved in Sardinia by a law of 2 December 1852,[22] a major U-turn in health policy similar to the one in France in the 1830s.[23] Nevertheless, anticontagionist regulations continued to be heavily criticised by the Genoese medical community, especially during the following cholera epidemic of 1854. Dr Bo was accused of concealing cases of cholera to protect Genoese commercial interests. Criticism was fuelled by the Hospital of Pammatone in Genoa, some of whose doctors recalled that Dr Bo had been a contagionist during the epidemics of 1844 and 1849, and that he 'saved Genoa' twice with quarantines.[24] However, it is also true that the distance between the port of Genoa and its new lazaretto in La Spezia had progressively increased quarantine costs:[25] in 1849, up to forty vessels coming from South America, where yellow fever prevailed, were transferred from Genoa to La Spezia, as Dr Bo recalled at the ISC (Session 27, 6 November 1851). Indeed, two kinds of protectionism (economic and sanitary) were actually at stake.

A new law of 13 April 1854, passed in the wake of another cholera epidemic, harmonised quarantine costs and above all consecrated the new *Direzione generale della Sanità Marittima* (Maritime Health Board) in Genoa as the executive institution for quarantine, though only the Minister of Maritime Affairs could really decide on its eventual application. The new and subordinate *Ufficio di Sanità Marittima* of Nice was empowered to admit in free circulation vessels from all destinations, including those arriving from the Levant and America, if they had been granted a bill of health and if no modification in the sanitary condition of the ship had been found during the voyage. This change was due to the *Ufficio* becoming a sanitary institution of first category, equivalent to those of Genoa, Savona, La Spezia and Cagliari.[26] In exchange for this higher sanitary status, Genoese authorities requested the end of the free port privileges for Nice and the reform of its customs duties, both things being implemented in 1854. Despite the fact that since 1847 the people of Nice had supported the *Risorgimento*, members of Parliament representing its interests could not prevent the loss of free port status.

This loss would be greatly influential in the rising of a pro-French party from 1851, since Nicean commerce could not do well without France. In the port of Villefranche, for example, 80% of commercial interchange was with France and only 11% with Sardinia.

Cholera in 1854 and 1855: revoking quarantine at the peak of epidemics

In 1854, once again, the danger of an epidemic for Nice came from Marseille, where cholera cases appeared from the end of June. However, the disease first struck Genoa. The rumour of an outbreak in this city had to be denied by the *Direzione generale di Sanità Marittima*. Certainly, a case of cholera had occurred in the Hospital Pammatone: a sailor arriving from the southern coast of France died on 14 June – though his body showed no clear proof of the disease. At the request of the king, Dr Bo was obliged to explain the admission into 'free circulation' of the Avignon ship carrying the patient, when he had dispensed of the sanitary regulations in force. The *Direzione generale* had to provide official explanations too: the *Official Journal of Genoa* published a retraction in its 25 June issue. Apart from this case, health conditions seemed to be satisfactory in both Genoa and Marseille. Information on the health situation in Marseille had been previously transmitted to Genoa by the Sardinian consul in that city by telegraph, and he also reassured the *Intendente* of the province of Nice by letter.[27] A circular dated 16 June 1854, signed by Dr Bo, allowed ships coming from France's southern ports to be admitted into free circulation after a simple medical examination, a quarantine of just five days being necessary if cholera was detected on board.

In spite of this, the *Ufficio di Sanità Maritima* of Nice took the initiative of placing in quarantine all vessels arriving from the south of France on the 13 July, suggesting that its stance on the matter was contagionist.[28] Ottavio della Marmora, *Intendente* of the province of Nice and President of the Provincial Council of Health, who was away until 31 July, was not in favour of these measures. His report to the Home Office at the end of the epidemic denounced 'the serious difficulties and unnecessary consequences caused by [...] the establishment of a lazaretto in Villefranche to put vessels in quarantine'.[29] Nice's commercial interests placed overwhelming pressures against quarantine too. The liberal and pro-French local press used the same arguments that Dr Bo had expressed in the ISC: quarantines were useless if land borders were unchecked (*cordons sanitaires* had been abandoned in Nice in 1842). Trade was just being diverted overland to other French ports. As *L'Avenir de Nice* put it in mid July 1854:

> We have argued, from the very beginning, that the quarantine imposed on ships arriving from France's southern ports was a vexation and a nuisance for commerce and that it would result in cabotage steamboats landing in the port of Cannes, from where travellers and merchandise would reach Nice by land. In effect, two paquebots bound for Nice have disembarked on Sunday at the port of Cannes a certain quantity of merchandise addressed to Nice and five or six hundred Genoese passengers, workers, porters, sailors, etc. on their way back home. If cholera were a contagious disease, as the use of quarantine let it be understood, wouldn't it be transmitted to our population by those travellers who arrive every day by land? In this case, for logical reasons, it would be necessary to establish a sanitary cordon along the border.[30]

In spite of this, Nice's health administration decided to strengthen quarantine after concern was raised in two cases: the death of a soldier from Marseille who was quarantined in the lazaretto of Villefranche; and, on 15 July, the death by measles of a young girl in the same place. 'It is fear and ignorance that trigger alarming rumours', the abovementioned journal argued.[31] But the report prepared by two doctors from the *Ufficio di Sanità Marittima* found both deaths had been actually caused by cholera.[32] On 17 July, the director of the civil hospital in Nice alerted the Vice President of the local board of health, Francesco Malaussena, that there was no more room to isolate contagious patients. Malaussena decided then to install a temporary hospital for choleric patients in the Episcopal Seminary. He also divided the city into districts and called for sustained political support for hygienic measures (27 July).[33] From a medical point of view, the setting up of specialised hospitals for cholera patients prefigured neoquarantinism, a sort of spatial isolation policy intermediary between the old lazaretto sequestration and the relaxed English system.

Two weeks later, *L'Avenir de Nice* informed the public that after Marseille, 'cases of cholera have been recorded in Genoa; there is no doubt about the existence of an epidemic in this city', but 'the epidemic which has made great havoc in Marseille, in Arles and in the other cities of the

French southern coast, and which reached Genoa, has not appeared in Nice'.[34] In Genoa, 'the population escapes from all sides. More than a thousand Genoese migrants arrived in Turin only on 25th July.' A lot of migrants moved to Savoy to seek refuge against the disease, the daily migration amounting to 'more than 10,000 people'. On 31 July, it was estimated that between 20,000 and 25,000 people had left Genoa.[35] The sea link between Nice and Genoa was interrupted because sailors had deserted.[36] A new circular, dated 31 July 1854 and signed again by Dr Bo, abolished, in agreement with the president of the Council of Ministers, the previous one of 16 June. The new order prescribed that all vessels arriving from infested countries would be admitted into free circulation after a medical examination, though those vessels were only to be 'cleared' in the ports of Genoa, Savona, La Spezia, Nice and the lazarettos of Villefranche and Varignano (in La Spezia).[37] Following this, the press in Nice denounced the contradictions found in the public health policy. According to *L'Avenir de Nice*, a hidden economic protectionism was being promoted under the pretext of health measures:

> When cholera broke out in Marseille, the Maritime Health Board of the Sardinian States imposed a quarantine on the arrivals from the Mediterranean ports of France. Today, when cholera strikes Genoa and not Nice, why should free practice be given for the arrivals from Genoa while those from France continue to be subject to so-called cautionary measures? We have already insisted how illogical it was to put maritime arrivals under quarantine while allowing stagecoaches free entrance [...] For our part, we confess we don't understand anything about the quarantine regulations that the different European states throw back at each other;[38] we do not see in those measures public health preservation but a measure of preservation of the large revenues collected by the sanitary administrations of those countries. The invasion of Naples by cholera seems to us to be an argument without reply against the efficiency of quarantines and sanitary cordons.[39]

Even Nice's conservative newspaper *La Verité* was surprised by these decisions:

> We have been assured that the paquebot arriving from Genoa on Sunday evening has provided us with sixty travellers who have been admitted in free practice. We cannot imagine how, after having showed such severity with paquebots arriving from France, those coming from Genoa have been treated so lightly, despite that city being at least as struck by the disease as Marseille.[40]

Thus, both newspapers demanded that either quarantine was revoked for Marseille's arrivals, or it was applied to Genoa's, as if in anticipation of the displacement of political borders which was already looming. The question of real and symbolic borders is a significant one here. It seemed more important for Nice's economic interests to restore trade relations with Marseille than to detain the ships arriving from Genoa. Finally, in contrast with the adjacent province of Oneglia (Liguria), where authorities tolerated the establishment of a *cordon sanitaire* in spite of the government's prohibition,[41] quarantine was for the first time revoked in Nice at the peak of an epidemic (3 August 1854). From that date, 'all quarantines against the arrivals from Mediterranean countries still affected by cholera were supressed'.[42] The same day, an official public proclamation was issued which, according to the *Intendente*, left an impact on the population. In addition, local authorities circulated an *Instruction populaire sur le cholera* published by the *Consiglio Superiore di Sanità* of Sardinia in 1849.[43] The port of Villefranche resumed its commerce of cabotage with Marseille and Genoa, which had been the hardest hit by cholera, while mortality in Nice remained low. *L'Avenir de Nice* decided to publish from 2 August the daily commercial movement of the port 'in the interest of local traders'. Vessels arrived in free practice from Marseille and Genoa, but also from Livorno, Rome, Barcelona, Monaco, Menton, Savona, Toulon, etc.[44]

Father Justin-Ignace Montolivo (1808–81), a local herbalist and librarian, described in his chronicles, *Storia Patriae*, the march of the epidemic and the inconsistency of the measures taken by the different administrations. He wrote that the captain of a French brig died while the health office was closed; the health authorities refused his burial and the body was thrown into the sea.[45] The lazaretto of Villefranche had a staff comprising only four agents. Montolivo was also surprised that ships from Nice and Villefranche were quarantined while those arriving from Marseille and Genoa were not.[46] He recalled that public opinion supported the dissolution of the local health board since the cholera outbreak was over and the temporary hospital closed.[47] He considered the epidemic over on 9 September, with the closure of the specialised hospital. The morbidity and mortality toll rose to 361 cases of cholera, including 219 deaths. Only a quarter of them was reported at the hospital.[48] Those figures show that the epidemic had been as intense as the one in 1835 – though very modest when compared with the cholera outbreak in France. On the other hand, Dr Francesco

Freschi (1808–59), hygienist, medical historian, professor at Genoa University, member of the *Accademia di Medicina* and occasional collaborator of Dr Bo, was shocked by the effect on the province of Nice. In his opinion, 'although in Genoa it was generally believed that the province of Nice could not be spared the intrusive epidemic, since it raged in Avignon, Arles, Marseilles and Toulon, and most other places in the south of France', it was nevertheless considered that the health precautions adopted by the local authorities and the slow progress of the epidemic would leave the city spared this time. The mortality figures had shown otherwise.[49]

Apart from sanitary and economic tensions, another serious dispute arose during the epidemic, between the Sardinian Government and the Catholic Church and regarding the so-called *affaire des couvents* (convents affair). In August 1854, in order to transform the convents into specialised hospitals for cholerics, the central authorities decided to confiscate church property. Initially only requisitioned, convents would be later confiscated by the law of 29 May 1855. Reacting to what he perceived as anticlerical laws, Pope Pius IX excommunicated King Vittorio Emanuele II and the President of the Council of Ministers Camillo Cavour. Catholic sectors came to consider liberals as 'auxiliaries of cholera'. Certainly, the cholera epidemic was used as a pretext to appropriate and convert a disproportionate number of monasteries into isolation hospitals: 139 convents owned by mendicant orders and another 334 of other orders were taken, while 5,400 monks were expelled, the bishop of Turin was exiled and recalcitrant monks were imprisoned. In Nice, by contrast, the Episcopal Seminary used as a hospital was later returned to its owner. Despite this, the anticlericalism shown by the Sardinian Government became one of the main reasons behind the position of the Nice clergy in favour of annexation with France.

In 1855, a new cholera outbreak erupted in Nice and Genoa as a consequence of the massive movement of troops heading from France and Sardinia towards the Crimean War. The Episcopal Seminary in Nice was again transformed into a specialised hospital, while the vessel *Il Dante* linking Genoa to Nice weekly was quarantined for six hours because of the cholera that broke out in the former city.[50] Quarantine, however, was kept only in name. By contrast, the use of a very different invention left a remarkable public impact. From 1853, following the telegraph convention between France and Sardinia, the Sardinian

Government had established telegraph lines connecting Torino and Chambery. A cable also connected the gulf of La Spezia to Cagliari, in Corsica, on 10 June 1853. That cable was one of the conditions that the law of 13 April 1854 demanded such that the *Direzione generale della Sanità Marittima* became the sole executive instance for sanitary matters. As a result of all this, during the cholera epidemic of 1855, health bulletins were sent by electric dispatches between the various provinces of the Sardinian states: Nice, Genoa and Oneglia had a telegraph station. In 1856, an International Telegraph Convention was signed between Sardinia, France, Spain, Switzerland and other European countries which reflected a prevailing spirit of international cooperation similar to the first ISC of 1851.

The renowned Marmora brothers would play important roles in the 1855 epidemic. General Alfonso della Marmora (1804–78), acting as Minister of War several times between 1849 and 1859 (and violently repressing the revolutionary uprising of Genoa in April 1849), was the head of the Sardinian troops sent to the Crimean War in 1855 that suffered the cholera epidemic like the rest of the armies participating in the conflict. His brother, Lieutenant General Alessandro della Marmora (1799–1855), actually died of cholera during the war in June 1855. He had visited Genoese hospitals during the 1854 outbreak and written a monograph on cholera in Genoa. The youngest brother, Ottavio della Marmora (1806–68), was, as mentioned, *Intendente Generale* of the province of Nice. In 1857, when the draft law on the transfer of the *Real Marina* from Genoa to La Spezia was being discussed in the House of Deputies, Alfonso was Minister of War and the Navy. Under his influence, transfer of the lazaretto of Varignano (La Spezia) to Villefranche was envisaged. Dr Bo, then a member of parliament, Alfonso della Marmora and the President of the Council of Ministers Cavour favoured the establishment of the State quarantine station in the province of Nice. However, the MP for Nice, the pro-Italian Dr Giovanni Battista Bottero (1822–97), opposed the project, arguing that foreigners who visited Nice for its climate would flee in fear, the local population would be frightened and the competition with other cities would turn out to be unfavourable; he also described the lazaretto of Villefranche as dilapidated and without the necessary equipment. Moreover, he asked: how can the Navy based in La Spezia purge the quarantine? It was always a question of yellow fever and plague, but never of cholera. This echoed the positions taken at the first ISC in Paris. The question of the usefulness of quarantine would be often brought back to the House of Deputies by Cavour himself[51] – who was a fierce anticontagionist – perhaps under the influence of Dr Bo.[52]

Conclusion: quarantine within states and neoquarantinism

Parliamentary debates on quarantine and the economy were heated on the eve of the annexation of the province of Nice to France. Would a more important role for the ports of Nice and Villefranche in the Sardinian states have changed things? What changed between 1818 and 1858 was the importance of foreign trade in Nice. And in any case, the bay of Villefranche found a new destiny. From the end of the Crimean War, Russia no longer had access to the Mediterranean Sea through the Bosphorus. Seeking to unblock this situation, the Russian imperial fleet was allowed to move into the Villefranche harbour in 1858. As *L'Avenir de Nice* celebrated: 'Villefranche would draw up a new industrial and commercial life that has long since lost, and Nice would finally be delivered from the sad vicinity of a lazaretto.'[53] The local authorities and press clearly no longer regarded the lazaretto as an advantage as they had done in previous decades. Already, in 1854, the Municipality of Nice, comparing the cholera mortality of Genoa and Marseille to Nice, boasted that the city was not only a haven against winter storms, but also against cholera. In order to reassure the growing numbers of foreigners, the administration was committed 'to dispel false rumours that envious malevolence poured against the health of the country'.[54]

Later, when in the midst of a new cholera epidemic Italy called into question its own legislation of *Sanità Marittima* (April 1866), it did so by taking into account the experience of the epidemic of 1854. On the one hand, it suppressed the *Direzione di Sanità Marittima*, and the dual system (land versus maritime measures; public hygiene versus quarantine) was merged into a single board of health. On the other hand, it criticised the deficiencies of the 1851 ISC regulations, particularly the optional quarantines against cholera in the context of neoquarantinism. The province of Nice had by then already changed its initial enthusiasm for Italian unification into that for annexation to France, which would be finally executed as a result of the Treaty of Turin of 24 March 1860.

The case of Nice has helped us show that difficulties in harmonising quarantine (regulations) did not only occur at the level of international cooperation but also, until the second half of the nineteenth century, within states; and it lends support to Peter Baldwin's criticism of Ackernecht's classic dualistic vision of the nineteenth-century debate between contagionism and anticontagionism. The division of the city of Nice into districts, the development of public hygiene and naval hygiene, the installation of specialised hospitals for cholera patients (already in 1835) do not suggest a clear-cut political dividing line between contagionism and miasmatism. Democratic, liberal, economic and health revolutions unfold with great complexity. To oppose in clear-cut fashion contagionism and anticontagionism around the issue of cholera quarantine measures can be reductive. Neoquarantinism actually involved both kinds of prophylaxis.[55] In the case of the province of Nice, it was less the geographical position than the pressure of traders and public opinion and the memory of the failure of stringent measures to prevent the first intrusion of cholera into the Kingdom of Sardinia, through the ports of Nice and Villefranche in 1835, that tipped the balance of sanitary regulations towards the field of anticontagionism.

Notes

1 D. Panzac, 'Pratiques anciennes et maladies nouvelles: la difficile adaptation de la politique sanitaire au XIXe siècle', *Bulletin et Mémoire de la Société d'Anthropologie de Paris* 10, 1, 1998, 53–66.

2 Erwin Ackerknecht, 'Anticontagionism between 1821 and 1867', *Bulletin of the History of Medicine* 22, 1948, 562–593.

3 Archives Départementales des Alpes-Maritimes, 2Q71/02, *Procédure d'amodiation en emphytéose de l'ancien lazaret de Nice* (1820).

4 Archivio Storico della Camera dei Deputati, *Tornata del 5 magio 1857*.

5 Richard Pankhurst, 'Europe's discovery of the Ethiopian Taenicide-Kosso', *Medical History* 23, 1979, 299.

6 A. Brayer, *Neuf années à Constantinople. Observations sur [...] la peste, ses causes, ses variétés, sa marche et son traitement: la non-contagion de cette maladie; les quarantaines et les lazarets [...]*, Bellizard, Barthès, Dufour et Lowell, 1836, 2, 368–372.

7 R. Tresse, 'Les débuts de la navigation à vapeur au Port de Nice (1830–1840)', *Recherches régionales des Alpes-Maritimes et des contrées limitrophes* 2, 1965, 39–55.

8 *Leggi e provvedimenti di sanità per gli stati di terraferma di S.M. il Re di Sardegna*, Torino, Per Cassone, Marzorati e Vercellotti, 1831, 247.
9 Ackerknecht, 'Anticontagionism between 1821 and 1867', 16.
10 *La Gazette médicale de Paris* 16, 16, 21 avril 1838, 242.
11 A. Bachemont, 'Cannes et les Anglais (1835–1930)', *Recherches régionales. Alpes-Maritimes et contrées limitrophes*, 197, 2011.
12 Janine Malaussena, 'Le Magistrat de Santé et la protection sanitaire à Nice au XIXème siècle', PhD thesis, University of Nice, 1983.
13 The report, entitled 'Histoire de la marche du choléra morbus à Nice', is published in A. Demougeot, 'Le choléra à Nice en 1835', *Nice-Historique* 1974, 103–113.
14 Ibid.
15 Archives Départementales des Alpes-Maritimes, 1FS432, *Choléra 1849*.
16 F. Hildelsheimer, 'L'administration sanitaire monégasque vue de Marseille (XVIII-XIXe siècles)', *Annales monégasques* 1, 1977, 111–122.
17 Ministère des Affaires Etrangères, *Procès-verbaux de la Conférence Sanitaire Internationale ouverte à Paris 27 juillet 1851*, Paris, Imprimerie nationale, 1852.
18 Francisco Javier Martínez, 'International or French? The early International Sanitary Conferences and France's struggle for hegemony in the mid-nineteenth century Mediterranean', *French History* 30, 1, 2015, 77–98.
19 Norman Howard-Jones, *The Scientific Background of the International Sanitary Conferences 1851–1938*, Geneva, World Health Organization, 1975, 15.
20 *Rapporto della commissione dell'Accademia medico-chirurgica di Genova incaricata di riferire sull'operato del Congresso Sanitario Internazionale riunito nel 1851 in Parigi, letto nella seduta generale del 26 luglio 1852*, Genova, Co'tipi del R.I. de' sordo-muti, 1852.
21 P. Bourdelais, 'L'épidémie créatrice de frontières', *Cahiers du Centre de recherches historiques* 42, 2008, 14.
22 'Legge, colla quale si autorizza il Governo a dare esecuzione alla Convenzione internazionale sanitaria e dall'annesso Regolamento firmati a Parigi il 3 febbraio 1852, 2 décembre 1852', *Raccolta degli atti del Governo di Suà Maestà il Re di Sardegna*, vol. 20, Torino, Dalla Stamperia Reale, 1852, 903.
23 Patrice Bourdelais and Jean-Yves Raulot, *Une peur bleue: Histoire du choléra en France 1832–1854*, Paris, Payot, 1987.
24 Próspero Pirondi, *Considerazioni sulla contagiosita del cholera-morbus asiatico precedute da una critica analisi delle due memorie del Signor Bo: le quarantene e il cholera-morbus*, Marsiglia, Arnaud e C[i], 1856.
25 M. Cevasco, *Statistique de la Ville de Gênes*, t.2, Gênes, Imprimerie Ferrando, 1840, 10. The author talks about 'indirect costs of quarantine' to

describe the specific situation in Genoa, with its old lazaretto of La Foce and its great lazaretto of Varignano in La Spezia. 'Ce qui augmente la dépense sanitaire à Gênes est la position de nos lazarets du Varignan et de la Foce. Il est prescrit par tous les Règlements Sanitaires des peuples civilisés qu'un bâtiment ne peut commencer sa quarantaine de rigueur, qu'après avoir débarqué ses marchandises. D'où il s'ensuit que les bâtiments ne pouvant aller au Lazaret de la Foce, à cause de sa position, l'on est obligé de débarquer la cargaison sur des bateaux [...]. Bien souvent le mauvais temps empêche ses embarcations d'approcher du rivage où est placé le lazaret de la Foce, et de là des frais encore plus prolongés de quarantaine à cause du non débarquement [...]. Il arrive que des navires sont frélés pour faire leur quarantaine dans le port de Gênes, et qu'à peine ils arrivent, ils sont obligés par le Magistrat de Santé d'aller au Lazaret du Varignan pour y purger leurs marchandises.'

26 Gio Battista Massone, *Manuale d'igiene medicina navale ad uso della marina mercantile italiana e specialmente sarda*, Genova, Presso Dario Giuseppe Rossi, 1856, 507.

27 Archives départementales des Alpes-Maritimes, FS 138/004, 14 juin 1854.

28 Jacques Ruffié and Jean-Charles Sournia, *Les épidémies dans l'histoire de l'homme. Essai d'anthropologie médicale*, Paris, Flammarion, 1995, 140.

29 Archives départementales des Alpes-Maritimes, FS 138/005, '*Relazione generale nel cholera 1854*', rédigée par l'Intendant Général de Della Marmora, brouillon daté du 24 septembre 1854.

30 *L'Avenir de Nice. Journal des Alpes-Maritimes*, 17 et 18 juillet 1854.

31 *L'Avenir de Nice. Journal des Alpes-Maritimes*, 17 et 18 juillet 1854.

32 Francesco Freschi, *Storia documentata della epidemia di cholera-morbus in Genova nel 1854*, Genova, Co' Tipi del R. I. de' Sordo-Muti, 1855, 61–65.

33 Archives départementales des Alpes-Maritimes, FS 138/004, 1FS 433.

34 *L'Avenir de Nice. Journal des Alpes-Maritimes*, 29 juillet 1854.

35 *La Vérité. Journal de Nice*, Jeudi 3 août 1854 et Mardi 8 août 1854.

36 '*Il Piroscafo il Dante, non è giunto questa mane da Genova, si dice che per tema della malattia i marinai sieno disertati e fuggiti*'. Abbé Montolivo, *Storia Patriae!* Registre no 337, 6 agosto 1854, Catalogue des manuscrits, Bibliothèque Municipale de Nice, 103.

37 Freschi, *Storia documentata della epidemia*, 24–25.

38 'The Maritime Health Board of Genoa has just ordered a quarantine against the arrivals from the Kingdom of the Two Sicilies' and 'the government of Naples has struck the arrivals from Malte with a quarantine of seven days'. Similarly, 'the Parmesan government has established a sanitary cordon in the border with the Sardinian States' and 'the health authority of Livorno has delivered foul bills of health because of the invasion of

epidemic cholera'. *L'Avenir de Nice. Journal des Alpes-Maritimes*, 30 juillet 1854, 4 août 1854, 5 août 1854.

39 *L'Avenir de Nice. Journal des Alpes-Maritimes*, 30 juillet 1854.

40 *La Vérité. Journal de Nice*, 1er août 1854.

41 Archives Départementales des Alpes-Maritimes, 1FS433.

42 Abbé Montolivo, *Storia Patriae!*, 102, 3 agosto 1854.

43 'Instruction populaire sur le choléra: sur les moyens de le prévenir et sur les premiers secours à donner aux malades, suivie de quelques avertissements sur la manière de ventiler et désinfecter les chambres des cholériques'. *L'Avenir de Nice. Journal des Alpes-Maritimes*, 3 août 1854.

44 *L'Avenir de Nice. Journal des Alpes-Maritimes*, août 1854.

45 Abbé Montolivo, *Storia Patriae!*, 107, 19 agosto 1854. 'Yesterday evening arrived in Vilafranca a French commercial "schooner" whose captain was sick on board. The health board was closed and the boat did not leave at the scheduled time waiting for the doctor [...] though the latter wanted to stay at length on a small boat. Around eleven o'clock the captain died. In the morning, a report was given to the Console di Marina, Mr. Ottavi, who ordered the corpse to be buried in the lazaretto's cemetery if local authorities did not oppose it. The commander did not agree and the corpse was thrown to the sea at some distance from the lighthouse. It is high time the government brings these procedures under control and give exact instructions to the commanders, whose acts of that kind arise widespread rejection.'

46 Abbé Montolivo, *Storia Patriae!*, 109, 27 agosto 1854. 'It seems the disease is close to disappear [sic]. In the present day, there was a single decease [sic]. That the boats arriving from Marseille, Genoa and other places infected with cholera morbus are admitted in free practice while those which depart from Nice, where cholera is virtually over, and touch the port of San Gioanni di Vilafranca, are under quarantine, these are absurdities I cannot understand.'

47 Abbé Montolivo, *Storia Patriae!*, 114, 15 settembre 1854. 'We have in Nice a *Consiglio di Sanità*, but the public opinion considers it would be better if it did not exist. For over fifteen days cholera has been completely absent from our city and territory, for many days the hospital for cholerics has been closed.'

48 Archives Municipales de Nice, I, 149. *Stato nominativo dei Ricoverati nello Spedale dei colerosi stabilito nel locale del Seminario e Movimento giornaliezo de medisini dal 29 Luglio a tutto il 9 setttembre 1854. Ricapitolazione.*

49 Freschi, *Storia documentata della epidemia*, 219–221.

50 *L'Avenir de Nice. Journal des Alpes-Maritimes*, 3 août 1855.

51 Archivio Storico della Camera dei Deputati, *Tornata del 5 magio 1857*.

52 Luigi Cesare Bollea, *Camillo Cavour e il colera del 1854–1855*, Torino, Tip. Pietro Cerbone, 1911.
53 *L'Avenir de Nice. Journal des Alpes-Maritimes*, 18 août 1858.
54 D. Bon, 'Nice et le cholera au XIXe siècle. Mesures sanitaires entre thèses contagionnistes et infectionnistes', *L'Etat et la mer. Environnements et usages. De l'Antiquité à nos jours. Du Rhône au Golfe de Gênes*, Monaco, Actes du Congress, IREP Come, 2008, 1–9.
55 P. Bourdelais, 'Comptes rendus', *Annales de demographie historique* 1, 2001, 213–242; Peter Baldwin, *Contagion and the State in Europe, 1830–1930*, Cambridge, Cambridge University Press, 1999; *Annales de démographie historique* 1, 2001, 213–242.

3

Mending 'Moors' in Mogador: *Hajj*, cholera and Spanish–Moroccan regeneration, 1890–99

Francisco Javier Martínez

Introduction

In the summer of 1896, two very different groups of people crammed into the tiny 500 × 300 metres uninhabited islet located in front of the Moroccan port of Essaouira (Mogador for Europeans, see Figure 3.1). The first and most numerous group consisted of the 1,653 *hajjis* (Muslim pilgrims) debarked in notoriously insanitary conditions from the French steamer *Gergovia*, owned by the *Compagnie Fabre et Cie* of Marseilles.[1] As the sultans of Morocco had allowed Mogador Island to be used as a lazaretto since 1866,[2] the pilgrims were quarantined in this site due to suspected cases of cholera. The second group was led by the Spanish army doctor Enrique Rebolledo, appointed director of the lazaretto by the Sanitary Council of Tangier, an international board to which the sultans had granted powers to fight the importation of epidemics since 1844. Rebolledo was accompanied by a team of eleven Spanish nurses and auxiliaries, plus seven Moroccan workers and eighty-seven Moroccan *askaris* (soldiers) for a total of 105 men[3] – with the final addition of Ricardo Álvarez, the Council's delegate in Mogador, who came and went between the islet and the coast with three Moroccan officials and eighteen sailors. In total, nearly 1,800 people occupied Mogador Island between 21 and 28 July 1896.[4]

This was not an isolated event. During the nineteenth and twentieth centuries, the saintly halo of *baraka* earned with the *Hajj* no longer prevented ever-increasing numbers of Muslim pilgrims from being

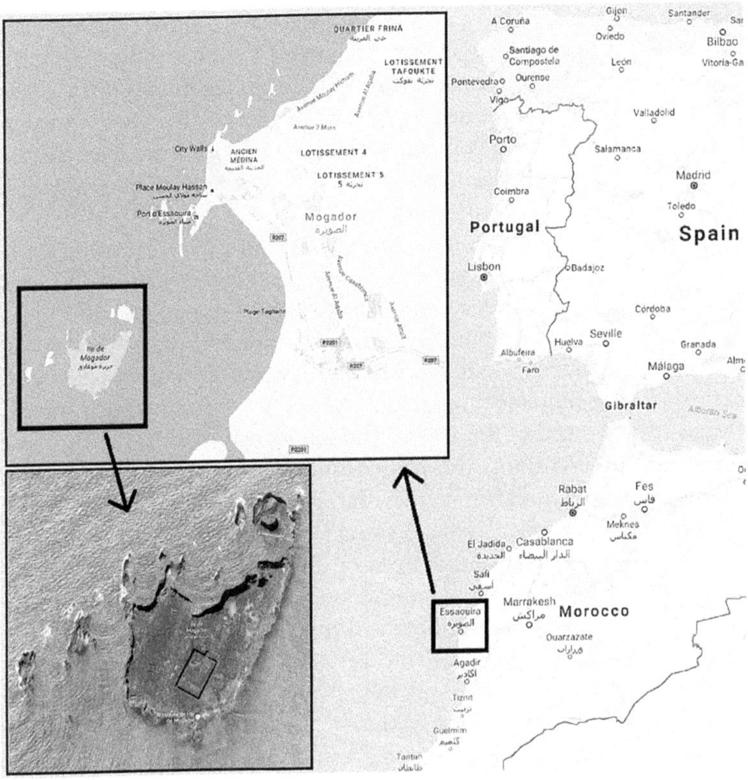

Figure 3.1 Location and present-day state of Mogador Island.

quarantined. The leading role of international health bodies and foreign doctors in this process has led to the belief that this was solely a consequence of European imperialism. Thus, Michael C. Low has argued that the real or perceived political and sanitary risks Europeans attached to the *Hajj* merged in a pathologising narrative of 'twin infection' by Pan-Islamism and epidemics which stood behind Europe's mounting intervention in Islamic countries in that period.[5] Actually, we think this narrative was also appropriated by local Islamic rulers whose modernisation plans could be equally hindered by either religious radicalism or incontrollable disease. Pilgrims were therefore suspected of importing ideas capable of triggering revolts not just against European imperialism, but also against the reforms promoted by those rulers (sultans, beys or khedives) and against their traditional religious authority. It was also believed that the disease they carried in their bodies would threaten not just Europe's strong containment efforts, but also the more fragile measures promoted by Islamic governments to protect their population against the ravages of cholera or plague.

In this context, the sanitary discourses and practices towards the Mecca pilgrimage had certain remarkable specificities in Morocco. This was probably due to the Alawite sultanate's peripheral status with regard to the *Hajj* and to European imperialism – as occurred in the case of Bosnia-Herzegovina, which Christian Promitzer analyses in Chapter 6 of this volume. Building on previous studies, we will study such specificities for the period of the 1890s. Though formally subject to multiple European interventions, the Moroccan *Hajj* became then mostly a Spanish-controlled affair, framed within a short-lived imperialist project of 'regeneration' by which Spain sought to acquire a hegemonic stand over the 'civilising mission' designs of their European rivals.[6] We will also analyse how such regeneration required the social production and protection of 'Moors', imagined as a modernised, Hispanophile and healthy elite eager to support, and actually expected to participate, in Spanish–Moroccan reforms – including public health reforms. This singular example of what Alison Bashford has dubbed 'imperial hygiene' – European domination of African and Asian societies by means of sanitation and cleanliness – had in the tiny Mogador Island one of its main material and symbolic sites.[7]

Regenerating Morocco into an 'African Spain'

Experts on Moroccan history, including many Spanish historians, usually assimilate, implicitly or explicitly, the nature of Spain's imperialism in Morocco into the one deployed by its more powerful competitors: Britain and France. The success of nineteenth-century British and especially twentieth-century French plans in the Maghreb therefore results in an image of Spanish initiatives oscillating between the ludicrous and the violent or, more often, in their being despised as largely non-existent or irrelevant – to such an extent that one might wonder how Spain ever managed to take hold of part of Morocco at all.[8] In our opinion, historiography has generally failed to grasp a fundamental contradiction in Spanish–Moroccan contemporary relations. Spain was a main European imperialist power in nineteenth-century Morocco, seriously challenging France and Britain for hegemony in the years following the Spanish–Moroccan War of 1859–60 and in the decade preceding the loss of Cuba and the Philippines in 1898; yet, Spain could only deploy specific, unconventional models of imperialist intervention owing to its modest economic and military power, its ranking as a secondary actor in international politics as well as its secular historical and cultural ties with Morocco.

During the 1890s, the second and last occasion in which Spain was well positioned to gain control over the whole of Morocco, Spanish policy relied mostly on a 'regeneration' project instead of the dominant 'civilisation' scheme which Great Britain and France wished to deploy in the Alawite sultanate – and were already practising in large parts of Africa and Asia.[9] The singularity of 'regeneration' as an imperialist model derived from its having been originally conceived for intervention in Spain itself. Since the 1870s, even earlier, regeneration had been put forward by some intellectual and political actors as an urgently required drive towards modernisation to end the country's centuries-long 'decay'.[10] Such a drive required deep changes in the political regime, the state administration, the army, agriculture, industry, education and science. In the beginning, advocates of regeneration called for the expansion of existing colonies and the acquisition of new ones as a necessary complement for reforms at home. However, by the mid 1880s, renowned personalities such as Joaquín Costa (1846–1911) saw that an eventual success of regeneration in Spain would closely depend on the ability to deploy a similar intervention scheme over non-European societies, in particular over Spain's southern neighbour. Costa argued in a famous rally held at the Alhambra theatre of Madrid in 1884 that Morocco was

> a country in decay, as we decayed too, and which, as ourselves, can regenerate itself and restore the splendour of those two African Athens: Fez and Marrakech. [We should help Morocco to] regenerate itself so completely that [it becomes] a virile, independent, cultivated nation, naturally allied with Spain.[11]

Costa's utopianism was bound to fail in real politics. However, the Liberal Party cabinet which rose to power in November 1885, with the regenerationist and 'Africanist' Segismundo Moret (1833–1913) as Minister of Foreign Affairs, sought to put into practice some pragmatic and feasible measures that the *Sociedad Española de Africanistas y Colonistas* (Spanish Society of Africanists and Colonists, SSAC) had picked up from the speeches of Costa and several other speakers in the Alhambra rally. As with Costa, the SSAC sought to encourage 'the regeneration of that country [Morocco] and its fraternal union with Spain',[12] but its ultimate goal, according to President Francisco Coello (1822–98), was to make of

> that rag of a nation a great people [...] fraternally united with Spain through the ties of education, a common mentality and the harmony of interests, as it already is by the ties of tradition, climate and blood, in such a way that, without losing its own personality, it substantially reproduces the features of the Spanish nationality, becoming a sort of African Spain.[13]

The creation of this 'African Spain' would not respect Morocco's sovereignty as much as Costa's proposals, but it would not imply a thorough dismantling of the Moroccan state, army, economy or education system either. Instead, it would build upon ongoing local reforms and modernisation projects of Sultan Hassan I (1873–94), who was decidedly following the steps of his predecessors on the Moroccan throne, as well as the pioneering example of the Ottoman Empire's *tanzimat* and of Muhammad Ali's reforms in Egypt. It is true that regeneration was to be led by an elite of Spanish experts (diplomats, army officers, physicians, engineers, teachers, entrepreneurs) occupying key power positions within the Moroccan state apparatus. Nonetheless, it also implied a commitment to the creation of local institutions to train an elite of modern experts who would play leading roles alongside Spaniards. In Costa's words, Spain:

> sought a foothold for reforms in Moroccan youth by training a generation of physicians, engineers, industrialists, army officers and jurists possessing all the tastes, the competences and the abilities of modern [European] culture.[14]

Although actual Spanish initiatives would not produce 'a generation' of Moroccan modern experts as Costa, again, hyperbolically imagined, they trained a non-negligible number of them. The most important projects were based in Tangier, the real 'centre of power' of late nineteenth-century Morocco[15] and the dreamed capital of the future 'African

Spain' (all Europeans imagined Tangier as the capital of their own colonial Morocco).[16] Largely forgotten today, several regenerationist projects were launched during the late 1880s and 1890s with the active collaboration of Moroccan authorities and elites. For example, a *Cámara de Comercio* (Chamber of Commerce), set up in 1888 for encouraging bilateral economic intercourse and composed of Spaniards and Moroccans – mostly Jews but some Muslims too. The army doctor Felipe Óvilo (1850–1909) (Figure 3.2), a member of the SSAC and close personal friend of Moret – who actually appointed him military attaché in Tangier in 1886 – was instrumental in its creation. During his ten-year term of office, Óvilo would intervene in many other projects. He founded and directed the *Escuela de Medicina* (medical school) in 1886, which turned into an official training centre for Moroccan army physicians four years later, with some fifteen to twenty students attending lectures until its closure in 1904.[17] He also set up a *Sociedad de Salvamento de Náufragos* (Lifeboat Society) in 1888 for shipwreck rescue in the Gibraltar Strait and took steps to create a Moroccan 'Red Cross' in the late 1890s.[18] He worked in the new Spanish Hospital (1888), built and managed by Franciscan friars, funded by the Ministry of Foreign Affairs and admitting European and Moroccan patients, and was co-founder and member of the *Comisión de Higiene* (Local Health Board) (1888) in which his colleague Severo Cenarro (1853–98), army doctor attached to the Spanish consulate, acted as permanent secretary.[19]

Óvilo and Cenarro were involved in two other ambitious projects. One was a hybrid *Academia Militar/Escuela de Artes y Oficios* (Military Academy/Technical School) for training both Moroccan military officers and civil technicians, and the other was an *Instituto de Enseñanza Secundaria* (High School) for Spanish and Moroccan pupils. Both would be interrupted around 1890.[20] Otherwise, the Franciscan Catholic Mission directed by José Lerchundi (1836–96) opened primary schools for girls and boys in the early 1880s, some of whose pupils and teachers were Moroccan. It also founded a 'Hispano-Arabic' printing house in 1880, constructed a working-class neighbourhood (San Francisco) in 1888, with adjacent factories employing residents, and built and managed both the old and new Spanish hospitals opened in 1881 and 1888 respectively. Lerchundi also set up an *Escuela de Estudios Árabes* (School of Arabic Studies) in nearby Tetouan in 1886 for the training of Spanish and Moroccan experts in Arabic language and culture.[21]

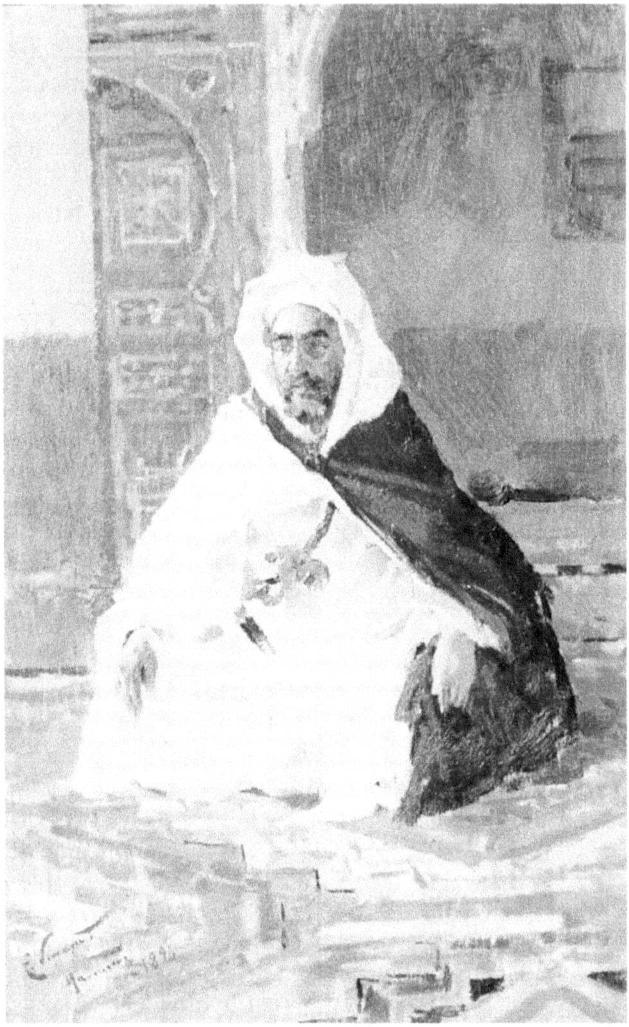

Figure 3.2 Portrait of Felipe Óvilo in 'Moorish' dress in Marrakech, by Enrique Simonet, 1894.

Finally, private entrepreneurs also made significant contributions to regeneration plans. Thus, Emilio Rotondo installed Tangier's first telephone network in 1887 (later, Larache's and Rabat's) operated by a staff comprising Moroccan Muslim and Jewish technicians, while Abelardo Sastre set up a large farm called *El Mediar* from where he annually exported hundreds of cattle heads to Gibraltar, Barcelona and Marseille and in which he employed Spanish and Moroccan workers.[22]

It should be pointed out that plans to turn Morocco into an 'African Spain' were not exclusively advanced by the progressive sectors in Spanish society. Conservative groups promoted an alternative understanding of that goal as well as alternative strategies for attaining it. Thus, Manuel Olivié, a lawyer and politician committed to overseas expansionism, argued that Spain should follow the nineteenth-century European trend of 'creating large states composed of a plurality of nations sharing strong ethnic, geographical and historical features'.[23] Spain had 'the duty of merging into a single [Spanish] state' Morocco, Portugal and Gibraltar.[24] With regard to the sultanate, 'there is no other option but to assimilate Morocco to us, so that the sentiment of a shared homeland extends from the Pyrenees to the sands of the Sahara'.[25] This would create a trans-Mediterranean polity occupying both sides of the Strait of Gibraltar, composed of a 'European Spain and [an] African Spain harmoniously tied by social assimilation'.[26] Olivié imagined this as a European-style state-building process rather than as an imperial enterprise – it would actually prevent the 'real' colonisation of Morocco by more powerful European countries. In his view,

> Spain, by extending its laws to the Atlas, undertakes a venture analogous to those of Germany and Italy, by redeeming Moroccans from the tyranny and anarchy in which they live, and from European influences, which regard that territory as a business haven.[27]

Olivié's projects, in contrast to regeneration, left little or no space for Moroccan agency in the creation of an 'African Spain'. They were more in tune with projects such as the establishment of a 'royal protectorate' over the Saharan coast south of Cape Juby obtained by Spanish agents in 1885. Despite all this, Spanish late nineteenth-century imperialism in Morocco, either progressive or conservative, did not demand such disrupting transformations as British and French civilising schemes did.[28] In this sense, although Khaled ben Shrir and other historians have ascribed the 'reforms' experienced by Morocco to British policy – during the long term of office of the diplomat John Drummond-Hay (1845–86)[29] – the main difference between British and Spanish reforms lay in the agency the latter allowed to local elites. The 'civilising mission' implied a systematic subalternisation of Moroccans in dependent roles under the lead of foreign experts monopolising knowledge and power. Spanish regeneration schemes, by contrast, committed themselves to train Moroccan experts and create modern local institutions, two things the British never attempted to do in Morocco, not even in nearby Gibraltar where dozens of Moroccans received only basic military or medical training. In addition, from the late 1880s, Britain openly despised reforms, its Moroccan policy consisting in lobbying the sultan and the higher government officials by way of influential agents, such as Sir Harry Maclean, in order to advance British economic and diplomatic interests.[30]

The Mogador Island lazaretto and Spanish–Moroccan sanitary borders

Public health reform was one important goal of Spanish regeneration in Morocco. Despite what many historians continue to argue, the country did not completely lack a modern sanitary administration.[31] Following general developments in the Arab-Islamic Mediterranean, especially in the Ottoman Empire and Egypt, an embryonic quarantine system had been put in operation during the nineteenth century as a combined outcome of local reforms and international pressure.[32] At the top of it stood the International Sanitary Council of Morocco (also known as the Sanitary Council of Tangier due to its being located in this town), to which Sultan Abderrahman ibn Hicham granted powers in 1840 to ensure 'the maintenance of public health over the empire's seaboard, to draft all regulations and take all measures to carry out this task'.[33] The Council had been preceded by a board called *Junta de Cónsules*, set up in 1792 – as Malika Ezzahidi points out in Chapter 4 – and it was composed of the diplomatic representatives of Britain, France, Prussia (later Germany), Spain, Piedmont-Sardinia (later Italy), Belgium, Portugal, Russia, Austria-Hungary, Sweden and the United States, who occupied its presidency in turns, and was a consultative body entitled to propose to the sultan (by way of his representative in

Tangier, the *naib*) measures against the importation and diffusion of 'exotic' epidemic diseases, originally cholera and, by the end of the nineteenth century, bubonic plague too. Council delegations were soon established in the ports open to international commerce (Tetouan, Larache, Rabat, Casablanca, Mazagan, Safi, Mogador) and doctors of several European nationalities began to act as *medicos de sanidad* or *consultores médicos* (medical advisors) of the Council and its delegations. From the end of the Spanish–Moroccan War until 1899 the head position in Tangier was monopolised by Spanish physicians, among whom were Óvilo (1877–78) and Cenarro (1884–97).

Certainly, this quarantine administration was insufficiently 'medicalised'. For example, the Council was not obliged to follow the technical advice of its medical advisors because only diplomats were official members. It was only natural that, as Óvilo explained in *De l'influence des pèlerinages marocains à la Mecque sur la propagation du choléra* (1882), 'in most occasions, the Council debates and takes decisions without the participation of its medical adviser'.[34] In the same vein, the sultan could always ignore the Council's suggestions for he had never turned over the executive authority on sanitary matters to foreign diplomats. Thus, in 1878, after Óvilo's proposed measures for preventing the diffusion of cholera from the interior of the country to the main ports (the ban on that year's pilgrimage to Mecca and the establishment of inland sanitary cordons and field lazarettos around the main ports) had been accepted by the Council and Hassan I, the sultan

> who backed the measures taken by the Sanitary Council, had deployed troops to execute them and had created a new tax 'for lazarettos', to provide funds for sanitary cordons, revoked these salutary measures through a *dahir* [decree] by the end of September and […] the whole edifice built with countless efforts crumbled in a single day.[35]

The weak medicalisation of Moroccan quarantines was also due to the lack of proper facilities and equipment. The only lazaretto existing in the country, Mogador Island, was inappropriate for the task. Sultan Mohammed IV had agreed to the site being used to confine suspect Mecca pilgrims in 1866[36] after projects and demands for sanitary use dating back at least to 1821.[37] Mohammed El-Bezzaz has explained how the serious threat posed by the fourth cholera pandemic, combined with Spanish pressure following the third ISC in Constantinople in

1866, led the sultan to allow quarantines in Mogador Island through a *dahir* issued on 18 November of that year.[38] However, the site had neither a disinfection stove, nor a barrack for the diseased, nor a pavilion where the healthy pilgrims might be lodged. According to Óvilo, pilgrims just spent 'from three to ten days on the [island's] reefs, after which they move to the mainland'.[39] There was no quay where ships could safely moor and unload their passengers and baggage regardless of weather conditions. The proximity to the coast and the city (less than a mile off) added to the risk of people escaping and spreading diseases inland. Last but not least, as the Irish doctor Arthur Leared pointed out, ships normally bound for Tangier were

> compelled […] to proceed to this place [Mogador Island], nearly four hundred miles further. This, and justly, has been considered a great grievance, though it is one which at present admits no remedy.[40]

To avoid this, ships that had been put under quarantine of observation in Tangier often escaped from the bay, rounded Cape Spartel and disembarked their passengers on various spots of the Atlantic coast.[41] It was only from 1890, when Spanish regeneration plans promoted the modernisation of the Moroccan sanitary administration, that the lazaretto was equipped and put to regular use. In September of that year, the French steamer *Gallia* arrived at Tangier with 700 pilgrims and a foul bill of health.[42] The Council's delegate visited the ship several times and noted the bad conditions on board, with hunger-stricken passengers crammed on deck. Cenarro and the British and French ministers in Tangier also approached the *Gallia*, and after dramatic scenes of panic and violence triggered by the distribution of 'an insufficient quantity of bread and a few olives' it was decided that the steamer should undergo a six-day quarantine at Mogador Island.[43] Cenarro appointed the Spanish doctor Gustavo Prieto, a regular visitor to Moroccan port towns from nearby Cádiz, as the lazaretto's director. Four *gardiens sanitaires* accompanied him, later joined by twenty-five soldiers sent by Mogador's *qaid* (military governor). A translator could have been used too, on this and on subsequent occasions – Hamed Romani, a physician trained by Óvilo in Tangier, who had taken care of Moroccan pilgrims travelling to Mecca in the previous year's *Hajj*.[44] Prieto was charged with the task of quarantining the pilgrims and disinfecting their luggage, for which purpose he took with him 'a well-supplied medicine chest and appropriate disinfectants'.[45] He was given a hard time. Military protection did not stop the pilgrims from revolting against disinfection procedures and threatening to attack him or swim to the coast. Things finally calmed down and no cholera outbreak occurred.

The quarantine procedure was continued and developed in the following years. Cenarro commissioned Prieto again in late August 1891 to deal with the pilgrims of the French steamer *Sahel*, arriving from Alexandria, who were suspected of cholera despite 'having undergone the quarantine and disinfection imposed on the arrivals from Arabia at the El Tor lazaretto'.[46] Again, no case of cholera was declared at Mogador Island. The following year the pilgrims posed no epidemic risk, but all alarms went off in 1893 after the 'greatest outbreak [of cholera] ever at Mecca since 1865'.[47] This time, Cenarro managed to get permission from the Council so that Prieto and another Spanish doctor, Sotero García de Mayoral, with *gardiens sanitaires* and disinfectants, were sent one month in advance of the expected arrival of pilgrims to organise the lazaretto and prepare the city of Mogador itself.[48] By the end of August, the French ships *Gallia* and *Lutetia* and the British *Afghan* disembarked 1,550 pilgrims.[49] Despite preparations, cholera broke out, causing eight deaths among the thirty-five declared cases.[50] This emergency obliged Cenarro to travel personally to the island, accompanied by two other Spanish physicians, Dr Jiménez and José Prieto (Gustavo's brother), plus eight Spanish medical auxiliaries.[51] The total Spanish and Moroccan staff reached 211 people, of which at least 100 were soldiers.[52] When quarantine was over, the British Vice-Consul in Mogador, Robert Lyon Nelson Johnston, criticised the shortcomings of the lazaretto in a report addressed to the British minister in Tangier. He believed the island had received too many people, was too close to the shore and proved too difficult to supply with water and food. Besides, Moroccan soldiers were reluctant to protect the medical personnel, threatened by pilgrims 'with violence if they persisted in the treatment of the sick, fumigation of clothes, etc.'.[53]

The year 1894 went by with no risk of cholera, but in 1895, following another serious outbreak in Mecca that 'reproduced in a smaller scale' the one that had occurred two years before,[54] the Sanitary Council appointed the Spanish army doctor Enrique Rebolledo as director of the lazaretto and sent him there in March to start preparations. He was expected to remain on Mogador Island until December of the same year.[55] But when the French ship *Maurice et Réunion* asked for permission to disembark 750 pilgrims in Tangier in late August, the Council surprisingly conceded after pressure from French authorities, who insisted that all passengers were in good health after having been inspected in Algier's Matifou lazaretto. Cholera broke out in Tangier, causing over 400 deaths, and subsequently spread to Tetouan, Fez and other cities.[56] In early October, Cenarro presented a report on the epidemic to the Council in which he suggested that cholera had been imported by the *Maurice et Réunion* and demanded the establishment of a permanent lazaretto at Mogador Island as the best way to protect the country against the disease.[57] In this way, Spain was trying to institutionalise the measures deployed in previous years, which had hitherto received no official sanction, neither by the sultan, nor by the Council. France opposed Spanish plans. The French minister denied the importation of the disease by the French ship based on reports drafted by Dr Spivakoff, director of the French Hospital in Tangier, and Dr Henri Soulié, director of the recently founded Pasteur Institute of Algiers, who had been sent on an official mission to Morocco to study the epidemic.[58]

The British also showed little enthusiasm for Mogador Island. However, the head of British diplomacy in Morocco, Sir Arthur Nicolson, visited the island in March 1896 accompanied by the Gibraltar-based Surgeon-Major MacPherson, to check the site's conditions before the new pilgrimage season.[59] The latter's report showed a significant improvement of facilities on the island over the previous years. A house had been built for the doctor and auxiliaries. The six artillery batteries on the island's perimeter had been repaired and equipped with underground water tanks for collecting rainwater. A baking oven had been set up in one of them. Three bigger water tanks had been additionally built in the centre of the island, while in its northwest corner an area had been allotted to serve as cemetery. As a result, and despite claiming for further works, MacPherson judged the island 'not unsuited for the purposes of a lazaretto' and capable of containing up to 3,000 people for two months.[60] This favourable opinion would be confirmed when the lazaretto was used later that year, as shown in this chapter's introduction.[61] Dr Rebolledo was sent again well in advance. A hundred conical tents for lodging healthy pilgrims were mounted, probably following a suggestion in MacPherson's report.[62] Infectious patients (with smallpox or dysentery, for no cases of cholera appeared) were treated in separate tents and assisted by separate staff. Pilgrims' clothes and luggage were disinfected with 'sulfuric vapours' in a stove installed in one of the batteries. After five days with no cases of cholera, quarantine was declared over,[63] the finest operation in the thirty years of existence of Mogador Island's lazaretto. On the basis of Rebolledo's experience, a *Projet de règlement général pour le service de quarantaine dans l'île de Mogador* was drafted, though it would never come into force (Figure 3.3).[64]

The weakening of Spain's position in Morocco after the onset of the last war for Cuban independence in February 1895 probably stood behind this failure – and behind the surprising decision of the Council that triggered the Tangier epidemic. Debility would bring more troubles for Spanish plans. In March of 1897, Sultan Abdelaziz (1894–1908) – actually Regent Ba Ahmed (the sultan was still a minor) – forbade the pilgrimage to Mecca due to the heightened risk of importing plague, which had broken out in Hong Kong in 1894 and was spreading rapidly towards Europe after striking British India and Mecca.[65] Such a radical measure had been attempted in Morocco only once since the times of Moulay Slimane (1792–1822) – by Óvilo in 1878, as we said before – because of the potential damage European interference in religious matters was likely to cause to the sultan's prestige.[66] This initiative was inconsistent with the strategy Spain had followed during the decade, and it is likely that it was promoted by France, which, according to Valeska Huber, 'often resorted to the complete prohibition of the pilgrimage' in its imperial possessions.[67] But Ba Ahmed sought to counterbalance the negative political effects of his unwilling decision by building a permanent state prison in Mogador Island.[68] Given that the ban on pilgrimage did not prevent a number of Moroccan *hajjis* from travelling to Mecca, the Council, after sending a medical advisor to the island, asked the regent to remove the prison so that the site was fully available in case of emergency.[69] Ba Ahmed opposed this and frictions escalated with the Council's refusal to admit in Moroccan ports (save for Tangier) any ship carrying pilgrims who could not prove fulfilment of certain strict formalities.[70] The measure was kept in force until 1900, though it was impossible in practice to force navigation companies to comply with it.[71]

These problems anticipated the abrupt end of Spanish plans for the Mogador Island lazaretto. The ban on the pilgrimage was lifted in early

PROJET DE RÈGLEMENT GÉNÉRAL
POUR LE SERVICE DE QUARANTAINE
DANS L'ÎLE DE MOGADOR.

I.

Le personnel de la station de quarantaine dans l'île de Mogador est composé de

1. un médecin en chef, délégué extraordinaire du Conseil Sanitaire, directeur de la station de quarantaine.
2. Deux médecins dont
(a.) un dirige le lazaret d'observation et
(b.) l'autre le lazaret d'infection.
3. Un aide pharmacien.
4. Un infirmier en chef.
5. 16 infirmiers.
6. Les soldats mis à la disposition du directeur par les autorités chérifliennes.
7. Un interprète attaché au médecin en chef

II.

(a.) Le médecin en chef est le représentant direct du Conseil Sanitaire vis à vis des autorités marocaines et de tous les habitants de l'île et est également le chef suprême de la dite île.

Il est de son devoir de s'informer continuellement et consciencieusement de tout se qui se passe sur l'île, de diriger l'administration entière de la station de quarantaine et de pourvoir à tout ce qui est nécessaire pour assurer non seulement la santé de tous ceux qui sont internés mais encore le fonctionnement regulier et correct du service établi. A cet effet il est chargé d'organiser ce service en indiquant à chacun les attributions de ses fonctions. C'est lui, qui, le cas échéant, ordonnera la mise en service du lazaret d'infection et designera le médecin qui devra le diriger.

De même il ordonnera la dissolution de cet établissement. Il visitera chaque jour et, en cas de maladies, plusieurs fois par jour toutes les habitations et autres locaux de la station pour s'assurer de l'état de santé et de l'ordre qui y régnent.

Chaque matin il réunira les médecins placés sous ses ordres ainsi que tous les gradés du personnel pour entendre leurs rapports rélatifs à tout ce qui concerne le service de chacun et leurs observations des dernières 24 heures.

C'est à lui de se prononcer sur les differends qui pourraient surgir entre les habitants de l'île quels qu'ils soient. A cet effet il recevra, après avoir entendu les rapports susmentionés, tous ceux qui auraient à lui soumettre une requête ou une plainte et qui devront lui être présentés par leurs superieurs.

Le médecin en chef est responsable vis à vis du Conseil Sanitaire de tout se qui se passe sur l'île, en consequence de quoi il est autorisé à donner tout les ordres qui lui paraitront nécessaires. Il addressera regulièrement des rapports hebdomadaires au Président du Conseil Sanitaire et si la peste éclatait dans l'île il devra dicter chaque jour et, s'il le trouve opportun, plusieurs fois par jour son rapport par le telephone au Délégué Sanitaire de Mogador, qui le transmettra au Président du Conseil Sanitaire

Pour faciliter la rédaction de ces rapports et assurer leur exactitude, il tiendra un journal "formulaire A" basé sur les rapports journaliers des

Figure 3.3 *Projet de règlement général pour le service de quarantaine dans l'île de Mogador*, 1896.

1898 as the risk of importing plague was low, but the new prison continued to deprive the Council of its only quarantine facility. The French negotiated on their own with the Moroccan Government so that the northern half of the island was used again for sanitary purposes.[72] Dr François was positive about this possibility after visiting the site in March and drew a map of the eventual partition (Figure 3.4).[73] However, after some give and take, Moroccan authorities decided on a further reduction of the space for an eventual quarantine. The Council's new medical advisor, the Spanish army doctor Joaquín Cortés, who had replaced Cenarro after his sudden death in January, travelled to Mogador Island in late 1898 to evaluate the new project, which he rejected.[74] In parallel, Ba Ahmed had proposed three alternative sites for a lazaretto: the island of Perejil/Turah, in the vicinity of Ceuta; the ruins of old Tangier (*Tanjah el-Bali*), in a secluded spot of the bay; and the village of Fedala-Mohammedia, close to Casablanca.[75] The Council judged none of them as suitable.[76]

At the end of 1898, bubonic plague struck Mecca again and, thus, threatened once more to reach Europe and North Africa. In February 1899, alarmed European diplomats in Tangier considered forcing Ba Ahmad to impose a new ban on the *Hajj*, but finally let go of the idea as most pilgrims had already left for Mecca.[77] They insisted, however, on the closure of the prison and, as Moroccan authorities refused, they even envisaged an eventual military occupation of Mogador Island.[78] Things would not go that far and finally, in June, Ba Ahmed agreed to shut down the prison and, in principle, to allow the building of a permanent lazaretto.[79] There was not much time left to have everything ready before the return of pilgrims, but the Council acted swiftly. Cortés, who had drawn for his own personal use a sketch of the 'whole facility',[80] arrived at the island on 4 August to supervise the works, which included the installation of twenty 'wooden sheds' fabricated in Tangier fit for lodging fifty pilgrims each.[81] He appointed the Spanish Navy doctor Alfonso Cerdeira as the lazaretto's director.[82] Nearly 44,000 francs of a projected 100,000 budget would be spent between July and September on the salaries of three physicians and dozens of auxiliaries and workers, plus the purchase and transport of 'a disinfecting oven'.[83]

A first group of 419 pilgrims[84] disembarked on 9 August from the Turkish steamer *Abdelkader* and endured quarantine with no cases

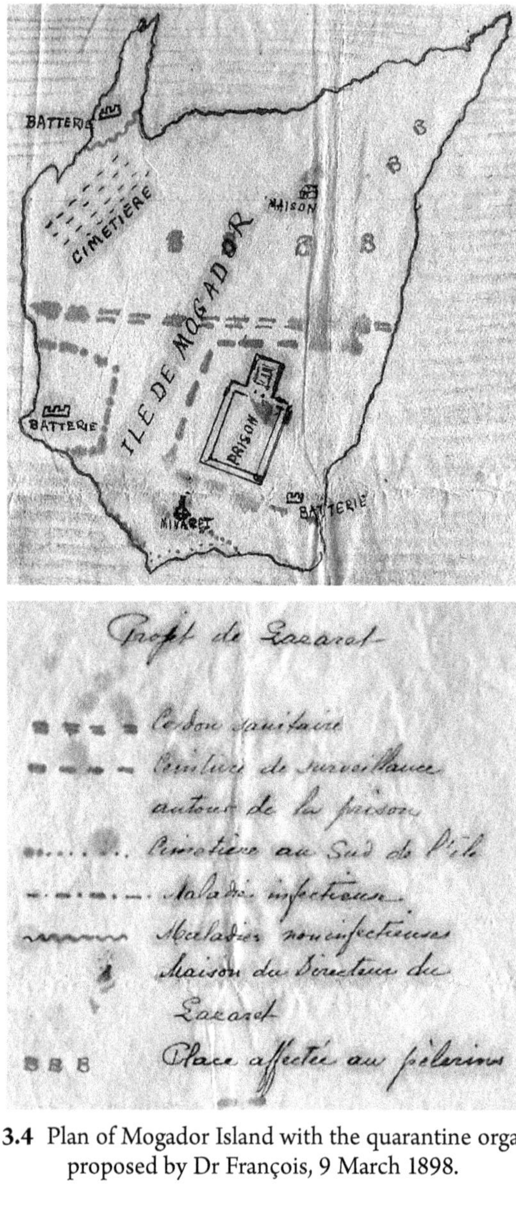

Figure 3.4 Plan of Mogador Island with the quarantine organisation proposed by Dr François, 9 March 1898.

of plague.[85] Before the expected new arrivals, works continued to fix various problems: the disinfecting oven had not been used for lack of a specific room; only a few sheds had been built. However, on 15 August, the *qaid* of Mogador ordered Moroccan workers to stop all activity and, on the 27th, his soldiers tore down the twelve wooden sheds already put up and forced Cortés to leave the island.[86] Although the French minister in Tangier condemned the 'arbitrariness' of Moroccan measures, the French consul in Mogador had complained about Cortés acting unilaterally and not providing information on the quarantine.[87] The French rose to the occasion and proposed that Cortés be 'removed' from all quarantine tasks;[88] he would be the last Spanish doctor to act as the Council's medical advisor. Ba Ahmed ordered that henceforth the directors of the lazaretto were to be physicians 'non-resident' in Morocco.[89] In practice, this opened the door for French doctors to replace Spaniards. Lucien Raynaud (1866–1931) of Algiers would be appointed in 1900 and consolidated France's increasing control of the Moroccan sanitary administration. Although Moroccan officials usually accompanied him – at least on one occasion by an army doctor trained by Óvilo in Tangier and on another one by Zubeir Skirej, a military engineer trained in England – he rejected or ignored them.[90] In his influential book *Étude sur l'hygiène et la médecine au Maroc* (1900), Raynaud ignored as well the quarantines organised by Spanish doctors during the 1890s, which he downplayed by affirming that after 1865 Mogador Island 'has hardly been used a dozen times'.[91] He did not mention the name of any of the doctors who had preceded him in the post.

The events of 1899 became the last and most serious attempt at building a permanent lazaretto on Mogador Island. For ten years, Spanish regeneration initiatives managed to put the site to regular sanitary use, appoint medical directors and auxiliary staff as well as construct facilities and install technical equipment. In general, Spain had significantly advanced its project of setting up a modern quarantine administration in Morocco, centralised in Tangier, with autonomous executive power based on medical personnel and sanitary facilities which intended to reach a good part of the country's maritime borders. All this effort should be understood, in any case, as part of the imperialist project of Spanish–Moroccan regeneration, whose ultimate goal would have been the articulation between the quarantine administrations of

'African Spain' and those of 'peninsular Spain', whose organisation was being accomplished in parallel. As Quim Bonastra shows in Chapter 1, an 1886 Royal Order creating the *Cuerpo de Sanidad Marítima* and another one in 1887 that fixed its *Reglamento* (regulations), culminated the process set off by Spain's 1855 Health Law. These regulations gave official status to the three foul lazarettos which were operating in practice on Spain's extensive seaboard: Mahón, in the Mediterranean Sea; San Simón, in the Atlantic Ocean; and Pedrosa, in the Cantabrian Sea.[92]

If lazarettos acted as maritime border-markers for states (as Daniel Panzac has argued sanitary cordons did for land borders),[93] these particular ones fixed the contour of Spanish national sanitary frontiers. It was, however, easy to see that the southern frontier was exposed, a serious and persistent problem owing to the presence of the British enclave of Gibraltar. Although Gibraltar applied stringent quarantines, as John Chircop explains in Chapter 8, they were not coordinated with Spain's; above all, Gibraltar prevented the establishment of a foul lazaretto in Algeciras that would have undoubtedly hindered the Rock's sanitary independence and commercial activity. The second sanitary border problem, of a rather different nature, concerned the Canary Islands, an archipelago located almost 1,000 km southwest of Spain, facing the Saharan coast beyond the Moroccan port town of Agadir. Canarian authorities had been demanding the construction of a foul lazaretto since at least 1811, when the archipelago had been struck by a massive yellow fever epidemic.[94] Subsequent epidemics (the yellow fever outbreaks of 1838, 1846–47 and 1862–63 and the cholera outbreak of 1851) showed, as I have argued elsewhere, that the Canary Islands were more linked from a sanitary and epidemiological point of view to Cuba than to Spain in that period.[95] This odd fact was nevertheless consistent with the singular relationship established between Spain and Cuba during the middle decades of the century, an intimate and weakly hierarchical link between an 'overseas Spain' and 'peninsular Spain' which served as a model for the late nineteenth-century 'African Spain' project. It was only when that particular relationship began to change, after the Ten Years' War (1868–78), that the Canary Islands moved towards reintegration within Spain's sanitary borders. A Royal Order of 10 February 1882 approved the creation of a fourth national foul lazaretto in Gando (Gran Canaria).

However, I argue/suggest that Spanish regenerationist plans for Mogador Island competed with Gando's project in subsequent years and became a decisive factor behind the latter's constant delays and ultimate lack of use. Gando's works did not start until 1887, the buildings were not finished until 1893, the equipment did not arrive until 1899, and the quay and road needed for the access of passengers and goods were never built.[96] As a result, when new *Sanidad Exterior* regulations were passed in 1899 and 1903, which substituted lazarettos for *estaciones sanitarias* following the new doctrinal orientations prevailing at the eleventh ISC held in Paris, Gando had not yet been used.[97] It would be just once in 1906, with unsatisfactory results, before being abandoned in 1911 in favour of the newly built *estación sanitaria* of the port of Las Palmas.[98] In our opinion, Gando and Mogador were mutually exclusive because they reflected the incompatible conservative and progressive approaches to the 'African Spain' project. Mogador's success would have made the archipelago dependent on Morocco in sanitary and epidemiological terms; Gando's supremacy would have turned the Canary Islands into an all-powerful and largely autonomous sanitary department with prerogatives over Morocco's Atlantic coast (including the Saharan protectorate). The options could not be more disparate for Canarian interests. Both of them implied, however, a close articulation of Spanish and Moroccan maritime sanitary frontiers that would have reduced the exposure of both territories to imported epidemic threats (Figure 3.5).

Constructing an elite of 'Moors'

Regenerationist projects in Morocco rested on a specific discourse about the local society and its inhabitants. To assimilate such a discourse automatically to the orientalist narratives produced by other European countries in that period would again be misleading. Edward Said affirmed in his ground-breaking book of the same title that 'orientalism' was 'a Western style for dominating, restructuring and having authority over the Orient'.[99] As such, it constructed a dualistic, irreducible opposition between the West and the East, which from the eighteenth century onward framed the former's humanistic, artistic and scientific views to help deploy and perpetuate its dominance over the latter. The origin and rise of orientalism were intimately associated with

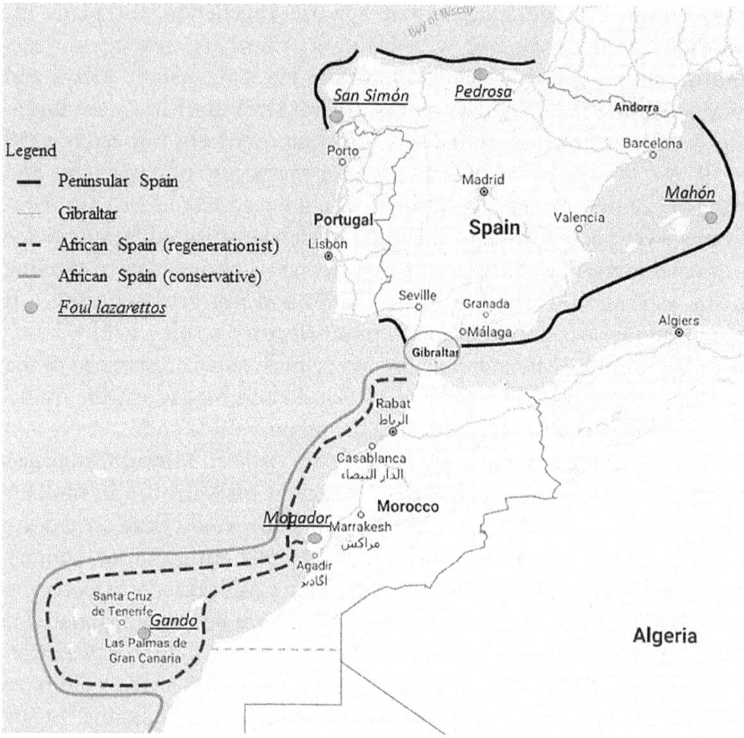

Figure 3.5 Map of the maritime sanitary borders of 'peninsular Spain' and 'African Spain', 1890s.

the second wave of colonial expansion that placed most of Africa and Asia under European rule. However, researchers have pointed out the existence of 'multiple orientalisms' (for example, the various national traditions in Europe) and the subsequent need for 'situating' them in 'time and space'.[100] Frederick Cooper has argued similarly for colonialism not to be taken as a universal, immutable reality, but as one intrinsically contextual and performative. In his opinion,

> The weighty -ity in such widely used words as coloniality or postcoloniality implies that there is an essence of being colonized independent of what anybody did in a colony […] Colonizer and colonized are themselves far from immutable constructs and such categories had to be reproduced by specific actions.[101]

Following Cooper, I suggest colonialism and orientalism showed significant variations according to the specific characteristics of each dominant power and each dominated society in a given historical period. Contemporary Spain was an example of such variability. Certain authors have already pointed out that Spanish nineteenth-century orientalism possessed distinctive features when compared to its European counterparts.[102] On the one hand, it was almost exclusively 'Arabist', with very minor production on the Ottoman Empire or the Far East – despite the proximity of the Spanish Philippines to China and Japan. On the other hand, such 'Arabism' paid less attention to contemporary societies over which Spain sought to impose colonial domination, than to the 'domestic Orient' or 'Spanish Orient' of Al-Andalus established on the Iberian Peninsula from the eighth century to the expulsion of the *moriscos* in 1609–14.[103] These specific features of Spanish orientalism were actually inseparable from those of Spanish colonialism. During the nineteenth century, Spain's expansionist expectations became essentially confined to Morocco, a neighbouring Arab country on whose northern coast Spain possessed several outposts and whose history, far from being exotic, was closely intertwined with that of Spain for many centuries. It was, thus, a 'domestic imperialism', deprived of most of the geographic and cultural displacement associated with colonial expansion.

An effect of all this was that modern Spanish discourses conceptualised Moroccan identity in a fairly balanced way when compared with other European countries' production on various Arab/Oriental societies. Without ignoring the elaboration of stereotyped negative images during the nineteenth and twentieth centuries, I argue there was a radical impossibility for modern Spaniards to define Moroccans as 'others'. This alterisation deficit, that is, the systematic recognition of the Spanish 'us' in the Moroccan 'them' (and vice-versa) would have been an outcome of 'domestic' orientalism and imperialism.[104] The proximity or confusion of identities was formulated in different ways over the course of the century. Regenerationism produced its own version, in which the polysemic category of 'Moors' was given a central role by redefining it in a very specific way. It is possible to analyse this in the works of Felipe Óvilo, despite the fact that his views on Moroccans changed significantly over time. In his early essays, Óvilo subscribed to ideas of older authors, especially the Basque traveller José María de Murga, who followed French discourses on Algeria when he identified five 'races' in

Moroccan society: Arabs, Berbers, Moors, Blacks and Jews.[105] However, while the French judged the dichotomy Arab–Berber as the defining feature of Algerian society, Murga highlighted the central role of the 'Moors' in Morocco. Following that trail, Óvilo considered the 'Moors' were 'the most educated, rich and powerful part of the Maghreb [...] all positions that entail honours and riches are occupied, in most cases, by these Moors, who exploit the members of other races only to be exploited themselves by the Sultan.'[106] They were descendants of 'Mauritanians [Berbers], mixed with Phoenicians, Syrians, Greek-Romans, Vandals, Arabs, Spaniards and Blacks' and their number had risen, especially in coastal cities, after the successive expulsions from Spain of Grenadines and *moriscos*.[107] Many 'Moors' had their origins in 'not few of our ancestors', and among those residing in towns 'the European type is so abundant and it is possible to see men so similar to those of our southern provinces that there is no doubt about it.'[108] If Óvilo blamed the Moors for having 'all the vices and the slyness' of the *razas mezcladas* (mixed races), judging them a 'race meant to disappear soon by consumption',[109] he affirmed nevertheless that only 'a tenth of their faults has its origin in their natural condition; the other nine parts owe to the pernicious organization and absurd regime which oppresses them.'[110]

It is evident that the centrality ascribed to the 'Moors' in Morocco by Murga and Óvilo was due to their perceived historical, cultural and racial links with Spain, to a Hispano-centric interpretation. However, while the former author actually considered Spanish 'renegades' that still existed in Morocco the ideal foothold for Spanish imperialist interventions, the latter assigned that role to 'Moors'. The key for Óvilo was their 'mixed' racial stock, which gave them a sort of proto-national potential for articulating a 'Moroccan' identity and nationality. Beyond the atomisation that characterised Murga's vision, 'Moors' were for Óvilo not just a race among others, but a 'Moroccan' elite that ruled the country. The study of that elite corresponded, thus, more to political analysis than to anthropology; Óvilo identified two groups of asymmetrical size bound together by opposite ideological affinities. Along a larger conservative section, he found that

> although very weak, there exists a group in Morocco which is not so reluctant to advances and progress as most of the powerful people of that country; this fraction, tied together by its friendship with and sympathy

> for the Great Vizir [Muhammad bin al-Arbi al-Jami'i], comprises Muhammad Dukali, Abdulkarim Brisha and their friends.[111]

In later works, published during his second stay in Tangier, Óvilo, while still making use of Murga's racial categories, stopped using them as analytical tools. His political inquiries focused now especially on the 'progressive' sector of the 'Moorish' elite, which had expanded in size and power and from which he chose his most important associates. To the individuals mentioned before, he now added detailed descriptions of two other members of the al-Jami'i family, the brothers Hadj al-Maati and Muhammad al-Saghir, who occupied various higher positions at the court and the government; of Si Faddul Gharnit, Minister of Foreign Affairs in various periods (Figure 3.6); of Sidi Muhammad Torres, *naib* in Tangier from 1885 to 1906; and of some high-level government and army officials (Ahmad al-Sueiri, al-Kerdudi, Muhammad al-Seffar, al-Belghuti).[112] The progressive group was still a minority and his influence restricted, but Óvilo believed its advance reflected the fact that Sultan Hassan I had started a 'regeneration drive' by designating

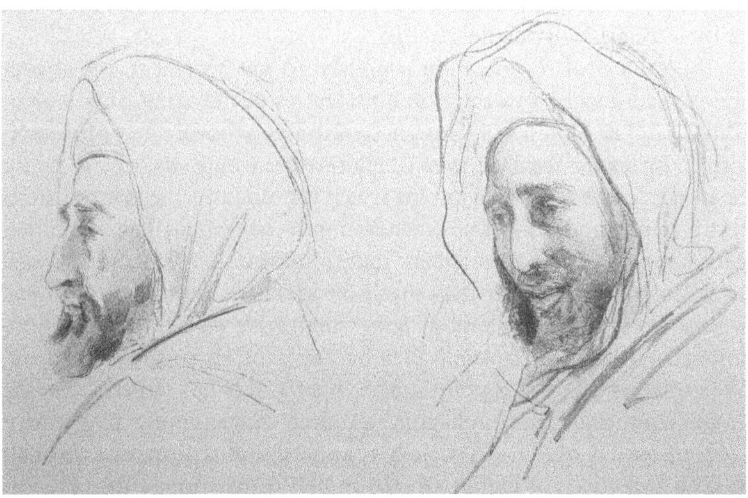

Figure 3.6 Portraits of 'Moors' Si Faddul Gharnit and Muhammad al-Seffar, by Enrique Simonet, 1894.

administration officials 'after personal merit instead of intrigue, hitherto sovereign in the Maghreb'.[113]

If progressive 'Moors' were to be co-opted for constructing the Spanish–Moroccan elite that would lead the process of regeneration, a discourse was required that emphasised the social, historical and cultural similarities on both sides of the Strait of Gibraltar. Thus, Óvilo began by defining the present state of Morocco as one of 'profound decay',[114] in line with the regenerationist diagnostic of Spanish society. Such a situation would have had its ultimate origin in the loss of the heritage transferred to Morocco from 'that feared and blooming Muslim state which passed over in Granada; [of] that Hispano-Arabic people who wrote such brilliant pages *of our glorious history*'.[115] The 'wreckage' and 'eclipse' of that heritage, within which the 'sciences and the remains of Hispano-Arabic art' had occupied an outstanding place, would have been aggravated by the decision of Spanish authorities to destroy and burn 'thousands' of books and documents rather than 'allowing their owners to take them' to North Africa. For Óvilo, this conduct that pleased 'the fanatics who applauded that action', had had negative consequences for Spain too.[116] In sum, Óvilo regarded Granada as a 'Hispano-Arabic' polity marking a zenith in the history of Spain *and* Morocco, its fall being detrimental for both countries, an inaugural sign of their longlasting parallel decline.

The project of regeneration promised to put an end to the above-mentioned decline by acting on both shores of the Strait of Gibraltar. Thus, it did not intend to construct a strongly subordinated Moroccan 'other'. Instead, a weak process of alterisation would distinguish those Spaniards *and* Moroccans joining hands for modernising reforms from those opposing them. The regenerationist 'us' would have included Moroccans and the immobilist 'them', Spaniards. (Actually, 'Moors' were not the only Moroccan group reserved an active role in those regeneration plans. An elite of Jews would have played an even more important role, based on equivalent narratives of 'Hispano-Sephardism'. We cannot develop this point further here as it is not directly relevant to the main topic of this chapter.) Modern, hispanophile, progressive 'Moors' would have been socially produced and reproduced through various initiatives of higher education and instruction, either civil or military; through foreign policy and commerce; through books and paintings. The competition of other European powers for hegemony in

Morocco and local opposition to the sultan's reforms endangered this process, including those threats pertaining to the field of public health.

Mending 'Moors' on Mogador Island

The pilgrimage to Mecca was one of the main political and sanitary threats to 'Moors' and regeneration. There were several reasons for this, which require a previous account of developments in the Moroccan *Hajj* before the 1890s. In that period, substantial transformations occurred in line with general developments in the Islamic world. The number of Moroccan pilgrims making the cherished once-in-a-lifetime visit to the Holy Sites showed a rising tendency, though with cyclical ups and downs. By the early 1880s, the yearly figures had reached 5,000/6,000 pilgrims, with ships usually carrying from 1,000 to 1,500 each.[117] The trip to Mecca had changed from the traditional caravan route across North Africa to the Egyptian Red Sea coast into a much faster journey by vessel first and steamship later, from Tangier to Alexandria, where the trip continued by caravan or ship. When the Suez Canal was opened, the direct journey from Morocco to the Hejaz ports became possible. British and French lines carried most pilgrims, too often in very unsanitary conditions due to overcrowding and a lack of medical staff on board.[118] Nonetheless, competition between shipping lines also made the journey more affordable and led to social diversification among pilgrims.[119] Finally, as already argued, European pressure on the sultans led to unprecedented bans on the pilgrimage when the risk of importing an epidemic from Mecca was too high, as occurred in 1897.

These changes increased the potential impact of the *Hajj* on Morocco. From a political point of view, pilgrims were exposed to European modernity, either in the ships that carried them to Mecca or during stops in French Algeria or British Egypt that put them in contact with Islamic societies transformed by European colonialism. Moroccan pilgrims were also exposed to ideologies of Islamic cultural and intellectual revival (*nahda*), Muslim religious reform (salafism, wahabbism), and national and transnational (Pan-Islamist, Pan-Arabist) patriotism, all of which encouraged self-esteem and a rejection of European domination over Islamic countries.[120] As Óvilo pointed out in 1881, 'a religious precept the sultans are unable to forbid, the pilgrimage to Mecca, pulls to pieces the precautions aimed at preventing the infiltration of certain ideas in the brains of Moroccans, who […] do not lack common sense and compare their condition with other peoples and make reflections which surely do not enhance the prestige of their own political organization.'[121] For example, Hassan bin Muhammad al-Rassal, the son of a Tangier's *amin* (custom inspector), who did the pilgrimage in 1897–98, praised in his travel diary the 'magnificent outlook' of Algiers and its 'huge stores filled with rich merchandises'; Malta's 'remarkably well built and carefully looked after' vegetable market and the 'superb' governor's palace equipped with 'state of the art cannons'; and the 'great development' of commerce in British-controlled Cairo, where 'streets are quite large and well-kept as they are in Europe'.[122] At the same time, Moroccan learned men were also bringing back home from their trip to Mecca 'the teachings of the famous Egyptian scholar Muhammad Abduh and his disciple Rachid Rida',[123] the fathers of Salafism. The renowned Abdallah ibn Idris al-Sanussi would be forced into exile during Hassan I's reign for his fervent defence of that doctrine.

From a sanitary point of view, the pilgrimage's effects intensified too. The growing speed of maritime communications implied now the risk of a direct and much faster importation of cholera from Mecca. The fourth pandemic that spread to Europe for the first time by sea from Alexandria in 1865 – and put the *Hajj* at the centre of discussions in the International Sanitary Conferences for the rest of the century, as Peter Baldwin has shown[124] – had already exposed Moroccan vulnerability by posing major threats in 1865 and 1866 (as said before) that brought about European intervention in public health, especially through the authorisation of quarantines on Mogador Island.[125] In 1878 and 1895, cholera brought directly from the Hejaz by *hajjis* struck the country, in marked contrast to the epidemics of the first two thirds of the nineteenth century, which had all been introduced by land from Algeria except the one that took place during the Spanish–Moroccan War of 1859–60, which arrived partly from Spain too.[126] Cholera, often in association with famine, could trigger social revolts capable of shaking the weak structures of the state and even the sultan's authority. As Óvilo commented for the 1878 epidemic, 'cholera and other calamities brought Morocco to such prostration that […] it was easy to foresee one of those historical cataclysms which mark the disappearance of a people'.[127] Otherwise, pilgrims grew familiar with modern quarantine facilities and procedures, especially at the lazaretto of El Tor in Egypt and Matifou in Algiers, such that they realised the sanitary backwardness of their country. But they could also become increasingly sensitised to sanitary interference in a religious, saintly affair, as the incidents on Mogador Island in 1893 and 1896 revealed.

All these reasons made the *Hajj* a threat for Spanish projects of regeneration and creation of a 'Moorish' elite. With regard to politics, the experience of British and French modernity in Algeria or Egypt and the fact that the journey was almost always made in British and French steamships could lead 'Moor' pilgrims to realise the modesty of Spain's projects in their country and its second-rank position in international politics, commerce or colonialism. On the other hand, they could be tempted to abandon their 'Hispano-Arabic' identity for a more attractive religious adscription as 'Muslims', ethnic condition of 'Arabs', cultural 'Islamic' background or political 'nationalism'. From a sanitary point of view, the pilgrimage threatened to discredit regeneration projects. Every time pilgrims imported or were suspected of cholera, the British and the French renewed their criticism of the Sanitary Council of Tangier and Mogador Island lazaretto despite Spanish-sponsored reforms. Epidemic risks justified their attempts at direct intervention in Moroccan public health or their plans for obliging Morocco to adopt international schemes. For example, in the convention resulting from the tenth ISC held in Venice in 1897, the French successfully included a plea to the sultan such that 'the Sanitary Council of Tangier adopts preventive measures against plague in harmony with the resolutions contained in the agreed convention.'[128] This strategy would be repeated in the following conference in Paris in 1903, where Lucien Raynaud was invited to present on the troubled state of Moroccan quarantines.[129] Finally, disinfection and isolation procedures imposed on pilgrims on Mogador Island were liable to trigger opposition against sanitary reforms from Morocco's conservative elites and popular masses.

For all this, regenerationist discourses and practices attempted to frame the Moroccan *Hajj*. The result was a loosely articulated vision that stood far from the 'twin infection' schemes already prevalent in French Algeria or British India at that time, as Luc Chantre and Saurabh Mishra have shown.[130] From an ideological point of view, as Óvilo argued in his study *El cólera en Tánger* (1895), the *hajjis* were believed by regenerationists to be 'moved by a religious idea and sanctified by it', that is, the pilgrimage was essentially regarded as an enriching and positive spiritual experience.[131] We may infer that Óvilo also saw it as a means of 'spiritual regeneration' for the elite of 'Moors', so that they developed a 'healthier' mentality and abandoned 'vices'. On the other hand, 'Moors' were considered as the central or characteristic actors of the Moroccan pilgrimage. Thus, the Spanish minister in Tangier was glad to inform the minister of foreign affairs in 1889 about the 'quality' of the 'considerable' number of *hajjis* leaving for Mecca that year.[132] Such 'quality' was marked by the presence of several important 'Moors', among which he mentioned the son of the *caid* of Meknes, accompanied by 'sixty relatives and friends' and Ahmed ibn Shucron, an army colonel who had been trained as an engineer in the Spanish Military Engineering School in Guadalajara in the late 1870s, who travelled in the company of 'five brothers'.[133] Medical care of the pilgrims was assigned to the previously mentioned Hamed Romani, of privileged social extraction too. All three were outstanding examples of 'Moors' targeted by, and actively involved in, regenerationist plans.

With regard to public health, Óvilo thought that the pilgrimage posed no essential risk of cholera epidemics and pilgrims were not sources of infection in themselves. On the one hand, he put the blame on the French and the British for the unsanitary conditions in which the *hajjis* travelled: they were just 'poor creatures that come back to their country after long sufferings [...] on board ships that profit and greed transform [...] into infamous stores in which passengers are carried and treated a thousand times worse than in those used for the *ebony traffic* [i.e. the slave trade]'.[134] On the other hand, he judged pilgrims not 'a very dangerous element by themselves, but just by their effects'.[135] As they had acquired some 'immunity' against cholera after being exposed to it in Mecca, it was unlikely that the disease would break out in their ranks during their return to Morocco. As a result, there was just one thing to be feared: if the germs pilgrims carried within their bodies or in their clothes and luggage spread to the general Moroccan population, the consequence would be a disastrous epidemic due to the latter's lack of immunity and bad health condition, as well as the precarious state of the sanitary administration beyond coastal areas. Óvilo acknowledged 'the lack of a good sanitary organization' in Morocco[136] and that it was 'not fair, from a sanitary point of view, to consider Morocco at the same level than other nations that march at the front of civilization'.[137]

It seems clear that, for Óvilo and the regenerationists, most 'Moors' were capable of dealing with the ideological and sanitary risks of the *Hajj* without much disruption for their modern, Hispanophile, identity and their rather healthy condition. However, it was also clear that a few of them would surely become 'dis-eased',[138] however surreptitiously, during the pilgrimage with the risk that they could trigger an epidemic if they came in contact with the general population. Thus, a site was needed for mending the dis-eased 'Moors' and protecting Morocco both in ideological and sanitary terms. Mogador Island was perceived as the best place from a regenerationist point of view. With regard to politics, it was highly symbolic that the site was located in front of Mogador, the most European city in Morocco. Mogador had been built anew in the 1750s and 1760s, during the reign of Sultan Mohammed III, who decided it would be the only port authorised for international commerce and promoted the settlement of Jewish and European merchants for that purpose.[139] Mogador was, so to speak, the Tangier of the eighteenth century and, as happened with the city of the Strait, Spaniards claimed to have played a decisive role in its development. According to Francisco Merry y Colom, Spanish minister in Tangier in 1860–72, Mogador had been 'designed and built' by Spanish renegades, its walls were similar to those of Cádiz and most of the cannons defending them had been given as a present by Spain.[140] The commercial prosperity of the city owed much to the 'fraternity' and 'friendship' between Carlos III of Spain and Mohammed III, the latter of whom tried, according to Merry, to 'regenerate' his country with Spanish support.[141] In sum, pilgrims isolated on Mogador Island were literally exposed to the earliest example of Spanish–Moroccan modernity. Staring at the city over the waves, they would feel reassured in their 'Moorish' mentality and forget any disruptive European, Muslim, Islamic or nationalist ideas acquired during the pilgrimage.

From a sanitary point of view, Mogador Island was established in the only suitable place for quarantine that existed in the whole Atlantic littoral of Morocco. Its tiny size and its proximity to the seaboard and the city – the usual reasons invoked for criticising its use – were actually very similar to the three foul lazarettos existing in Spain. San Simón Island in the fiord of Vigo, Pedrosa Island in Santander Bay and the Lazaretto Island in Mahón Bay were similarly small and close to the mainland and/or nearby cities. The only real difference was that it was far easier to disembark passengers and luggage in them because they were completely protected from the open sea. But there were no protected sites on the Atlantic coast of Morocco and those that were closer to fulfil this and the rest of the required conditions in the Mediterranean were Spanish outposts. In sum, Mogador Island was suitable as a lazaretto and Spanish-led reforms further improved this status. Besides, in front of it there was a city in the design of which public health had played a central role. As the British traveller Joseph Thomson put it in 1889, Mogador was 'the best-built and cleanest-kept place in Morocco'.[142] Its medina (old town) was made of 'spacious houses, clean squares and straight streets' and it had the 'unique distinction' of having been built with 'a partial sewage system'.[143] While staring at the city over the sea, Moroccan pilgrims would be reassured of the relevance of Spanish–Moroccan sanitary initiatives, which neither religion should oppose, nor European criticism could downplay.

Conclusion

In March 1900, Moroccan authorities recruited Lucien Raynaud to organise the quarantine on Mogador Island. When he arrived there, most pilgrims had already come back from Mecca, so just thirty would be confined in the island and no more would arrive during the summer.[144] The following year, Raynaud, joined by Dr Gagé, repeated the operation, with 177 pilgrims undergoing quarantine this time.[145] During the rest of the decade, however, when the risk of epidemic existed, either the pilgrimage was banned or the quarantine of Moroccan pilgrims was performed in Algiers' Matifou lazaretto. In spite of a French doctor being assigned to Mogador Island at least until 1911, the site was neither used nor modernised.[146] Instead, Raynaud lobbied the Sanitary Council and Moroccan authorities so that a modern lazaretto was built in Tangier. An international commission searched for the best location in 1901 and two projects were drafted for a complex in Malabata Point by two different private enterprises, but nothing was actually done.[147] The abandonment of quarantines when a comprehensive public health system was still a distant project resulted in small foci of plague striking the country from 1909 in anticipation of a massive outbreak in 1911 – which caused 10,000 dead in Dukkala – with minor episodes recurring in the newly established French and Spanish protectorates in subsequent years.[148] Plague brought by pilgrims and commerce but, above all, extended through the continuous and extensive military operations of France and Spain, would remain a severe threat for Morocco at least until 1929.

Parallel to this, the *Hajj* stood behind the wave of Islamic reformism that swept through Morocco in the first decade of the twentieth century. According to Etty Terem, some Moroccan scholars 'were exposed to Muslim reformers while on the pilgrimage to Mecca; others came under the influence of *hadith* scholars in Egypt and the Hejaz while on the pilgrimage'.[149] For example, in 1903–04, the *ulema* Muhammad ibn Abdalkabir al-Kittani did the pilgrimage with expenses paid by his 'old friend the sultan'.[150] His family had been opposed to the rise of European influence in Morocco during the nineteenth century, but a further step was taken when, after his return from Mecca, al-Kittani became a pioneer of the Salafiya movement in the country, campaigned against French reform proposals and even called for *jihad* against foreigners.[151] In 1908, the new Sultan Abdelhafid invited Abu Shuaib al-Dukkali to return to the country from Mecca. Dukkali, a scholar trained in Cairo's Al-Azhar University, where he became a follower of Salafiya, had moved to Mecca to work for the Wahabite sharif Awn al-Rafiq. In Morocco, Dukkali reformed the syllabus of the Qarawiyin University in Fez, 'was largely responsible for the spreading of Salafiyah doctrines among intellectuals' and, through his disciples, influenced the origins of the Moroccan national liberation movement.[152]

Plague and Salafism were precisely the risks Spanish regeneration projects in Morocco, and more particularly those regarding the control of the Moroccan pilgrimage to Mecca, had tried to prevent during the last decade of the nineteenth century. Their appearance and diffusion in Morocco in the first years of the new century showed how quickly such projects had become a failure after the fall of Spanish prestige in the country following the loss of Cuba and the Philippines in 1898. The new situation of the 1900s resembled more closely the realities and narratives of the 'twin infection' associated with the pilgrimage to Mecca in British India or French Algeria – though the limitation of French hegemony due to the participation of Spain in the division of Morocco and the international status granted to the city of Tangier still made the Alawite sultanate an unconventional case. When in operation during the 1890s, Mogador Island had become a key material and symbolic site of regeneration projects which, building on local modernising reforms promoted by the sultans, aimed at transforming Morocco into an 'African Spain' closely attached to 'peninsular Spain' and producing an elite of modern, healthy, Hispanophile 'Moors'. Much faster than expected, however, these projects became distant, blurred memories for both Spain and Morocco.

Notes

This chapter has been written within the frame of UID/HIS/00057/2013 (POCI-01-0145-FEDER-007702) – FCT, COMPETE, FEDER, Portugal2020 and also with the support of an Investigator contract and the project IF/00835/2014CP1232/CT0002 of the *Fundaçao para a Ciência e a Tecnologia* of Portugal.

1 *Rapport du Dr. Rebolledo au Conseil Sanitaire de Tanger. Mogador, 17 Octobre 1896.* Centre des Archives Diplomatiques de Nantes (CADN), Fonds Tanger A, Carton 167.

2 Mohamed Amine El-Bezzaz, 'Les débuts de la réglementation sanitaire du pèlerinage marocain à la Mecque (1831–1866)', *Hesperis-Tamuda* 22, 1984, 67–77.

3 *Rapport du Dr. Rebolledo au Conseil Sanitaire de Tanger. Mogador, 17 Octobre 1896.* CADN, Fonds Tanger A, Carton 167.

4 Ibid.

5 Michael Christopher Low, 'The twin infection: pilgrims, plagues and pan-Islam under British surveillance, 1865–1924', *International Journal of Middle East Studies* 40, 2008, 269–290.

6 Francisco Javier Martínez-Antonio and Irene González González (eds), *Regenerar España y Marruecos. Ciencia y educación en las relaciones hispano-marroquíes a finales del siglo XIX*, Madrid, CSIC-Casa Árabe, 2011.

7 Alison Bashford, *Imperial Hygiene: A Critical History of Colonialism, Nationalism and Public Health*, London, Palgrave-MacMillan, 2004.

8 Edmund Burke III, *Prelude to Protectorate. Precolonial Protest and Resistance, 1860–1912*, Chicago and London, The University of Chicago Press, 1976; Charles-André Julien, *Le Maroc face aux impérialismes, 1415–1956*, Paris, Éditions J.A., 1978; Charles R. Pennell, *Morocco since 1830. A History*, London, Hurst & Company, 2000; Víctor Morales Lezcano, *Historia de Marruecos*, Madrid, La Esfera de los Libros, 2006; Susan G. Miller, *A History of Modern Morocco*, Cambridge, Cambridge University

Press, 2013. A harsher critique should, in any case, be made of those historians – especially in Spain – that regard Spanish intervention in Morocco as non-imperialistic or disinterested or just focusing on spiritual and cultural matters with no alleged desire for political control or economic gain.

9 Francisco Javier Martínez-Antonio, ' "Dos dedos de una misma mano": propuestas para un nuevo análisis de las relaciones hispano-marroquíes a finales del siglo XIX', in Francisco Javier Martínez-Antonio and Irene González González (eds), *Regenerar España y Marruecos. Ciencia y educación en las relaciones hispano-marroquíes a finales del siglo XIX*, Madrid, CSIC-Casa Árabe, 2011, 21–58.

10 Ramón Villares and Javier Moreno Luzón, *Restauración y dictadura. Historia de España. Josep Fontana y Ramón Villares, Volumen 7*, Barcelona and Madrid, Crítica-Marcial Pons, 2009, 307–364.

11 *Intereses de España en Marruecos*, Madrid, [n.p.], 1947, 28.

12 Ibid., 81.

13 'La política del statu quo en Marruecos', *Revista de Geografía Comercial* 47, 19 October 1887, 541.

14 *Intereses*, 1947, 35.

15 Mohammed Kenbib, *Les protégés: contribution à l'histoire contemporaine du Maroc*, Casablanca, Najah El Jadida, 1996, 92.

16 Francisco Javier Martínez-Antonio, 'L'année de la peste: santé publique et impérialisme français au Maroc', *Mélanges de la Casa de Velázquez* 44, 1, 2014, 265.

17 Francisco Javier Martínez-Antonio, 'The Tangier's School of Medicine and its first physicians: a forgotten initiative of medical education reform in Morocco (1886–1904)', *Journal of the International Society for the History of Islamic Medicine* 10–11, 19–22, 2011–12, 80–88.

18 Francisco Javier Martínez-Antonio, 'Resilient modernization: Morocco's agency in Red Cross projects from Hassan I to the Rif Republic (1886–1926)', *Asclepio* 66, I, 2014, 3.

19 Francisco Javier Martínez-Antonio, 'El doctor Severo Cenarro y los proyectos médico-sanitarios de la España africana (1884–1898)', *Cuadernos del Archivo Central de Ceuta* 19, 2010–11, 255–296.

20 *Propuesta hecha por el ministro de Estado para la creación de varios organismos religiosos y seglares*, Archivo Histórico Militar de Madrid, África, Légajo 1, Carpeta 24.

21 Ramón Lourido Díaz, 'José Lerchundi y las relaciones culturales hispano-marroquíes de finales del siglo XI', *Hesperis-Tamuda* 30, 1, 1992, 39–66.

22 Alberto España, *La pequeña historia de Tánger*, Tánger, Distribuidora Ibérica, 1954, 34.

23 Manuel Olivié, *Aspiraciones nacionales. Marruecos*, Barcelona, Imprenta de Heinrich y Cía, 1893, 237.
24 Ibid., 242.
25 Ibid., 247.
26 Ibid., 248.
27 Ibid., 249.
28 Alice L. Conklin, *A Mission to Civilize: The Republican Idea of Empire in France and West Africa 1895–1930*, Stanford, Stanford University Press, 1998.
29 Khaled Ben Srhir, *Britain and Morocco during the Embassy of John Drummond-Hay (1845–1886)*, London and New York, Routledge-Curzon, 2006, 206–263.
30 Ibid.
31 Mohammed Ghoti, *Histoire de la medècine au Maroc. Le XXe siecle (1896–1994)*, [n.p.], Ibrahim Saad Eddin, 1980; Daniel Rivet, *Lyautey et l'institution du Protectorat français au Maroc, 1912–1925*, Paris, L'Harmattan, 1996, vol. II, 223–240; Ellen J. Amster, *Medicine and the Saints. Science, Islam and the Colonial Encounter in Morocco, 1877–1956*, Austin, University of Texas Press, 2013.
32 Oleg Schepin and Valdemar Yermakov, *International Quarantine*, Madison, International Universities Press, 1991.
33 Mohamed Amine el-Bezzaz, 'The International Sanitary Council of Morocco, 1792–1929' [in Arabic], PhD thesis, University Mohammed V, 1992; Francisco Javier Martínez-Antonio, 'La sanidad en Marruecos a mediados del siglo XIX', *Medicina e Historia*, cuarta época 2, 2005, 1–15.
34 Felipe Óvilo, *De l'influence des pèlerinages marocains à la Mecque dans la propagation du choléra*, Madrid, Typographie de Manuel G. Hernández, 1882, 20.
35 Ibid.
36 Michel-Pierre Roux, *Mogador-Essaouira. Acteur et témoin pour l'histoire de la santé*, Marrakech, El Watanya, 1996, 30.
37 Lucien Raynaud, *Étude sur l'hygiène et la médecine au Maroc*, Alger, Léon, 1902, 64.
38 El-Bezzaz, 'Les débuts de la réglementation sanitaire', 77.
39 Óvilo, *De l'influence des pèlerinages marocains*, 16.
40 Arthur Leared, *Morocco and the Moors*, London, Sampson, Low, Marston, Searle & Rivington, 1876, 84.
41 Ibid., 15.
42 Regreso de los hadjes, *Al Mogreb al-Aksa*, 21 September 1890.
43 Ibid.

44 *Informe del ministro de España en Tánger al ministro de Asuntos Exteriores. Tánger, 28 de junio de 1889*. Archivo Provincial de Pontevedra, Colección Solla, 198–199.
45 Ibid.
46 Ecos y rumores, *Al Mogreb al-Aksa*, 30 August 1891.
47 Saurabh Mishra, *Pilgrimage, Politics and Pestilence. The Haj from the Indian Subcontinent, 1860–1920*, New Delhi, Oxford University Press, 2011, 113.
48 Weekly notes, *Al Mogreb al-Aksa*, 26 August 1893.
49 *Situation sanitaire de l'île de Mogador d'après les rapports du Dr. Prieto, médecin du lazaret*. CADN, Fonds Tanger B, Carton 500.
50 Ibid.
51 'L'état sanitaire à l'île de Mogador', *Supplement au Reveil du Maroc*, 4 Septembre 1893.
52 *Situation sanitaire de l'île de Mogador*.
53 *Extracts from despatches from M. Vice-Consul Johnston, 1893*. The National Archives (TNA), Foreign Office, 99/374.
54 Mishra, *Pilgrimage, Politics and Pestilence*, 113.
55 *Rapport du Dr. Rebolledo au Conseil Sanitaire de Tanger. Mogador, 17 Octobre 1896*. CADN, Fonds Tanger A, Carton 167.
56 Felipe Óvilo. *El cólera en Tánger. Memoria acerca de su aparición en Marruecos*. Tánger, Imprenta de A.J. Lúgaro, 1895, 13.
57 *Rapport lu à la séance du 17 Octobre 1895 par le médecin-consulteur, Mr. le docteur Severo Cenarro*. CADN, Fonds Tanger A, Carton 167,
58 *Rapport de M. le docteur Soulié, sous-directeur del'Institut Pasteur d'Alger en mission à Tanger. Tanger, le 8 Octobre 1895*. CADN, Fonds Tanger A, Carton 167.
59 *Sir Arthur Nicolson to the Foreign Office. Mogador Island. Morocco City, April 13th 1896*. TNA, Foreign Office, 99/374.
60 Ibid.
61 *Rapport du Dr. Rebolledo au Conseil Sanitaire de Tanger. Mogador, 17 Octobre 1896*. CADN, Fonds Tanger A, Carton 167.
62 Ibid.
63 Ibid.
64 *Projet de règlement général pour le service de quarantaine dans l'île de Mogador, 1896*. CADN, Fonds Tanger B, Carton 501.
65 *Avis. Conseil Sanitaire du Maroc. Tanger, le 15 Juin 1897*. CADN, Fonds Tanger B, Carton 500.
66 Following the outbreak of plague in 1818, triggered by pilgrims from Mecca (including the sultan's own two sons) who were allowed to disembark in Tangier, Moulay Slimane banned the pilgrimage. The ban

allegedly lasted until 1827 or 1828 (El-Bezzaz, 'Les débuts de la réglementation sanitaire', 69).

67 Valeska Huber, 'International Bodies: The Pilgrimage to Mecca and International Health Regulations', in Eric Tagliacozzo and Shawkat M. Toorawa (eds), *The Hajj: Pilgrimage in Islam*, Cambridge, Cambridge University Press, 2016, 180.

68 James Richardson, *Travels in Morocco*, London, Charles J. Skeet, 1860, II, 300; *Conseil Sanitaire du Maroc. Memoire. Tanger, 21 December 1898.* NA, Foreign Office, 99/374.

69 Ibid.

70 Ibid.

71 Ibid.

72 *Chargé d'Affaires de France à Tanger au ministre des Affaires Etrangères. Tanger, 19 janvier 1899.* CADN, Fonds Tanger B, Carton 501.

73 *Dr. François au ministre de France à Tanger. Mogador, 9 Mars 1898.* CADN, Fonds Tanger B, Carton 501.

74 *Chargé d'Affaires de France à Tanger au ministre des Affaires Etrangères. Tanger, 19 janvier 1899.* CADN, Fonds Tanger B, Carton 501.

75 Ibid.

76 *Conseil Sanitaire du Maroc. Memoire. Tanger, 21 December 1898.* TNA, Foreign Office, 99/374.

77 *Chargé d'Affaires de France à Tanger au ministre des Affaires Etrangères. Tanger, 19 janvier 1899.* CADN, Fonds Tanger B, Carton 501.

78 *Résolution prise par le Conseil Sanitaire en vue de l'occupation éventuelle de l'île de Mogador. Tanger, 24 Avril 1899.* CADN, Fonds Tanger B, Carton 501.

79 *Le ministre de France à Tanger au ministre des Affaires Etrangères. Tanger, 30 Septembre 1899.* CADN, Fonds Tanger B, Carton 500; The lazaretto, *Al Mogreb al-Aksa*, 17 June 1899.

80 *Le docteur Joaquín Cortés au Consul Général des Etats-Unis. Tanger, 18 Octobre 1899.* CADN, Fonds Tanger B, Carton 501.

81 Weekly notes, *Al Mogreb al-Aksa*, 5 August 1899.

82 Ibid.

83 Ibid. *Frais anticipés par le Conseil Sanitaire de Tanger pour le lazaret de l'île de Mogador. Juillet-Septembre 1899. Ministre de France à Tanger au ministre des Affaires Etrangères. Paris, 6 Juillet 1899.* CADN, Fonds Tanger B, Carton 501.

84 *Copie d'une lettre du délégué sanitaire. Mogador, 12 Aout 1899.* CADN, Fonds Tanger B, Carton 501.

85 *Dr. Joaquín Cortés al ministro de Francia en Tánger. Mogador, 13 de agosto de 1899. Consul de France à Mogador au Ministre de France à Tanger. Mogador, 13 Aout 1899.* CADN, Fonds Tanger B, Carton 501.

86 *Consul de France à Mogador au Ministre de France à Tanger. Mogador, 23 Aout 1899. Consul de France à Mogador au Ministre de France à Tanger. Mogador, 31 Aout 1899.* CADN, Fonds Tanger B, Carton 501.
87 *Consul de France à Mogador au Ministre de France à Tanger. Mogador, 13 Aout 1899.* CADN, Fonds Tanger B, Carton 501.
88 *Ministre de France à Tanger au ministre des Affaires Etrangères. Tanger, 13 Novembre 1899.* CADN, Fonds Tanger B, Carton 501.
89 *Conference Sanitaire International de Paris 10 Octobre – 3 Décembre 1903: Procès-verbaux*, Paris, Imprimerie nationale, 1904, 410.
90 Jamal el-Himer. *Las expediciones educativas en tiempos del sultán Muley Hassan I* [in Arabic], Salé, 2015, 107.
91 Raynaud, *Étude sur l'hygiène*, 64.
92 'Reglamento orgánico provisional de Sanidad Marítima para el servicio de las dependencias', *Gaceta de Madrid*, 25 June 1887.
93 Daniel Panzac, 'Politique sanitaire et fixation de frontières: l'exemple ottoman (XVIII-XIX siècles)', *Turcica* 31 (1999), 87–108.
94 Manuel Ramírez Muñoz, *El lazareto de Gando, 1893–1998. De complejo sanitario a establecimiento aeronáutico*, Las Palmas, Ediciones del Cabildo de Gran Canaria, 2001, 61.
95 Francisco Javier Martínez-Antonio, 'La problemática dimensión imperial de la Sanidad Exterior española a través del cólera, la fiebre amarilla y la peste (1833–1931)', in María Isabel Porras Gallo, Bertha G. Rodilla, Mariano A. Sanz and Jaime de las Heras Salord (eds), *Transmisión del conocimiento médico e internacionalización de las prácticas sanitarias. Una perspectiva histórica*, Ciudad Real, Facultad de Medicina/SEHM, 2011, 273–277.
96 Ramírez, *El lazareto de Gando*, 118–130.
97 Ibid., 132.
98 Ibid., 133.
99 Edward Said, *Orientalism*, New York, Berghan Books, 1976, 3.
100 Lisa Lowe, *Critical Terrains*, Ithaca, Cornell University Press, 1992; Coopan Vilashini, *Worlds Within: National Narratives and Global Connections in Postcolonial Writing*, Standford, Stanford University Press, 2009; James Hodkison and John Walker, *Deploying Orientalism in Culture and History. From Germany to Central and Eastern Europe*, London, Camden House, 2013.
101 Frederick Cooper, *Colonialism in Question. Theory, Knowledge, History*, Berkeley, Los Angeles and London, University of California Press, 2005, 17.
102 Pedro Martínez Montávez, 'Sobre el aun "desconocido" arabismo español del siglo XIX', in *Ensayos marginales de arabismo*, Madrid, Instituto de Estudios Orientales y Africanos, 1977, 3–22; Bernabé López García,

'Arabismo y orientalismo en España: radiografía de un gremio escaso y apartadizo', *Awraq* 11, 1990, 35–69.

103 José Antonio González Alcantud (ed.), *El orientalismo desde el sur*, Sevilla, Anthropos, 2006; Fernando Rodríguez Mediano and Mercedes García Arenal, *Un Oriente español. Los moriscos y el Sacromonte en tiempos de Contrarreforma*, Madrid, Marcial Pons, 2010.

104 Francisco Javier Martínez Antonio, 'Un viaje a ninguna parte: discursos científicos y proyectos políticos de médicos españoles en Marruecos', *Hesperis-Tamuda* XLIII, 2008, 23–60.

105 José María de Murga, *Recuerdos marroquíes del Moro Vizcaíno*, Madrid, Miraguano Ediciones, 2009, 147–261. For French authors such as Pascal Duprat, there existed five races in Algeria: Berbers, Arabs, Turks, Koulouglis and Jews (Patricia Lorcin, *Imperial Identities. Stereotyping, Prejudice and Race in Colonial Algeria*, London-New York, I.B. Tauris, 1995, 150).

106 Felipe Óvilo, 'Estudios políticos y sociales sobre Marruecos', *Revista Contemporánea* 1881, 61–62.

107 Ibid., 58.

108 Ibid., 60.

109 Ibid., 58.

110 Ibid., 63.

111 Ibid., 76.

112 Felipe Óvilo, *Intimidades de Marruecos*, Madrid, Librería de Fernando Fé, 1894, 39–47.

113 Felipe Óvilo, *Estado actual de Marruecos*, Madrid, Librería de Fernando Fé, 1888, 29.

114 Ibid., 3.

115 Ibid., 3–4 (italics are mine).

116 Ibid., 4–5.

117 Emilio Bonelli, *El imperio de Marruecos y su constitución*, Madrid, Imprenta y Litografía del Depósito de la Guerra, 1882, 88.

118 Firmin Duguet, *Le pèlerinage à la Mecque au point de vue religieux, social et sanitaire*, Paris, Les Éditions Rirder, 1932; El-Bezzaz, 'Les débuts de la réglementation sanitaire'; Luc Chantre, 'Le pèlerinage à La Mecque à l'époque coloniale (v. 1866–1940): France, Grande-Bretagne, Italie', unpublished PhD thesis, University of Poitiers, 2012, 240.

119 Sylvia Chiffoleau, 'Le pélerinage à la Mecque pendant la période coloniale: matrice d'une opinión publique musulmane?', in Sylvia Chiffoleau and Anna Madœuf (eds), *Les pèlerinages au Maghreb et au Moyen-Orient* [en ligne], Damas, Presses de l'Ifpo, 2005.

120 Sylvia Chiffoleau has argued that radical political and religious exposure was indeed very restricted by the end of the nineteenth century, but

acknowledges its existence for the case of rich and cultivated pilgrims (Chiffoleau, 'Le pélerinage à la Mecque').

121 Óvilo, 'Estudios políticos y sociales sobre Marruecos', 70.

122 Hassan bin Muhammad al-Rassal 'Voyage de Tanger à La Mecque par El Hasan Ben *Mohamed* El R'assâl, traduit par A. Rezzouk', *Revue du monde musulman* 1, 1908, 2–3, 5.

123 Pennell, *Morocco since 1830*, 141.

124 Peter Baldwin, *Contagion and the State in Europe, 1830–1930*, Cambridge, Cambridge University Press, 2005, 226–236.

125 Francisco Javier Martínez Antonio, 'International or French?', *French History* 30, 1, 2016; Raynaud, *Étude sur l'hygiène*, 87.

126 Ibid.; Francisco Javier Martínez Antonio, '*La otra guerra de África. Cólera y conflicto internacional en la olvidada expedición militar de Francia a Marruecos en 1859*', Ceuta, Archivo General, 2010.

127 Óvilo, *Estado actual de Marruecos*, 11.

128 Raynaud, *Étude sur l'hygiène*, 68.

129 *Conference Sanitaire International de Paris*, 1904, 102.

130 Luc Chantre, 'Entre pandémie et panislamisme. L'imaginaire colonial du pèlerinage à la Mecque (1866–1914)', *Archives de Sciences Sociales des Réligions* 163, 2013, 163–190; Mishra, *Pilgrimage, Politics and Pestilence.*

131 Óvilo, *El cólera en Tánger*, 8.

132 *Informe del ministro de España en Tánger al ministro de Asuntos Exteriores, Tánger, 28 de junio de 1889*. Archivo Provincial de Pontevedra, Colección Solla, 198–199.

133 Ibid.

134 Ibid., 21–22.

135 Ibid., 4.

136 Óvilo, *El cólera en Tánger*, 8.

137 Ibid., 16.

138 We use the term 'dis-ease' to indicate that the disruption triggered by a certain situation, in this case, the pilgrimage to Mecca, affected the physical, psychological and social dimensions of individuals. Examples of this use can be found in Anne Pérez-Hattori, *Colonial Dis-Ease: US Navy Health Policies and the Chamorros of Guam, 1898–1941*, Honolulu, University of Hawai'i Press, 2004; Bennett Kravitz, *Representations of Illness in Literature and Film*, Cambridge, Cambridge Scholars Publishing, 2010.

139 Daniel J. Schroeter, *Merchants of Essaouira. Urban Society and Imperialism in Southwestern Morocco, 1844–1886*, Cambridge, Cambridge University Press, 2009, 7–20.

140 Francisco Merry y Colom, *Relación del viaje a la ciudad de Marruecos*, Madrid, Imprenta Nacional, 1864, 28.

141 Merry, *Relación del viaje a la ciudad de Marruecos*, 8; Rafael Mitjana, 'Viaje a la corte del sultán de Marruecos', *La España Moderna* 13, 145, 1901, 138–139.
142 Joseph Thomson, *Travels in the Atlas and Southern Morocco. A Narrative of Exploration*, London, Georg Philip & Son, 1889, 67.
143 Ibid., 68.
144 *Lazaret de Malabata* [unsigned report]. CADN, Fonds Tanger B, Carton 504.
145 Roux, *Mogador-Essaouira*, 35.
146 Francisco Javier Martínez-Antonio, 'Double trouble: French colonialism in Morocco and the early histories of the Pasteur Institutes of Tangier and Casablanca (1886–1932)', *Dynamis* 36, 2, 2016, 324.
147 *Projet d'établissement d'un lazaret a la pointe de Malabata. Tánger, Imprenta Abrines, 1901*. Archivo General de la Administración, Fondo Histórico de Marruecos, Caja M-21.
148 Martínez-Antonio, 'Resilient modernization'.
149 Etty Terem, *Old Texts, New Practices. Islamic Reform in Modern Morocco*, Stanford, Stanford University Press, 2014, 52–54.
150 Pennell, *Morocco since 1830*, 131.
151 Ibid.
152 Robin Bidwell, *Dictionary of Modern Arab History*, London and New York, Routledge, 2012, 129.

II

Identity

4

Quarantine in Ceuta and Malta in the travel writings of the late eighteenth-century Moroccan ambassador Ibn Uthmân Al-Meknassî

Malika Ezzahidi

Introduction

Interest in public health on the southern littoral of the Mediterranean Sea began to decline by the end of what is considered as the golden age of medieval Islamic medicine between the eighth and the thirteenth centuries. Before this occurred, hospitals (*bîmâristâns*) had played a central role in the treatment of the sick in major Islamic cities.[1] In the case of Morocco, for example, Marrakech and Fez hospitals flourished during the Almohad (1147–1269) and the Marinid (1269–1465) eras. The same applies for Egypt's Qalawun Hospital in Cairo, built in the 1280s, which could provide care for up to 8,000 patients. Separate quarters in these hospitals were reserved so that the people with contagious diseases could be isolated from other patients. Many Islamic cities had been also equipped with sophisticated water supply and sewage systems, while the so-called *ḥisba* administration dealt with the supervision of food weight, price and quality in markets, the control of the sacrifice of animals in slaughterhouses and the organisation of street cleansing – keeping a close eye on public morality too.[2] Finally, the great Islamic physicians enjoyed a wide reputation throughout Western Europe, where their influence was spread by an abundant literature that testified to the vitality of Arab-Muslim medicine.

In contrast with Islamic decline, in Europe strict and stringent sanitary measures were pioneered following the Black Plague – measures which had an enormous demographic impact on the entire

Mediterranean area during the fourteenth century and beyond. Yet it was only from the seventeenth century that maritime quarantine – generally understood as an isolation period for men, vessels and cargos – came to be seriously applied in almost all Mediterranean ports of Europe.[3] This helped to limit the number of epidemic cycles and later contributed to the disappearance of the plague, which by contrast continued to be widespread throughout the East until the 1840s.[4] Certainly, maritime quarantine was also known and implemented from the eighteenth century in various Islamic countries, as European commercial expansionism began to be felt and local rulers sought to stop the epidemic risk associated with its progression. As Nancy E. Gallagher has shown for the case of Tunisia, the beys refused entry of foreign vessels arriving from countries struck by plague to local ports from at least 1722 and armed conflicts developed occasionally with states such as Venice over disagreements on quarantine measures.[5] But, in practice, maritime quarantine in Islamic countries was neither widespread geographically, nor uncontroversial beyond minority groups favourable to modernisation.

Only a handful of first-person accounts of Muslims who were subjected to quarantine in the eighteenth century have been identified by historians. This chapter analyses those contained in the travel writings of the Moroccan ambassador Ibn Uthmân Al-Meknassî (d. 1799). Al-Meknassî acted as a prominent agent intervening in the multiple and complex foreign policy affairs that characterised the reigns of the sultans Muhammad III (1757–1790) and Moulay Slimane (1792–1822).[6] His diplomatic activities explained his frequent travels throughout the Mediterranean to Spain, Italy, Malta or the Ottoman Empire, which served as the basis for three classic travel diaries (*rihlas*). In them, Al-Meknassî devoted only a handful of paragraphs to his experiences on quarantine, but they nevertheless give an invaluable account of the reactions of a Muslim and a diplomat to the anti-epidemic measures routinely imposed on the northern shores of the Mediterranean. Through the analysis of these short excepts, referring to the quarantine he endured at Spain's Ceuta and Malta's Valletta, I will try to show how the Moroccan ambassador was alive to the political as well as the medical implications of quarantine either in the relations with European countries, or within Moroccan society and power elites.

A glimpse of epidemics and quarantine in eighteenth-century Morocco

During the eighteenth century, Morocco, like the rest of the Islamic countries, remained hesitant and somewhat inattentive to the development of sanitary measures needed to protect the population from the importation of 'exotic' epidemics. Throughout this century, the Alawite sultanate had to face cycles of plague[7] which limited demographic and economic growth and provoked crises of which chroniclers left accurate descriptions.[8] After the severe outbreak during Moulay Ismail's reign, which struck in the years 1678–80, Morocco showed signs of recovery, despite the fact that the disease was still diffused in Algeria and Tunisia until the end of the century. However, the epidemic reappeared again in March 1742, coming across the eastern border with Algeria, first striking Taza (a small city in the northeast) and subsequently spreading to all of the main northern cities including Tetouan, Asilah and Tangier. Due to the civil war waged between the Alawite crown princes from Moulay Ismail's death in 1727 until the late 1740s, the armies, moving from Tetouan and Tangier toward Fes, contributed to the propagation of the epidemic in other regions of the country.[9] Taking the city of Tangier as an example, its chroniclers narrated how it was savagely hit by plague between 1742 and 1744, with the number of victims ranging between thirty to forty persons a day and rising up to seventy during summer, according to Henri-Paul Joseph Renault, a French doctor who carried out research on the history of Arab and Islamic medicine, especially in Morocco.[10] Nonetheless, the most serious plague epidemic which struck the country occurred in 1799–1800, during Moulay Slimane's reign.[11] The city of Marrakech, for example, lost 50,000 of its 60,000 inhabitants according to the French hygienist Lucien Raynaud, who published a classic book on the history of medicine and public health in Morocco.[12] The Spanish traveller Domingo Badía/Ali Bey el Abbasi, during his visit in 1803, would describe the city as 'deserted by the scourge of plague', estimating its population as a meagre 30,000 people.[13] Ibn Uthmân Al-Meknassî would himself die in the course of this epidemic, as I will mention later.

In these tragic circumstances, the *makhzen* (central government) often took practical measures to reduce the risk of contagion: the isolation of patients, sometimes the incineration of contaminated buildings, but also the evacuation of cities, without forgetting, of course, the ample use of traditional and 'religious medicine' (the so-called 'medicine of the Prophet').[14] Everything showed that these measures were not as effective as those applied in the European quarantine systems. However, when political stability returned to Morocco during the reign of Muhammad III, the first steps were slowly taken to develop a similar system in the country. For example, the Peace and Commerce Treaty signed with Spain in 1767 established that the Moroccan vessels arriving to Spanish ports would undergo quarantine 'unless Spanish consuls [in Morocco] have given security of its perfect health condition'.[15] But it would only be at the beginning of Moulay Slimane's reign that the European consular representatives in Tangier set up in 1792–93 a *Junta de Cónsules* (consular board) to discuss all kinds of affairs which affected them in common, including the eventual quarantine measures that would be advisable to take against the arrival of epidemics to the city and the country in general.[16] The *Junta* succeeded, for example, in forcing the sultan to set up a sanitary cordon on the border with Algeria in 1793[17] and around the cities of Melilla and Tetouan in 1799.[18] One of the forts of Tangier was designated in April 1799 as a site for the observation of passengers debarking in the city.[19] The consular board preceded the International Sanitary Council that was set up in Tangier on the 28 April 1840, an organ which received a delegation of Sultan Moulay Abderrahman ibn Hicham for 'maintaining the public health upon the coast of this Empire, to make all rules and take all measures to reach this end'.[20] Over the following years, the board extended its activities to the rest of the Moroccan ports open to foreign trade, with the appointment of a health inspector charged with monitoring incoming ships and especially those carrying pilgrims.[21]

Quarantine in Ibn Uthmân's travel writings

During the second half of the eighteenth century, a new sultan, Muhammad ibn Abdallah, took power in Morocco, ruling the country from 1757 until 1790. The period under his administration is known as the 'quiet period' by medical historians, given the remarkable decline in the frequency of epidemics – especially of plague – experienced by the population. This was just another effect of the main aim of the sultan, which was to restructure the state on a new basis.[22] His attention was directed mainly to increasing tax revenues and strengthening the economy, so he developed an ambitious foreign trade policy for which he deployed an active diplomacy towards the European powers, particularly those of the Mediterranean because of their geographic proximity and close historical relations.[23] To achieve his objectives, he first had to overcome obstacles that prevented the normalisation of these bilateral relations, such as the old troublesome issues of piracy and captives. For this purpose, he signed treaties with France, Spain, Portugal, Venice, Sweden, Denmark and the Netherlands, through which he achieved a relevant position for himself and Morocco in the international sphere – though this did not prevent him from launching military campaigns against the Spanish and Portuguese enclaves located in the Atlantic and Mediterranean coasts of the sultanate. As historian Ramón Lourido summarised, Muhammad III succeeded in 'taking his country away from the chaos and isolation in which it found itself, both in relation to the European and the Muslim world'.[24]

In this context of diplomatic negotiations, Muhammad III appointed the *makhzen* official Muhammad Ibn Uthmân Al-Meknassî to visit the court of King Carlos III of Spain in 1779. The son of a religious scholar, Ibn Uthmân Al-Meknassî was born in the old imperial city of Meknes in the first half of the eighteenth century and received a classical higher education at the prestigious Qarawîyîn University of Fez. He later managed to hold an office of secretary in the palace of the sultan, by whom he would be appointed ambassador three times. After the death of Muhammad III in 1790, Ibn Uthmân used his experience in the service of Moulay Al Yazid (1790–92) and his successor Moulay Slimane. He became very popular among Europeans; the sources testify that the French consul in Tangier, Louis de Chénier,[25] wrote in a letter to his ambassador that the death of Ibn Uthmân was a great loss to all the nations of Europe because he was a loyal friend. This letter came just after Ibn Uthmân had reached the zenith of his diplomatic activities through his intervention in the signing of the Treaty of Meknes with Spain on 1 March 1799, one of the most important agreements in Moroccan history due to its lasting impact on the sultanate's relations with Europe during the nineteenth century.[26]

The main tasks of Ibn Uthmân during his first diplomatic mission as ambassador to Spain in 1779 were to obtain the freedom of Muslim captives held in that country, all of them Algerians, as well as to negotiate a new treaty of peace and commerce which restored the good bilateral relations after the Moroccan siege of Melilla in 1774–76 had interrupted them. He carried out his diplomatic mission in Aranjuez, the summer residency of King Carlos III located south of Madrid. The treaty was signed on 30 May 1780.[27] Two years later, Ibn Uthmân was chosen again for a double diplomatic mission, this time to proceed to Malta for talks with the Grand Master of the Order of the Knights Hospitaller of St John, Emmanuel de Rohan, who ruled over the island,[28] and also to Naples as ambassador to the court of King Ferdinando IV (1759–1825), son of Carlos III of Spain. The Neapolitan king eagerly waited for him to negotiate a peace and commerce treaty similar to that signed in Aranjuez, which would be signed in Naples on 18 October 1782.[29] The visit to Malta aimed to obtain the liberation of Muslim captives, but was also in connection to the devolution by the sultan of Morocco of merchandise captured by Moroccan pirates to Maltese merchants in 1779.[30]

The diplomatic activities of Ibn Uthmân are not, however, the main subject of this chapter: I have written about them elsewhere.[31] My main purpose here is actually to analyse the ambassador's personal experiences of the quarantine he underwent in two Mediterranean port cities, first in Spain's Ceuta in 1779, then in Valletta, the main port of Malta, in 1782. Ibn Uthmân became widely known for his travel books in eighteenth-century Europe. He was among the few Moroccan ambassadors who produced those literary texts known as *rihla* (travel diaries). As he left Morocco for the first time in 1779 and began to learn about different countries and cultures, he started writing his first book *Al Iksir Fî Fîkak Al Asîr* (Elixir for the captive's release), in which he reported everything he saw and witnessed in Spain.[32] He would also leave a valuable travel account that traced his adventure and his diplomatic experiences in Malta in 1782, as well as in the Kingdom of the Two Sicilies, where he visited Naples and spent a few months in Sicily. This second book is entitled *al Bâdr as-Sâfir lî Hidâyat al-mûsafîr* (The full moon guiding the traveller to release captives from the infidel enemy).[33] In both these publications, quarantine is shown as the first medical–cultural practice which the ambassador was forced to confront in his travels to European countries. So how did he perceive it? A couple of pages from his writings allow us to analyse this man's response – which embodies Islamic culture on the one hand, and the Moroccan *makhzen* elite's views on the other – to the sanitary measures taken in Europe to protect the health of the population and the merchandise of commercial interchange.

The Moroccan ambassador left the imperial city of Rabat, located on the Atlantic coast, to reach Ceuta (*Sebta*), the Spanish enclave on the Strait of Gibraltar, on 13 November 1779. Ibn Uthmân's first remark in his writings is about the military fortifications that the Spanish authorities had built around the city during the time of Moulay Ismail's siege. To enter the walled city, he had to cross a suspended wooden bridge attached to chains separating Ceuta from the rest of Morocco. To his surprise, he was then subjected to quarantine for a period of fourteen days.[34] Local authorities granted him the privilege of undergoing isolation in a villa, which he described as being among the most beautiful residences of the king of Spain in the city. He began his narration by giving the following general definition of quarantine, as well as some details about its actual implementation:

> This quarantine, according to them, means that anyone who comes to them should reside for forty days in a place they have prepared for this purpose. He can neither go out nor receive anyone to avoid contagion because they suspected our country – may God protect it – being hit by the epidemic. However, that was not the case; they establish the quarantine prudently for fear of doubt during this period. Anyone contaminated will not be allowed to enter their territory and a doctor comes to examine him. Once declared free, he can then access the city and get in touch with locals. Among their provisions too, if one of their citizens encounters a person from a foreign country and is suspected to be contaminated, he is also obliged to undergo quarantine … Frankly, they are too strict in this matter, even food is served from a distance to avoid physical contact.[35]

In reality, the health measures applied to Ibn Uthmân in Ceuta were not that severe, as the ambassador was entitled to receive daily visits from important figures, such as the governor of the city, General José Orcasitas. His experience was of a sort of a 'semi-quarantine' endurance because the Spanish authorities were keen on showing their respect to the representative of the sultan of Morocco, a constant during the whole duration of the ambassador's travel.[36] It is not said in the diary if his entourage received the same privileged treatment or had to endure a stricter confinement. In any case, Ibn Uthmân spent fourteen days at the villa and twenty-seven days in Ceuta before departing for Cádiz in mid December, from where he reached Madrid on 12 January 1780. He walked around the city and described the military fortifications. He also wrote about military parades which he watched from his residence every day. Muslim captives went to visit him and he promised to free them from their imprisonment.

In 1782, the ambassador Ibn Uthmân would again be subjected to a period of quarantine, this time in the port of Valletta, in Malta. His ship left Tangier's bay on 19 March bound for the Spanish port of Cádiz. The authorities of this city may have exempted him from quarantine, as nothing else is mentioned in his narrative other than that he was allowed to disembark upon arrival in port. He described the ceremonies and the warm welcome the local authorities granted him. In his opinion, such fine treatment was due to the friendly relations he had struck with the Spanish authorities during his first mission there in 1779–80.[37] Ibn Uthmân stayed in Cádiz for twenty-six days; then, he boarded a Spanish ship for Malta. He devoted a few pages of his book to narrate his crossing of the Mediterranean Sea, the risks encountered in the Strait of Gibraltar and the strong currents of the Gulf of Lion.[38] After twenty-two days of trying navigation, the ambassador and his entourage landed in Valletta, Malta's main port. Upon verification of his identity, the Malta port authorities obliged all of them to undergo a twenty-day quarantine, which Ibn Uthmân only reluctantly accepted, as shown in the dialogue with someone who came to meet him on behalf of the Grand Master:

> He said: You must purge the quarantine. I replied: Why are you forcing us to do it while we have come directly from Spain? Contrary to your suspicion, our country is safe and sound! If it had been otherwise, the Spaniards would have prohibited us from entering their territory before you. He replied: It is an obligation for all those who come to us because you have certainly met the Spanish warships, which in their turn had contacted a ship from a suspected country ... Now you stay under quarantine for twenty days in a mansion prepared for you. I replied: I refuse to go down and will spend the twenty days on board of my ship.[39]

Ibn Uthmân also wrote in his diary that the Maltese authorities assigned a servant to him because of his status as ambassador, a Christian agent who was sent on board his vessel, specifically to take care of his personal needs. But he did not approve of this act since, according to the laws of quarantine, from the first contact with the ship's crew and passengers, this servant would not be allowed to disembark again. Actually, he suspected that 'this Christian was there to spy on us and see if we had a patient we hid on board'.[40] To describe Malta's quarantine, Ibn Uthmân used the same quotation I extracted from his first travel book, adding a few particular details about some purification methods applied by the Maltese health personnel to passengers 'during quarantine'. He described, for example, how they subjected them to a process of fumigation, with a kind of incense made out of sulphur with a composition seemingly made of 'dog and cat waste'. Also, when a quarantined person wished to send a letter, they got hold of it by using a wooden stick, and before opening and reading it, the letter was soaked in vinegar and then 'fragranced'.[41] Once his period of quarantine was finally over, Ibn Uthmân went ashore and the Maltese authorities prepared for him a residence which was 'worthy of his person'. After three days of rest, he presented his letter of appointment to the Grand Master, for he was eager to begin the negotiations for the purchase of Muslim captives.[42]

Quarantine and Ibn Uthmân's identities

The few precious pages on quarantine contained in Ibn Uthmân's travel writings, which present the first-hand testimony of a person from the southern shore of the Mediterranean Sea in the eighteenth century, allows us to draw the following conclusions. First, despite his status of *makhzen* official and his title of ambassador, Ibn Uthmân was not exempted from quarantine, especially in Malta. He himself wrote that the strict Maltese quarantine regulations *in vigore* at the port of Valletta were never breached, reinforcing in this way the reputation of Malta's lazaretto at that time as a place where the most strict quarantine was implemented – as John Chircop argues in his Chapter 8 within this volume.[43] With regard to the special treatment that the Spanish authorities granted him in Ceuta (only fourteen days of 'semi-quarantine') and Cádiz (exempted), it seems to us that this was not only due to the respect they had for the sultan of Morocco, as Ibn Uthmân argued in his narrative, but also because they were well informed about the epidemic situation in his country of origin, which had been free from plague during the period 1778–82. It is true that historical sources confirm the existence of a 'great famine' during those years[44] – the worst of the century in the country according to Raynaud[45] – so the European consuls feared the outbreak of a serious plague epidemic at any moment, and this would finally occur in 1786. But at the time of Ibn Uthmân's travel to Malta, the plague was absent from Morocco.

Second, Ibn Uthmân was the first Moroccan traveller to leave his readers an account of quarantine in Europe. For a long time before him, especially during the seventeenth and early eighteenth centuries, numerous Moroccans travelled to Europe as emissaries or ambassadors, some of them leaving records and chronicles of their travel experiences.[46] However, neither Muhammad ben Abd Alwahab al Ghassani, ambassador of the Sultan Moulay Ismail in Spain in 1690, nor Ahmad al Mehdi Al Ghazzal, ambassador of Sidi Muhammad ibn Abdallah in the same country in 1766, nor others mention quarantine.[47] For us, this raises the question of the actual standpoint of the *makhzen* elite of Ibn Uthmân's time in relation to some aspects of Christian Europe's 'modernisation'. During the eighteenth and nineteenth centuries, a division arose between those who rejected any Western influence and those who encouraged the state to adopt novelties developed in Europe – including those in medicine and public health. Such division was mainly due to the dominance of Islamic thought in all spheres of Moroccan society and administration at that time, especially through the intervention of the *ulama*[48] (religious experts), given the crucial role they played in Muslim society – having the power to issue *fatwas*.[49]

For example, with regard to quarantine, in the eighteenth century, Ahmed Ibn Ajiba (1748–1809), a contemporary of Ibn Uthmân, was among the first who refused all protection measures against epidemics, and especially quarantine. In his manuscript *Sîlk ad-dûrar fî dîkr al-qadâ wâ al- qâdâr,*[50] he explained his rejection of all measures taken by 'man' to escape 'one's fate', based on the widespread interpretation of the plague as a punishment from God for human misconduct. Accordingly, 'man' would have no other recourse against the disease but God. In spite of this, when the plague struck Morocco in 1799, he refused to follow the advice of the authorities and fled from Tetouan, while all his children succumbed to the epidemic. He himself would die of plague in 1809. Yet, we often notice that in the eighteenth century the view of the *ulama* was the same as that of *makhzen* officials – and Ibn Uthmân was one of them – since they had all attended the same religious schools in the big cities of Morocco (Marrakech, Rabat and

Meknes) and, of course, the famous Qarawîyîn University in Fez. In this high institution of learning, the curriculum had remained unchanged for centuries, revolving around religious studies while scientific knowledge was downplayed – merely a shadow of the golden age of Arab-Islamic science.[51]

Moreover, Ibn Uthmân's writings reflect considerable concern and dissatisfaction with quarantine, especially in Malta. In his opinion, quarantine was an obstacle that came to delay a diplomatic mission he considered as being particularly 'noble' and important because it aimed to release Muslim captives from the hands of 'infidel enemies', and more precisely from the island of Malta, at the time being perceived as a 'nest of pirates' – such was the expression used in his narrative.[52] From this point of view, quarantine assisted Maltese piracy practices that targeted shipping/commerce – particularly that flying the Muslim flag – throughout the Mediterranean. This position continued to prevail even during the second half of the nineteenth century. Muhammad An-Nasiri (1835–97), a renowned Moroccan historian and statesman, wrote about quarantine:

> Today, if we look at this quarantine, it is clear that it has material and religious advantages and disadvantages. On the one hand, it contributes to the protection of the countries that use it against the damage caused by the epidemic, and we notice that this objective is not always achieved. On the other hand, quarantine touches so obviously and blatantly the interests of traders and travellers, it also comes to disturb the confidence and beliefs of people in their destiny ...[53]

To summarise the abovementioned points, I would argue that quarantine, on the one hand, acted as a marker of otherness by which the Moroccan ambassador Ibn Uthmân Al-Meknassî was identified as a Muslim, though significant differences existed in the degree of alterity experienced in Spain and Malta due to the diversity in quarantine procedures and the state of bilateral relations – among other factors. His subjective opinion on quarantine, on the other hand, was also one of the means through which Ibn Uthmân situated himself within the *makhzen* elite at a time when a division between those who declared themselves in favour of European-style modernisation and those who advocated a rejection of European novelties was already visible. In this sense, although he criticised and loathed the isolation practices he was obliged to endure, he seems to have regarded quarantine as a sanitary measure indicative of the modern era. To understand why he did not express the need to see it implemented in Morocco we should nevertheless take into account that his travel diaries were originally written at the request of the sultans themselves, and for this reason they avoided any real criticism of existing measures in Morocco and refrained from proposing any changes to things as they were. Somewhat paradoxically, Ibn Uthmân would die in Marrakech in 1799 during the great plague epidemic of 1799–1800.[54] The introduction of the disease in Morocco was possible because Sultan Moulay Suleiman refused the suggestion of the *Junta de Cónsules* of Tangier to impose sanitary isolation on the ships carrying pilgrims returning from Mecca. It would not be the last time, since he allowed the Moroccan *hajjis* to disembark in 1818, this time because among them there happened to be his two sons; plague ravaged Morocco again as it had done two decades earlier.[55] The conflict between quarantine and the religious and class identity of the larger sector of the *makhzen* elite was often resolved at the expense of the former, symbolically overruling those who, as Ibn Uthmân, had been used to the practice of compromise between his beliefs and ideas and those of the Europeans.

Notes

1 Bel Kamel Al bidaouia, 'ALwadaâ Tîbî Saâdi' in *Al maarîfa Tîbîa watarikh Al Amrad fî Al Maghreb* (Conference proceedings), Casablanca, King Abdul-Aziz ibn Saud Foundation – Editions Okad, 2011, 32.

2 Caroline Stone, 'The Muhtasib', *Saudi Aramco World*, September/October 1977, 22–25; R.P. Buckley, 'The Muḥtasib' *Arabica* 39, 1, 1992, 59–117; Cl. Cahen, M. Talbi, R. Mantran, A.K.S. Lambton and A.S. Bazmee Ansari, 'Ḥisba', in *Encyclopédie de l'Islam*, Brill, http://referenceworks.brillonline.com/entries/encyclopedie-de-l-islam/hisba-COM_0293 (accessed 2 April 2017).

3 The Valletta lazaretto complex was constructed in 1643 on an *isolotto* named Manoel Island, although one must mention that quarantine was already being used in the Valletta harbour in the 1520s and that during the 1592 plague one finds evidence of a makeshift lazaretto set up on this island. It was Venice which was the first to set up a lazaretto in 1403. Marseille's lazaretto was built in 1526, Livorno's in 1590–95, Naples' in 1626 and Ragusa's in 1642. Anne Brogini, *Malte, Frontière de la Chrétienté*

(1530–1670), Rome, École Française de Rome, 2006, 567; Daniel Panzac, *Quarantaines et Lazarets*, Aix-en-Provence, Édisud, 1986, 34.

4 Elizabeth Longuenesse, Silvia Chiffoleau, Nabil Kronfol and Omar Dewachi, 'Santé publique et métiers du médecin au monde arabe: vue historique', in *Al Mustakbal Al Arabi*, 2014, Fasc. Unique, 11.

5 Nancy Elizabeth Gallagher, *Medicine and Power in Tunisia, 1780–1900*, Cambridge, Cambridge University Press, 1983, 23–24.

6 On Morocco's foreign policy in this period, see Jacques Caillé, *Les accords internationaux du sultan Sidi Mohammed ben Abdallah: 1757–1790*, Paris, Librairie Générale de Droit et de Jurisprudence, 1960; Ramón Lourido, *Marruecos y el mundo exterior en la segunda mitad del siglo XVIII*, Madrid, Instituto de Cooperación con el Mundo Árabe, 1989.

7 For a chronology of the main outbreaks of plague and cholera and of the famine crisis until the end of the nineteenth century, see Louis Raynaud, *Étude sur l'hygiène et la médecine au Maroc*, Alger, Léon, 1902.

8 Mohammed Kenbib (ed.), *La Grande Encyclopédie du Maroc, Histoire*, Rabat, GEM, 1987, 109–113. The main chroniclers of this period are: Abu Al Kasem Zayanî, *Attûrjomân Al Mûghreb*, trans. Houdas, 1886; and Al Duayyîf Rîbatî, *Tarikh Al Dawla Saaida*, Rabat, Dar Al maturate, 1986.

9 Mohammed Amine El-Bezzaz, *Tarekh al majâa wa al awbîae bi al Maghreb* [History of famines and epidemics in Morocco in 18th and 19th centuries] [in Arabic], Rabat, Université Mohammed V, 1992, 54.

10 Henry-Paul-Joseph Renaud, 'Les pestes du milieu du XVIIIe siècle', *Hespéris* XXVI, 1939, 293–319.

11 Henry-Paul-Joseph Renaud, 'La peste de 1799 d'après des document inédites', *Hespéris* I, 1921, 160.

12 Raynaud, *Étude sur l'hygiène*, 81.

13 Domingo Badía/Ali Bey, *Viajes de Ali Bey*, Madrid, Compañía Literaria, 1996, 170.

14 Driss Moussaoui and Michel Roux-Dessarps (eds), *Histoire de la médecine au Maroc et dans les pays arabes et musulmans*, Casablanca, Najah el-Jadida, 1995.

15 Alejandro del Cantillo, *Tratados, convenios y declaraciones de paz y de comercio que han hecho con las potencias extranjeros los monarcas españoles de la casa de Borbón desde el año 1700 hasta el día*, Madrid, Imprenta de Alegría y Charlain, 1843, 506.

16 Mohammed Amine El-Bezzaz, *The International Sanitary Council of Morocco, 1792–1929* [in Arabic], Rabat, Université Mohammed V, 2000, 85–87.

17 Ibid., 48.

18 Raynaud, *Étude sur l'hygiène*, 63.
19 Michel-Pierre Roux, *Mogador, Essaouira. Acteur et témoin pour l'histoire de la santé*, Marrakech, El Watanya, 1996, 29.
20 El-Bezzaz, *The International Sanitary Council of Morocco*, 151–186; Mohammed Amine El-Bezzaz, 'Les débuts de la réglementation sanitaire de pèlerinage Marocain à la Mecque (1831–1866)', *Hesperis-Tamuda* XXII, 1984, 94.
21 Ibid.; Francisco Javier Martínez, 'La sanidad en Marruecos a mediados del siglo XIX', *Medicina & Historia* 1, 2005, 1–15.
22 Kenbib, *La Grande Encyclopédie du Maroc*, 111–112; Jacques Caillé, *La petite histoire de Rabat*, Rabat, Université Mohammed V, 2012, 132–133; Jaques Caillé, *Les Accords Internationaux de Sidi Mohammed Ben Abdallah*, Rabat, Librairie Génerale de Droits, 1960.
23 Lourido, *Marruecos y el mundo exterior*, 145.
24 Ibid., 717.
25 Jacques Caillé, *Le Consulat de Tanger (des origines à 1830)*, Paris, Pedone, 1967.
26 Jean-Louis Miège, *Le Maroc et l'Europe (1830–1894). Tome II. L'ouverture*, Paris, Presses universitaires de France, 1961, 19–38.
27 Vicente Rodríguez Casado, 'La embajada del Talbe Sidi Mohamed ben Otman en 1780', *Hispania* 3, 1943, 598–611.
28 This Grand Master was of French origin. He ruled the Maltese island from 1775 to 1797 as the penultimate Grand Master of the Order of the Knights Hospitallers in Malta. Ibn Uthmân devoted a few pages to his relationship with him in his diary *Al Badr asâfir*.
29 Lourido, *Marruecos y el mundo exterior*, 504.
30 Ibid., 525.
31 Malika Ezzahidi, 'Le rachat des captifs Musulmans à Malte en 1782, d'après le récit de voyage d'Ibn Uthmân Al Meknassî', *Cahiers de la Méditerranée* 87, 2013, 221–228; 'Le voyage diplomatique en Europe, Rihlatu "al badr asâfîr" comme modèle', in *Proceedings of the symposium Al Rihla entre l'Orient et L'Occident*, Rabat, Université Mohammed V, 2003, 110, 159–170.
32 Ibn Uthmân Al-Meknassî, *Al Iksir Fî Fîkak Al Asîr*, Mohammed Al Fassi edition, Rabat, University Centre for Scientific Research, 1965.
33 Ibn Uthmân Al-Meknassî, *Al Bâdr as-Sâfir lî Hidâyat al-Mûsafîr ila Fâkâk al-Asârâ mina al-'Aduww al-Kafir*, Malika Ezzahidi edition, Mohammedia, Université Hassan II, 2005. This work won the 'Ibn Battuta Award' (dedicated to travel literature in the Arab and Muslim world), awarded by the Center Irtîyad al Afak, based in Abu Dhabi and London (2nd edition, 2013).
34 Ibn Uthmân, *Al Iksir Fî Fîkak Al Asîr*, 9.

35 Ibid., 10.
36 Lourido, *Marruecos y el mundo exterior*, 444.
37 Ibn Uthmân, *Al Iksir Fî Fîkak Al Asîr*, 10.
38 Ibn Uthmân, *Al Bâdr as-Sâfir*, 126.
39 Ibid, 130.
40 There were two quarantine sites in Valletta: one in the Grand Harbour under the ramparts of the city, for those who could not or did not want to spend quarantine on board their vessels. The other was the lazaretto at Marsamxett at the western part of the Grand Harbour. The ambassador might have spent his quarantine in the latter according to his account. Ibid., 140.
41 Ibid., 131.
42 Ezzahidi, 'Le rachat des captifs Musulmans', 130.
43 Carmen Depasquale has claimed that 'no one was exempt from [Malta's] quarantine; ambassadors, ministers, consuls, knights, all should submit to it' (author's translation). 'La Quarantaine à Malte au XVII et XVIIIe siècles dans les mémoires, journaux et récits de quelques voyageurs', *The Northern Mariner/Le Marin du Nord* XIX, 2, 2009, 159.
44 Zayanî, *Attûrjomân Al Mûghreb*, 82–83.
45 Raynaud, *Étude sur l'hygiène*, 75.
46 Abdelmajid Kaddouri, *Moroccan Ambassadors in Europe, 1610–1922* [in Arabic], Rabat, Université Mohammed V, 1995.
47 Ahmed Ben Kassem Al Hajari, *Naser Addin Aalaalqawm al kafirîn*, Mohamed Razouk edition, Casablanca, 1987. Al Ghassani was ambassador to the King Carlos II of Spain in 1690 and Al Ghazal was ambassador to the King of Spain Carlos III in 1766: Muhammad Ben Abdelwahhab al-Ghassani, *Rihlat al-wazir fi iftikak al-assîr*, Abderrahim Benhadda edition, Tokyo, Research institute for Languages and Cultures of Asia and Africa, 2005; Ahmed al-Mehdi al-Ghazal, *Natijât al ijtihad fi al mohadana wa al-Jihad*, Ismail al-Gharbi edition, Bayrut, Dar al-Gharbal-Islami, 1980.
48 The *ulama* were scholars of the religious sciences who saw themselves as the guardians of the faith and jurisprudence (*shari'a*). In the absence of a formal Muslim clergy, they represented a sort of religious aristocracy whose acquiescence was necessary not only for the religious but also for the secular policies of the sultan. Mohammed El Mansour, 'Les Oulemas et le Makzen dans le Maroc précolonial', in Jean-Claude Santucci (ed.), *Le Maroc actuel*, Aix-en-Provence, IREMAM, 1992, 3–15.
49 'Fatwa' in Islam is a legal opinion given by an expert of Islamic law on a particular issue. The opinion is often issued following the request of an individual or a group of people.

50 Jeans-Louis Michou, *Le Sofi marocain Ibn Ajiba (1746–1809) et son Mi'raj* [n.p.], 1990.
51 Lulat, Y.G.-M., *A History of African Higher Education from Antiquity to the Present: A Critical Synthesis,* Westport and London, Praeger, 2005.
52 Ibn Uthmân, *Al Bâdr as-Sâfir,* 28.
53 Ahmed Ben Khaled An-Nasiri, *Al istiksa, Li Akhbar Doualî Al-Maghrib Al-Aksa,* Casablanca, vol. 5, 1997, 184.
54 Renaud, 'La peste de 1799', 160.
55 Raynaud, *Étude sur l'hygiène,* 82.

5

Policing boundaries: quarantine and professional identity in mid nineteenth-century Britain

Lisa Rosner

Introduction

As the British imperial presence spread across the world's inland seas and oceans from the late eighteenth through the nineteenth centuries, so too did deadly diseases like yellow fever, cholera and dysentery. Management of these diseases invariably created disputes between medical men in Royal Navy ships and those at the ports they visited, over whether specific diseases were communicable and, thus, whether there was any purpose to quarantine. As Mark Harrison has argued forcefully in *Contagion: How Commerce has Spread Disease*, 'the resolution of such disputes [...] owed more to diplomacy than to the force of scientific logic'.[1] Harrison made his comment in connection with what became known as the *Éclair* tragedy, in which a devastating outbreak of yellow fever on Boa Vista, in the Cape Verde Islands, had been linked to a steam-powered Royal Navy ship. This became an international incident, as controversy raged over where blame should be apportioned, both for the initial infection and for subsequent deaths. Was the disease yellow fever? If so, was yellow fever contagious? Had the naval vessel brought it? Or had it originated on Boa Vista? Was it the responsibility of officials – whether in the Azores or in London – to have instituted measures to halt the epidemic? Or of the medical men in attendance, whether military or civilians?

Harrison's own conclusion can be found in his subtitle, in that he sees commerce as the ultimate cause, not only of the outbreak on Boa

Vista, but also of the global spread of disease in the modern world. By commerce, he means more than just the global exchange of goods, or even the technologies, like steam-powered vessels, that transported microorganisms across longer distances in a shorter period of time than the world had ever seen. Instead, his focus is on the government policies regarding empire, and the concrete mechanisms they instituted to create, develop and maintain it. As Harrison has recently argued, 'The 1800s saw the greatest redistribution of pathogens the world has ever known. Human, animal, and plant diseases circulated in many directions, with enormous social and political ramifications. This global picture usually appears as a dimly illuminated backdrop to a local or national story. It is therefore necessary to think more deeply about the connections between these apparently disparate events.'[2]

Like many recent commentators on Harrison's work, I agree with virtually all his major contentions, while wishing to leave room for a more nuanced discussion of specific historical factors affecting movement of pathogens, ideological positions and local responses.[3] In this chapter, I will argue that any discussion of nineteenth-century British conflicts over contagion and quarantine must take into consideration the lived experience of the medical men who had to live with and, frequently, die from them. The mortality rate on the Royal Navy West African squadron, charged with suppressing the Atlantic slave trade by patrolling the coast of West Africa, could exceed 50%,[4] including many surgeons and assistant surgeons; the disease on the *Éclair* killed four medical men and the ship's captain. If anyone had asked these men what they were dying for, it is unlikely they would have responded 'commerce', or even 'empire'. Instead, it is most probable that they would have referred to the professional ethics that required them to stay with their patients and with their ship.

This chapter will further argue that naval experience in the Mediterranean was crucial to the formation of this professional identity, particularly with respect to quarantine regulations. Young British medical officers during the first decades of the nineteenth century acquired their first experience of quarantine and contagious diseases through the Mediterranean ports of Gibraltar and Malta. This experience was extended through their Atlantic voyages, as they called at ports governed by Mediterranean powers and regulated, at least in principle, by Mediterranean models of quarantine. Yet they entered a maritime hierarchy that regarded each ship as its own floating village, with the naval surgeon as chief public health officer. Quarantine, like disease, was assumed to come from outside the ship; believing otherwise would have created the kind of cognitive dissonance that often ended a naval career.

During those same decades, the rise of British medical journalism created an opposing professional identity, one that pitted the land-based medical observer against the lived experience of the naval surgeon on the spot. Medical writers emphasised independence and impartiality in their definition of 'professional'. By their definition, a naval surgeon – or Physician-General of the Navy – who had to defend his actions in a public forum could not be truly independent and, therefore, could not be truly professional.

Defining professions

We can see this process in a book review that appeared in 1849 in the *Edinburgh Medical and Surgical Review*. The book under review was by Sir William Pym (1772–1861), then Superintendent of Quarantine, and it was a re-issue of his earlier book on yellow fever, which argued that the disease was contagious.[5] A book review that begins, 'It is quite unnecessary to say, that we regret to see the present work published', is unlikely to be favourably disposed to the work under discussion and, indeed, the reviewer made clear his displeasure. It was not so much the contents that offended him, though he noted that all Dr Pym's opinions 'have been stereotyped for the past thirty-five years'. But what he found truly distasteful was the manner in which Pym expressed his opposition to other medical writers. The book 'contains language', he wrote,

> which ought not to be spoken by one member of the profession of another. Nothing ... should have induced the author to express himself in the manner in which he has done; and nothing, either in his own professional character or the official situation which he holds, can furnish either an excuse or a defense of such language. It is impossible to review further a work containing statements of this nature ...[6]

This brief non-review refers twice to something that the reviewer calls a 'profession'. In the first usage, referring to language 'which ought not to be spoken by one member of the profession of another', the reviewer is implying that there is one unifying profession that all medical men belong to, and within which certain codes of civility apply. There are other things implied by this idea of a profession, as sociologists have identified for this period: a common training, a common emphasis on science, on logic, on sifting of evidence, on dedication to public welfare. At first glance, it might seem that the second use of 'professional character' means the same thing. But there is a subtle difference: by 'professional character', the reviewer meant Dr Pym's own personal 'professional experience and reputation', just as by 'official situation' the reviewer meant Pym's position as superintendent of quarantine. Pym might believe that both of those set his opinions apart from, and above, the rest of the medical profession. But that attitude, to the reviewer, belonged to the Old Regime of medical preferment, which his generation was determined to reform.

We can also see that this reviewer is making his own claims to professional authority: this is implied in the designation of journals like the *Edinburgh Medical and Surgical Review* as the 'professional press'. Not only were these written by and for doctors, but also their goal was the encouragement of 'temperate discussion', in order to mobilise 'enlightened public opinion'.[7] That is, they used calls for professional behaviour to advocate for medical reform: reform of licensing institutions, so that provincial medical practitioners were freed from the jurisdiction of the Society of Apothecaries, and reform of navy medical positions to bring them to parity with opportunities in the Army and Indian Medical Services. The idea of a universal medical profession that transcended mere 'position' or 'office', that was as respectable and respected on land as at sea – indeed, anywhere in the British Empire – was a powerful tool on behalf of numerous institutional reforms, and a powerful weapon in numerous medical controversies. Reviewers for the professional press juxtaposed their own impartiality, their own ability to sift through numerous reports and to discern the kernel of truth, against the claims for professional authority made by individuals with first-hand experience in the field or aboard ship, or those with government appointments.

Creating professional identities

To understand that first-hand experience, and explore professional mores among navy surgeons, we can start at the very beginning of a navy career, with the experiences of James Williamson, who in January 1829 visited Gibraltar in his very first appointment as surgeon on the *Duke of York* packet, on his first trip to the Mediterranean. Fever had been raging at Gibraltar, and at first he was afraid he would not be able to get ashore. But on the very day the *Duke of York* arrived, the fever was declared over, and Williamson's ship was given a clean bill of health. As he wrote,

> the present diminished mortality is attributed to the attention paid to cleanliness – ventilation – fumigations, and the separation of the healthy from the diseased. It is now thought that the result of this fever, which seems to have resembled the yellow Fever of the West Indies will set at rest the great question so long agitated by medical men of all countries, as to whether this and other fevers are contagious or non-contagious. The medical officers here decide it in the affirmative, and substantiate their opinion by bringing forward the circumstances that those who were completely debarred from the patients were quite free from the fever, whilst the attendants and visitors of the sick, were almost all seized with the fever in their turn. A Dr Pym who came out here about two months ago, has the merit assigned to him of having first ameliorated, and then stopped the ravages of the dreadful disorder – and some men say, that had he been present at the first attack, he would have put a stop to it immediately.

That was 17 January, and on the 28th the *Duke of York* arrived in Malta. Alas for young Williamson, the ship received a very different reception. Williamson wrote that 'Valetta is one of the most romantic and finest cities I have yet seen', but he could only view it through a spyglass for the ship was

> immediately upon our arrival, put into strict Quarantine. None of the Ships Company were permitted to land – and in order to insure the strict observance of this regulation two Quarantine officers came on board and one of them always accompanied our boat, when it was necessary to take the mail ashore, or bring it on board … In addition to all this, we were obliged to hoist a yellow flag at the foremast head, as a public signal that we were tabooed.

Williamson thought these precautions

> laughable – yet how … and you may be sure, that we did not at all recognise the propriety – much less the necessity of them in our own individual case. Till now I had always thought it just and right to be rather over prudent in regard to contagious fevers – but the rigid surveillance, in which we were held, altered the character of my opinions not a little.

That is, within the space of three weeks, and on his very first voyage, Williamson had gone from being firmly convinced of the value of quarantine measures in protecting the health of the public, to questioning their 'propriety, much less' their 'necessity'. Williamson was indignant on behalf of his ship and his captain, and his scepticism continued for the rest of his career. Convinced that his own ship was 'sweet' – that is, 'that there was nothing in her to generate disease' – he had no scruples about occasionally flouting quarantine if he thought he could get away with it. On subsequent voyages, including voyages across the Atlantic in the heart of the pathogen exchange, he deliberately misled quarantine authorities, on occasion hiding a sick sailor on board ship so as to be allowed to land, or exploring a populated area even while under quarantine. Williamson provides an excellent example of the value of quarantine regulations from the point of view of the native population: unless there were guards posted to observe him, he used his own medical judgement about whether the regulations were necessary.[8] His criterion was not the health and safety of the population, nor even his own health and safety, but rather his perception of the interest of the ship and the approval of its captain.

What we can see from Williamson's journal is the formation of boundary lines between the 'professional character' (meaning 'professional experience and reputation') of the young naval surgeon and the 'professional character' of the quarantine officer. It is likely that young Williamson did not long retain his positive view of William Pym, because it was axiomatic in the navy that Sir William Burnett, Inspector General of Naval Hospitals and Fleets, had 'completely disproved many of Dr Pym's statements'.[9] Very few naval medical personnel sided with 'Dr Pym' in print, unless they were on the verge of leaving the navy. Indeed, naval surgeons on active service were much more likely than their civilian counterparts to publish articles indicating that diseases located near ports – leprosy, for example – were not communicable.[10] Men we might now regard as medical professionals clearly did not make common cause as professional brethren.

Crossing boundaries: from naval surgeon to epidemiologist

We can further explore the tensions by examining another naval surgeon who switched sides in the boundary dispute, but this time in the other direction. James Ormiston McWilliam started his career as a navy medical man in 1829, like Williamson. Though it is not clear whether he had early experience in the Mediterranean, his first set of ships certainly did: they were sailing vessels, several of which had been deployed in the sea battles of the Napoleonic Wars.[11] It may well have been with a great sense of satisfaction that in 1841 he secured the position of senior surgeon to an expedition to the Niger region, whose hybrid purpose was to help end the slave trade and demonstrate the power of the Royal Navy, by surveying the coast and Niger basin, transporting missionaries to Liberia and convincing African coastal rulers to switch to legal trade. The *HMS Albert,* on which McWilliam was stationed, as well as the two other ships, the *Wilberforce* and the *Soudan,* were under McWilliam's direct supervision and fitted out with the latest in ventilation and sanitation equipment. Like young Williamson, McWilliam had a close relationship with, and full support of, his commanding officer, in this case Captain Trotter.

And yet fever broke out, with more than 130 men affected and 40 deaths. The mortality was highest on McWilliam's own ship, with an especially high death rate among medical officers. McWilliam himself behaved very heroically, at one point having, with the geologist on board, effective command of the *Albert.* Though he was very circumspect in his account, it seems clear it was on his strong recommendation that the expedition was abandoned and the ships headed for the open sea. He himself was very ill by the time the voyage ended, and spent some months recovering.

McWilliam wrote a report of the voyage, cogently titled *Medical History of the Expedition to the Niger ... comprising an account of the fever which led to its abrupt termination.* It is a clear exposition of what we can consider professional mores among naval surgeons, with numerous references declaring his allegiance to naval medical etiquette. He dedicated the book to Sir William Burnett; he criticised Sir William Pym's theories on yellow fever; he provided page after page of evidence that the expedition had been well run, well planned, exemplary in attention to the health and safety of officers, men, civilians on board and local communities, whom they vaccinated for smallpox. He stated, clearly, that 'No fact' came under his observation 'affording the slightest evidence that the disease was communicable from one person to another'.[12] What comes through in the account is McWilliam's pride in his own ship, and in his professional character, particularly his efficacy as a sanitary engineer. Each 'floating village', under his care was as healthy, as sweet, as modern scientific knowledge could make her.

After the Niger expedition in 1843, the *Albert* was thoroughly cleaned and returned to West Africa, but it was never again a sweet ship. Fever broke out on its next voyage, killing the captain and some number of others. In July 1845, it was in Sierra Leone. Its own crew had been paid off, and so the cleaning was done by men from HMS *Éclair*, back from what had been a very unhealthy and unsuccessful service. Ten men had already died by the time the *Éclair* met the *Albert*; another eighteen died between Sierra Leone and Boa Vista, in the Cape Verde Islands; thirty-one died at Boa Vista; and another twelve on its way back to Britain. Among the dead, as mentioned earlier, were four medical men and Captain Estcourt. The arrival of the *Éclair* in Britain became the *cause celebre* that occasioned the controversy with which this chapter began. Those on the ship, sick and well, were convinced it was the *Éclair* itself that was unhealthy and desperately wanted to get off; Pym, as Superintendant of Quarantine, diagnosed the disease as yellow fever and enforced strict quarantine. There were several more deaths. There was outrage, much of it directed against the inhumanity of quarantine regulations; Pym reissued his book and used intemperate language in defending his diagnosis and quarantine decisions; the professional press was divided on the *Éclair* and yellow fever but agreed that such language was unprofessional.

Meanwhile, back at Boa Vista, a deadly disease was spreading. There was international outcry: wasn't this yellow fever? Hadn't it come from that plague ship, the *Éclair*? Why had the *Éclair* been allowed to land if it had so obviously been 'pest-smitten', as Pym claimed? No less a public authority than Sir William Burnett asked McWilliam to investigate the outbreak. He might well have assumed that McWilliam would, once again, come up with an account that carefully and scientifically supported naval interests, that the fever had nothing to do with the *Éclair*, and that it was of local, land-based origin and had not come from the ship. If that was his assumption, he was disappointed. McWilliam in fact concluded that 'connecting the whole of the circumstances attending the arrival and stay of the "Eclair" at Boa Vista with those under which the disease appeared on the small island, and afterwards on Boa Vista itself, leaves no doubt of its having been introduced by the Eclair'.[13]

McWilliam arrived at this conclusion through what is, by modern standards, a model epidemiological study, anticipating John Snow's *On the Mode of Communication of Cholera* by almost a decade. In carrying out the study, he also documents the obstacles to enforcing Mediterranean standards of quarantine in the Atlantic archipelago. As he notes, when the *Éclair* left the west coast of Africa there was already documented illness on board. For that reason, the Government of Goree, located off the Senegal coast, did not permit her to land. When, on the *Éclair*'s approach to Boa Vista on 21 August 1845, the British consul on the island sent a boat to meet her, Captain Estcourt refused all communication and indicated that quarantine might be necessary. No Portuguese medical man was available, and so Dr Kenny, a British surgeon resident on Boa Vista, was commissioned to go on board and examine the patients. He concluded that the disease 'was the common endemic fever of the African coast, which was not of a contagious or infectious nature'. At that point, the *Éclair* was allowed 'free intercourse with the shore'.[14]

We need not attribute Dr Kenny's diagnosis to the insouciance that led James Williamson to flout quarantine regulations. Almost certainly it was compassion allied with a realistic appraisal of the likely outcome, for the *Éclair*'s men and officers, if they had been forced to put out to sea. It was not possible, in the Cape Verde islands, to create the conditions of a Mediterranean quarantine, where sick sailors could be disembarked with humanity and the ship provisioned a safe distance from harbour. Still, Dr Kenny's decision was one that he, as well as the authorities at Boa Vista, English and Portuguese, had ample reason to regret. Within four days the number of the *Éclair*'s sick had increased to such an extent that they were moved into the captain's cabin, while the captain himself moved in with a British official. By 31 August, more than sixty men had contracted the fever, and all the seamen were moved to a small island about half a mile away from the chief port, Porto Sal Rey. The sick and well were lodged in separate sections of the Fort Duke of Braganza (see Figure 5.1). It was hardly an ideal lazaretto. 'The whole building,' McWilliam wrote, 'is in a state of disrepair, if not of dilapidation ... Some sheds and huts in a ruinous state extend along each side of the yard, and were ... assigned to the healthy part of the crew.' The sick were marginally better housed. As McWilliam noted, 'The house in which the sick were lodged consists of two floors. The upper

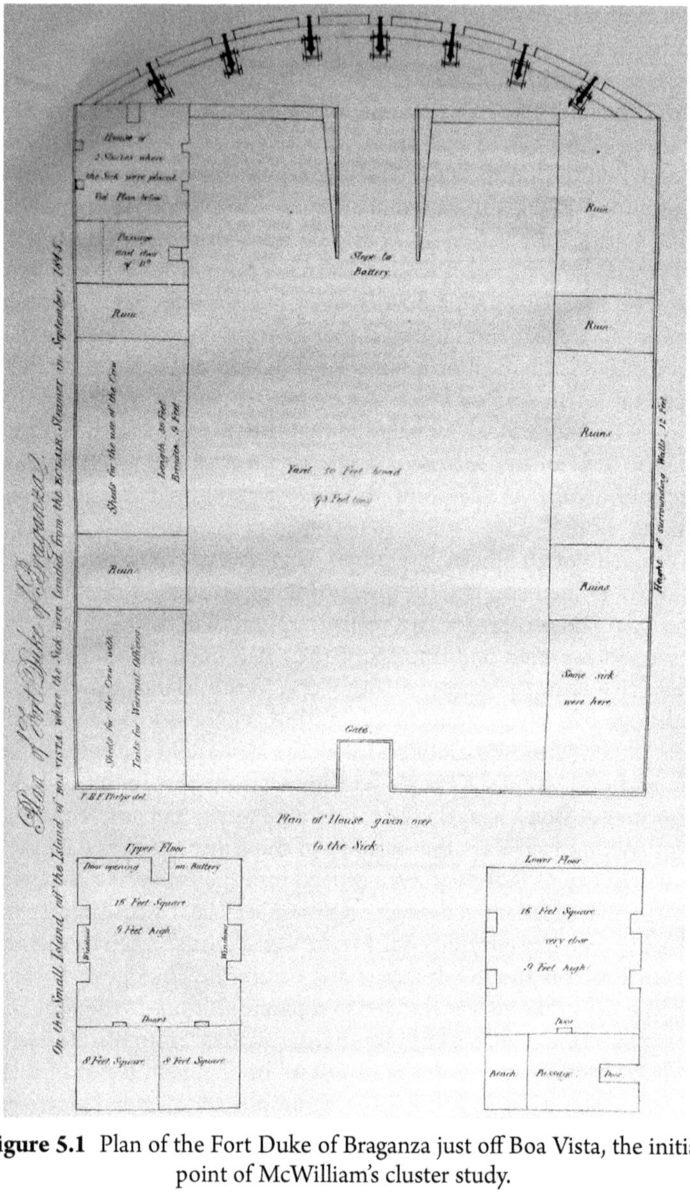

Figure 5.1 Plan of the Fort Duke of Braganza just off Boa Vista, the initial point of McWilliam's cluster study.

floor … is well provided with windows, and is exposed to the breeze.' However, 'The whole of [the] lower floor is close, hot, and miserably ventilated.'[15]

The focus of McWilliam's investigation, however, was not the care of the sick, but instead the impact of frequent and unrestricted contact between civilians and sick seamen. It started with John Jamieson, British storekeeper, who took the soiled linen from the ship's officers and distributed it to seventeen washerwomen from the town. 'Do you know the names of the washerwomen to whom the clothes were given to be washed?' Jamieson was asked. Yes, he responded, and proceeded to give the names. 'Can you bring the above-named washerwomen here?' McWilliam continued. 'Yes, with exception of the last-named four, who are dead', he replied.

And yet, when McWilliam questioned the remaining thirteeen women, it became clear that the soiled linen could not have been the culprit. The women ranged in age from 17 to 60, and were variously described as 'mulatto', 'dark mulatto' or 'negress'. Either they, or close family members, had come down with fever and black vomit, in some cases leading to death.[16] Yet the linen had been washed, ironed and returned to the *Éclair* in three days, long before the ship had sailed in September, while the fever had appeared much later in the season, December or January. By that time, many residents had died – including Dr Kenny – and anyone who could fled from the increasingly unhealthy Porto Sal Rey to neighbouring villages or adjacent islands. If the source of contagion had been carried to shore in the soiled linen, wouldn't the disease have struck those most closely associated with it? 'So that in none of these cases,' McWilliam concluded, 'can the occurrence of the fever be fairly attributed to infectious matter conveyed by the linen.'[17]

The same logic could be applied to the ship itself. As was common practice, local labourers were hired to assist the seamen in cleaning the *Éclair*, as well as providing fresh water and coal. McWilliam was told that 'natives' were not required to work below the upper deck. Nevertheless, he reported, 'of the forty who were employed upwards of a week on board, hoisting in coal-bags and water-casks, several assisted in cleaning, whitewashing and bestowing the holds; most of them were, during some period, on the lower deck; and nearly the whole, including the launchmen, were on board the day the ship siled, and after the sick had returned from the Fort'.[18] Still, none of them developed any illness.

There was thus no evidence to suggest that *HMS Éclair* was the source of the contagion.

From then on, McWilliam's investigation has its closest parallel with Snow's, as he mapped the infection from the Fort Duke of Braganza on the 'small island' as it spread across Boa Vista from west to east (see Figure 5.2). The fort was no longer in general use – which explained its dilapidation – but a corporal and two privates were generally stationed there as part of their tour of duty on the island. The three soldiers on guard duty when the sick seamen were transferred there completed their service without any noteworthy illnesses, and so did the second guard. The third guard, however, were not so fortunate. 'By the evidence of [Private] Miguel Barbosa, the only survivor of this guard,' McWilliam noted, 'it appears that he and his comrades were at the Fort several days before and after its evacuation by the sick of the Eclair.' They had served as orderlies to the sick before the *Éclair* sailed; they were also ordered to sweep out the rooms once the ship had departed. The two other guards were attacked with a fever, delirium and black vomit within a few days, and died shortly thereafter. Two more guards were ordered to Fort Duke of Braganza to look after the sick soldiers, and subsequently to bury them. When they, in turn, became ill, their commanding officer would not admit them to the barracks, located in Porto Sal Rey's lower town, but instead sent them to be lodged in the Beira district, consisting of four houses on the northern end of the city. By that time, a fourth guard had been assigned to the Fort. One of their number had been 'taken ill in the course of two days', McWilliam noted, 'and, strange to say, was at once conveyed to the barracks in Porta Sal Rey'. When two soldiers in the fifth guard in turn became ill, 'the commandant resolved for a while to withdraw the guard altogether from that fatal post'. Both those soldiers likewise returned to the barracks.[19]

As McWilliam's map shows, by 15–16 September, a deadly disease with the symptoms of fever, delirium and black vomit – symptoms identical to those found among *Éclair*'s seamen and medical officers – had appeared among the military guard stationed on the 'small island' where those seamen and medical officers had fallen sick and died. Sick soldiers had been transferred to the military barracks in the heart of the port, as well as to lodgings in Beira. There was no attempt at any kind of quarantine: the soldiers at Beira had many visitors, and cooking and washing was done by local women with no particular concern

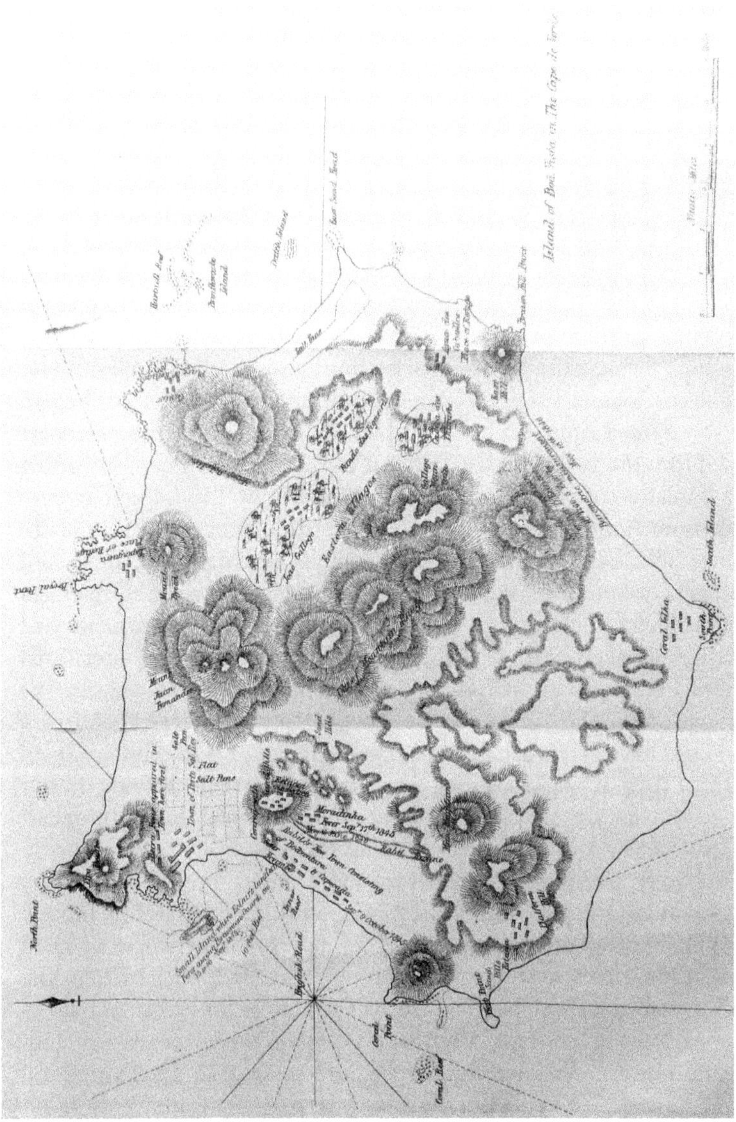

Figure 5.2 Map documenting the spread of the fever to villages of Boa Vista Island, Cape Verde.

for any kind of contagion. It is of the greatest importance, McWilliam wrote, 'that every circumstance connected with their stay here, be carefully noted, as it afterwards turned out that the very first case of fever in the town appeared in the room adjoining that in which the soldiers were lodged'.[20]

That first victim was Anna Gallinha, described by the soldiers as 'a Portuguese woman, who cooked for us'.[21] She lived in the same house as the soldiers, in the room next door, and seems to have visited frequently. By early October, the soldiers were well enough to have returned to their duties, but Anna Gallinha 'was attacked with fever in the course of three or four days after the soldiers left Beira, and died with high fever, delirium, and black vomit', around mid October.[22] Her neighbour, Joanna Texeira, 'was also constantly in the house'.[23] She and her son nursed Anna Gallinha, and fell ill in turn, though both recovered. From there, the disease radiated outward across Beira, spreading to a 'mulatto native called Manoel Affonso, who lived about twenty yards from Anna Gallinha's house', to Gertrude Bent, 'a native mulatto woman, who had visited both Anna Gallinha and Manoel Affonso, and lived next door to the latter', to Antonio Perica 'who arrived at Boa Vista from Madeira, a few days after the departure of the "Eclair," and had occasionally seen Manoel Affonso during his illness, and afterwards carried his corpse as well as that of Anna Gallinha to Rabil, for the purpose of burial'.[24] Again, McWilliam was careful to note, the disease could not have been spread by inanimate objects, for the soldiers testified that they 'brought nothing from the Fort but the clothing on our backs. The first day we came to the house we stripped this clothing off' and gave it to a local woman 'to be washed'.[25]

The fever radiated outwards from the barracks into 'Porto Sal Rey proper' at around the same time, that is, around mid October, though McWilliam could not trace its spread from person to person in as much detail. From mid November 1845 through January 1846, he wrote, 'the disease was at its height in Porto Sal Rey, sometimes six and seven persons dying in one day'.[26] Wealthy residents of the lower town, including the Governor-General and most of the English merchants and public officials, left Boa Vista for other islands in the Cape Verde archipelago, and the entire island put under quarantine. The upper portion of Porto Sal Rey, 'occupied by the lowest classes … mere hovels, rudely built, much crowded together, and with few exceptions, dirty', was left largely to fend for itself.[27] This seems to have been the period when the four washerwomen who had attended to the *Éclair* officers' linen contracted fever and died, and when the fever appears to have attacked one after another of the survivors' households.

In mid November, a British resident, Mr Pettingal, returned to Porto Sal Rey with his wife and daughter. Two female servants became ill; one went home, while the other remained for three days, cared for by Miss Pettingal, the daughter of the house. She in turn became ill and died of fever, delirium and black vomit within a week. An English housekeeper and steward, who had remained on Boa Vista to look after their employers' interests, helped nurse her, subsequently dying of the fever. Dr Kenny, who had also remained on the island, treated Miss Pettingal and died of the fever. An American sea captain who had visited Miss Pettingal also became ill and died. Mr and Mrs Pettingal left Boa Vista after the death of their daughter, but Mr Pettingal died on board ship within a week. Mrs Pettingal had no choice but to return to Boa Vista, where she remained until mid January. On her arrival at the Cape Verde island of San Nicolao, she was placed in quarantine.[28]

McWilliam identified a secondary source of contagion that arose in the village of Rahil, south of Porto Sal Rey, by mid September of 1845. Luis Fortes Pathi, a labourer on the *Éclair*, had returned to his home in the most crowded part of Rahil, the Cabeçada district, consisting of '120 small hovels, rudely constructed of sandstone, and much crowded'. McWilliam described the inhabitants as 'very poor, earning a livelihood as labourers when there is shipping in the port, carrying water, and cultivating patches in the ravine'. Pathi became ill with a fever within a few days of working on the *Éclair*, though he eventually recovered. However, his wife, two daughters and a son died within a few days with symptoms of high fever, suppression of urine and black vomit: 'such was the ominous commencement of the fever in the populous district, Cabeçada'. McWilliam traced the spread of the fever from Pathi's household outward, reaching the neighbouring district of Boaventura by November. The smaller villages to the south along the coast were more fortunate: they suffered outbreaks of fever, but few deaths.[29]

Having traced the fever down the western coast of Boa Vista, McWilliam turned to the three eastern villages. He may well have considered this the most convincing part of his argument. As the map indicates, the three villages are a substantial distance from Porto Sal Rey and its environs. 'João Gallego, the north-westernmost, or that nearest to Porto Sal Rey,' he wrote, 'is situated in the middle of a large plain, which is covered with sand, volcanic debris, and fragments of basalt … Fundo das Figueiras lies at three-quarters of a mile to the south-east … on a rising ground of sandstone … Cabeça dos Tharafes … also stands on a sandy elevation.' That, is, according to all known medical theory, there was no reason to expect a deadly fever to arise from the external environment. The villages were 'exposed to the trade breeze', and not far from the sea. They were not marshy or swampy. They had no previous history of deadly fever. The inhabitants 'cultivate a little corn, beans, and other vegetables; fish; and occasionally work as labourers in the ships at Porto Sal Rey'.

The first case of fever did not come from those labourers, however, but instead from a young girl, daughter of a local ship captain, who had been living in the house of one of Porto Sal Rey's fever victims. Her mother and sisters took care of her, and were themselves attacked by fever. They recovered, but the fever spread throughout the village, with at least four fatalities. João Gallego was, McWilliam wrote, 'in a state of perfect health on the 1st of November, when Pedro Moraes and Ignacio da Cruz Silva, soldiers, came from the barracks in Porto Sal Rey, where the fever was raging, to the houses of their relations'. Once again, the disease spread outward, first to their families and then to their neighbours. From there, 'the disease seemed to radiate in all directions through the town'. At least the village was the last place to fall victim to fever. By the end of April, the outbreak had subsided; no new cases were reported.[30]

The British professional press was delighted with McWilliam's *Report*. Its logic was impeccable, noted a reviewer, for it showed how 'every village, then, gradually receives the disease, and in every instance its introduction is traced to an individual, and its propagation from this individual as a centre'.[31] It is possible that McWilliam himself did not see this as switching sides in the professional dispute over quarantine, but rather as continuing the research begun in his *Expedition to the Niger*. He placed at the top of his list of 'main conclusions' that 'the fever on board the "Eclair" was primarily the remittent of the African coast, which is not a contagious disorder'. It clearly could not be yellow fever, as Pym had claimed; indeed, he criticised Pym's subsequent handling of the quarantine when the *Éclair* arrived in British waters.[32] It is even possible to read his entire line of investigation, as well as his conclusions, as placing the blame squarely on decisions taken by local authorities, rather than on the Royal Navy.

But if McWilliam's goal was to please Burnett, he did not succeed. In transmitting the report to the Secretary of the Admiralty, Burnett wrote that 'Dr McWilliam appears to have taken considerable pains to gain information; but after a careful perusal of the papers he has sent I am compelled to say that I cannot conscientiously arrive at the conclusion the Doctor has done, viz., "That the fever was occasioned by the intercourse with the 'Eclair'"'.[33] And while modern readers may praise McWilliam's careful questioning of Boa Vista washerwomen, soldiers and labourers for making visible the local experience of quarantine often obscured by official medical reports, Harrison has noted that British opponents of quarantine condemned him for relying on testimony of the 'lower orders of society'.[34]

Both *The Report of the Fever at Boa Vista* and the Navy's response made McWilliam a hero to his civilian medical audience, and they were very clear why: it was precisely because he had crossed the boundaries that others were so concerned to police. 'Commencing his inquiry into the fever at Boa Vista, Dr McWilliam did not let his prepossessions [from his previous voyage] to bias his inquiry'; wrote one reviewer. On the contrary, 'confident that Truth was the goal, no matter in what region she might dwell, he has given the undistorted results of a most laborious and difficult inquiry. We can give him no greater praise.'[35] In praising McWilliam's undistorted pursuit of 'Truth', the *Journal* was praising its own truth and rigour as well. But the reviewer is making an additional rhetorical point: while it might be the province of on-the-spot observers like McWilliam to travel to far-off regions and collect information, it was the province of the professional press to sift the evidence and choose the victor in all disputes. And it implied dangerous epidemics were things that arose in other parts of the world, somewhere out in the Empire or on the high seas, articulating an insular sense of medical geography that would continue to inform both the professional and popular press.

Conclusion

This chapter has argued that the lived professional experience of British medical practitioners was a crucial component of mid-century quarantine debates. British navy surgeons, responsible for the healthcare of their ships, regarded them as 'floating villages', and followed best practices for sanitary reform. This was particularly noteworthy in the new, up-to-date steam vessels, like the *Albert*. Fitted with every modern convenience for fresh air and clean water, the ships were as 'sweet' as scientific practices could make them. They simply could not be vectors of infection, insisted Navy medical staff, even as their own numbers were decimated by disease.

Medical practitioners with primarily land-based experience saw those same ships through a different lens. A ship appeared in a harbour, and disease spread on land, in clusters that followed the movements of sick people. Quarantine practices that had developed over hundreds of years of sail-based travel in the Mediterranean could prevent isolated outbreaks from spreading, but only if they could be applied under the vastly different conditions of global steam-based trade routes. When those practices proved inadequate, British medical professionals came into conflict on quarantine practices, calling into question the very nature of a single, unified, medical profession.

We can pursue the ongoing impact of those conflicts in the professional history of the best-documented of our protagonists, James Ormiston McWilliam. After the *Éclair* affair, he left the Royal Navy and became medical officer of the Custom House, where his views on the communicability of disease from ships to shore were a better fit for his position. He also became the perpetual secretary of the new London Epidemiological Society, where he joined professional colleagues like John Snow in mapping epidemics throughout Great Britain and around the globe. The Epidemiological Society included professional men from all sides of the quarantine controversy – and we know they are 'professional' men, because they allowed no hint of any disagreements to infiltrate the medical journals. Indeed, the officers of the new society were at pains to correct the public's impression that there were disagreements among the universal medical profession for which they advocated. 'That there are conflicting views upon some points, and especially on the subject of contagion, is fully admitted' one of the early presidents wrote, 'but it deeply concerns the public welfare that it should be well understood, that all practitioners are completely in accord ... as to practical measures' such as sanitation and hygiene. There were only a 'few' exceptions, he concluded, 'for the most part relating to international communication' of diseases.[36] The boundary dispute over quarantine, in other words, was far from over.

Notes

1 Mark Harrison, *Contagion: How Commerce Has Spread Disease*, New Haven, Yale University Press, 2012, 106.
2 Mark Harrison, 'A global perspective: reframing the history of health, medicine, and disease', *Bulletin of the History of Medicine* 89, 2015, 651.
3 See the discussion of Harrison's 'A global perspective' by Alison Bashford, 'Bioscapes: gendering the global history of medicine', J.R. McNeil, 'Harrison, globalization, and the history of health, medicine, and disease', and Kavia Sivramakrishnan, 'Global histories of health, disease, and medicine from a "zig-zag" perspective', *Bulletin of the History of Medicine* 89, 2015, 690–704.
4 Cited in Harrison, *Contagion*, 81.
5 There is a substantial scholarly literature on nineteenth-century theories of contagionism. For a summary view of the older literature, see Edwin Ackerknecht, 'Anticontagionism between 1821 and 1867', *Bulletin of the History of Medicine* 22, 1948, 562–593. Recent studies that put contemporary debates in a broader cultural context are Thomas Appel, *Feverish Bodies, Enlightened Minds: Science and the Yellow Fever Controversy in the Early American Republic*, Palo Alto, Stanford University Press, 2016; Peter Baldwin, *Contagion and the State in Europe, 1830–1930*, Cambridge, Cambridge University Press, 2005.
6 'Review of Observations upon Bulam Fever ... by Sir William Pym', *Edinburgh Medical and Surgical Review* 71, 1849, 482–485.
7 *The case of the Medical Officers of the Army fairly stated, in a letter to the Right Hon. Earl de Grey and Ripon*, London, Charles Griffin and Company, 1864.
8 Williamson, James, *Packet Surgeon's Journals*, National Maritime Museum of Cornwall, www.nmmc.co.uk/index.php?/packet_surgeons_journals/ (accessed 2 May 2016).
9 James Ormiston McWilliam, *Medical History of the Expedition to the Niger*, London, John Churchill, 1843, 183.
10 See Rod Edmond, *Leprosy and Empire. A Medical and Cultural History*, Cambridge, Cambridge University Press, 2006, 61–109; Gavin Milroy, *Report on Leprosy and Yaws in the West Indies*, London, Clowes, 1873.
11 The National Archives, *Records of the Admiralty*, ADM 196/8/219.
12 McWilliam, *Medical History of the Expedition to the Niger*, 181.
13 James Ormiston McWilliam, *Report of the Fever at Boa Vista*, London, Presented to the House of Commons, 1847, 111.

14 Ibid., 78.
15 Ibid., 78–79.
16 Ibid., 13–18.
17 Ibid., 82.
18 Ibid., 81.
19 Ibid., 83–84.
20 Ibid., 85.
21 Ibid., 24.
22 Ibid., 85.
23 Ibid., 24.
24 Ibid., 85.
25 Ibid., 24.
26 Ibid., 86.
27 Ibid., 84.
28 Ibid., 86–87.
29 Ibid., 88–91.
30 Ibid., 92–93.
31 'On the Contagion of Yellow Fever', *British and Foreign Medical and Chirurgical Review* 1, 1848, 60.
32 McWilliam, *Report of the Fever at Boa Vista,* 111.
33 Cited in McWilliam, *Report of the Fever at Boa Vista,* 3.
34 Harrison, *Contagion,* 100.
35 'On the Fever of Boa Vista in 1845', *British and Foreign Medical and Chirurgical Review* 2, 1848, 171.
36 Benjamin Guy Babington, 'Presidential Address', *Transactions of the Epidemiological Society* 1, 1860, 5.

6

Prevention and stigma: the sanitary control of Muslim pilgrims from the Balkans, 1830–1914

Christian Promitzer

Introduction

The fight against plague and cholera allegedly or actually communicated by Muslim pilgrims from India and Southeast Asia while on the *Hajj* (pilgrimage to Mecca) has been the object of sustained research in the field of medical history. A recent contribution, Stefan Winkle's book *Cultural History of Epidemics*, explains how intensified maritime traffic over the course of the nineteenth century made the region of the Hejaz on the Western coast of the Arabian Peninsula a hotspot for the outward diffusion of cholera. This region – which is now part of Saudi Arabia – belonged to the Ottoman Empire until the end of the First World War and comprised the central sites of Muslim pilgrimage: Mecca and Medina. In parallel, when cholera was identified as a water-borne disease, the holy Zamzam well in Mecca was considered a major source of contagion as thousands of pilgrims immersed their burial gowns in the open water, drank from it and filled small bottles to take it back to their relatives, friends and the sick in their native lands.[1]

In his authoritative work on the influence of contagious diseases on the public health policies of the major European powers, Peter Baldwin identifies the fourth cholera pandemic as the decisive moment when attention was focused on the Ottoman Empire and Muslim pilgrims as possible vectors for the spread of the disease. Baldwin pointed out that in 1865 pilgrims from Java and Bengal communicated cholera to fellow Muslims from other countries on their arrival to Mecca. From

Hejaz the epidemic spread via Suez to Egypt, and from the port of Alexandria throughout the Mediterranean. Within weeks, the whole of Europe was infected. An ISC – the third after those held in Paris in 1851 and 1859 – was convened in Constantinople the following year. During this international conference, the representatives of the main European powers asked the Ottoman Porte and Egypt to implement severe measures of control and quarantine upon the Muslim pilgrims coming from and going through their territories.[2]

The first time that cholera made its way from India and modern-day Iraq to Mecca had been in 1831, during the second pandemic, killing around 3,000 pilgrims.[3] In 1846, cholera, again from the Indian subcontinent, reached Mecca for the second time, claiming nearly 15,000 victims, the majority of whom were pilgrims.[4] However, in marked contrast to the subsequent pandemic of 1865, the geographic reach of the epidemics of 1831 and 1846 passing through Mecca was limited to the Near East and Northern Africa. To be sure, on those occasions the European continent was not left unaffected, but the disease would actually arrive via Russia. This means that from the European point of view, until 1865, Mecca was only a secondary route in the transmission and spread of cholera.

In 1883, the *Hajj* found itself again in the midst of the international struggle against cholera. In that year, pilgrims returning from Mecca triggered a severe epidemic outbreak in Egypt that would cost the lives of more than 50,000 people. The European public became highly concerned, since this was the first outbreak in the region after the opening of the Suez Canal in 1869. Some contemporaries accused British ships carrying the Egyptian pilgrims of having brought the disease on board on their return from India. In any case, the hospitals of Alexandria saw the activities of various national teams of medical doctors sent from Europe that wanted to detect the causal germ of cholera. As is well known, the German bacteriologist Robert Koch would seize the prize.[5] From that moment until the First World War, Egypt and the Ottoman Empire would be subject to stronger surveillance by the 'European Concert' with respect to their actual commitment to exert various forms of sanitary control and quarantine measures upon Muslim pilgrims based upon the new scientific findings provided by bacteriology.[6]

In my opinion, the fact that most of the existing historiography on the relation between the Muslim pilgrimage and cholera concentrates on Western Europe, the Middle East and British India is responsible for a most interesting part of the story remaining completely ignored. I am referring to the question of Balkan Muslims, and also in part to the role of the Habsburg Empire (Austria-Hungary), in the control of the *Hajj* from 1867. With regard to the question of Muslims in the Balkans, which – apart from those in the Caucasus – were and still are the only autochthonous Muslim population in Europe, it is surprising that no relevant study has yet been conducted on their *hajjis*. As late as the Congress of Berlin of 1878 that put an end to the Russo-Turkish War, estimates pointed to more than 4 million Muslims living in the European provinces of the Ottoman Empire, which meant circa 35% of the total Balkan population. After the war, 'Turkey-in-Europe', i.e. the Ottoman possessions in the Balkans, would be reduced to Albania, Kosovo, Macedonia and Thrace. As a result, in 1878, half a million Slav Muslims living in Bosnia-Herzegovina would fall under Austro-Hungarian administration and later, in 1908, came to be integrated into the Dual Monarchy. The autonomous principality of Bulgaria (which in 1908 became an independent monarchy) was also home to a considerable number of Muslims of Slavic, Turkic and Roma descent. Finally, small Muslim minorities lived in the independent states of Montenegro and Romania.[7]

With regard to the role played by Austria-Hungary, it is evident that it was already losing its status as a Great Power in a process accelerated by the military defeat against Prussia in 1866 in the struggle for preponderance in the German Bund. In spite of this, the Habsburg Monarchy remained – in competition with Russia – a potent actor in southeastern Europe that still managed to exert some significant influence in the affairs of the Ottoman Empire. Taking into account this double background, this chapter will begin by addressing the general circumstances surrounding the annual displacement of Muslim pilgrims from the Balkans to Mecca from 1878 until the Balkan Wars of 1912–13. This will be followed by an examination of the methods of disinfection and quarantine that Balkan *hajjis* had to undergo on their return home. Focus will be on the cases of Bosnia-Herzegovina and Bulgaria, taking into account the fact that the latter country had to deal not only with its own Muslim pilgrims but with Serbian and Bosnian *hajjis* passing through its territory (preferring the use of the railway to navigation).

Muslim pilgrims from the Balkans and the establishment of Ottoman quarantines (1830–78)

Throughout the nineteenth century, male Muslims from the Balkans participated in the pilgrimages to the holy places of Islam on the Arabian Peninsula. Since the mid 1830s travellers from the Eastern Balkans – Bulgaria – could use steamships that were routinely plying the lower course of the Danube and the Black Sea in order to get to Constantinople. From this port, they could connect to international travel routes. With regard to pilgrims from the Central Balkans – Kosovo, Macedonia and Western Thrace – they would embark at the port of Salonika for Alexandria. Their fellow pilgrims from the Western Balkans – namely those from Bosnia-Herzegovina, Montenegro and Albania – relied on the vessels provided by the 'Austrian Loyd' steamship company. The latter would leave from the ports of the Eastern Adriatic coast – with Trieste as the main point of departure – and arrive either in Beirut or in Alexandria, from where the difficult land route had to be taken on camel caravans. This information, the only such available on the transport of Balkan *hajjis,* has been taken from an 1868 article on the global itineraries of Muslim pilgrims written by the Austrian doctor Jacob Eduard Polak (1820–91). Polak, who in the 1850s became court physician to the ruler of Persia Naser-al-Din Shah, wrote this work – whose main subject was the role of pilgrims in the spread of cholera – in his capacity as Austrian delegate to the third ISC held in Constantinople.[8] By contrast, Ottoman sanitary records, including those preserved in the archives, as well as the unpublished records of foreign consular offices in the Balkans, remain largely unexamined by historians.

Since the late 1830s, the Ottoman Empire had established sanitary offices in all of its districts. Maritime and terrestrial quarantines were enforced in the event of plague and cholera outbreaks. Actually, an epidemic of plague, which struck both Constantinople and the European part of the empire in 1836 and the following years, was the *raison d'etre* for this innovation, putting an end to the traditional religious opposition to such public health measures. Despite this, the Muslim population – like that of European countries one or two centuries before – had to undergo what Martin Dinges has called 'a learning process' before accepting that the imposition of quarantine was meant to protect them from epidemic diseases.[9] Still, 500 Muslim women protested against the introduction of quarantine in the Bulgarian port of Varna in 1840 and threatened the life of the newly installed director of the local sanitary office.[10] It is worth noting that with the imposition of quarantines, the plague retreated from the European part of the Ottoman Empire for good. Apart from internal repercussions, the implementation of quarantines in the Ottoman Empire was also of international significance. Thus, a high Ottoman official duly presided over the Supreme International Sanitary Board in Constantinople, but most of the members of this body were diplomatic representatives of the European great powers and medical doctors from these same countries.[11] This reflected how Western medicine had infiltrated the vast field of healthcare in the Ottoman Empire, while the recently founded Imperial Medical School still needed some time to produce native doctors of relevance.[12]

The geo-epidemiological meaning of quarantines in the Ottoman Empire seems evident: due to the intensification of international trade the European powers had a vital interest in reducing maritime quarantine in their own ports and for their ships abroad and for this they needed the Ottomans to develop a reliable sanitary administration. These were the same reasons why pruned – 'contingent' or otherwise attenuated – variants of contagionism or even the outright anticontagionist miasma theory, particularly in Britain, became popular over a timespan which the renowned medical historian Erwin Ackerknecht assessed between 1821 and 1867.[13] But this was also the period when quarantines – for the adherents of traditional contagionism the ideal instrument to prevent plague and cholera – were introduced in the Ottoman Empire. With regard to plague and cholera, the Ottoman Empire was considered a major threat to the Christian part of Europe, and for reasons of self-defence the concepts of attenuated contagionism and miasma theory had to end at the ports and borders of the Western European powers. European observers consequently held the view that quarantines in the Ottoman Empire – a country they perceived as lagging well behind the standards of Western civilisation and hygiene – would be of great use because of their protective character for the emerging capitalist economies of the European continent.[14] Therefore, the anti-miasmatic turn ascribed to the 1866 ISC in Constantinople, when the delegates of the European Great Powers reconsidered quarantines, was not perceived as such by the representatives of the Ottoman Empire. For them, it rather meant that the pressures imposed on them since the 1830s were only being intensified. At that juncture they realised that the issue of Muslim pilgrims was no longer an internal affair but also an international matter and that the West – at least in part – asked for its share in controlling the itineraries of the *hajjis* in the Red Sea and Egypt, which was formally subject to the Ottoman sultan, but in practice increasingly under French and British influence.[15]

In this emerging scenario of imperialism and epidemic threat, the scarce and casual information on the autochthonous Muslims in the Balkans throughout the entire period is puzzling – though analogous to other peripheral Islamic localities such as Morocco, as Francisco Javier Martínez has shown in Chapter 3. Balkan Muslims played a negligible role in the proceedings of the International Sanitary Conferences, although this group, of all possible vectors of cholera, was the one positioned geographically closest to the heart of the Danube monarchy, and thereby of Europe. The alleged responsibility of Muslim pilgrims for the spread of cholera to the Mediterranean and Western Europe, brought forward by the European delegates at the Constantinople Conference, did not take those pilgrims into consideration. In other words: a new international sanitary policy which increased pressure on the Ottoman Empire by associating the threat of cholera with a religious ritual – the Muslim pilgrimage to Mecca – was put in place in 1866, and a culprit – the *hajjis* – was found, but, curiously enough, at the same time, this scheme was not applied to the local framework of the Ottoman Balkans, the closest Ottoman possessions to Europe. The fact that this negligence was not followed by any harmful effects over the subsequent years, reveals, at least in part, that the new sanitary policy did not only rest on scientific, but also on ideological, pillars, the latter undoubtedly targeting the unhygienic consequences attributed to Muslim religious practices and these in turn being used as a justification for keeping the *hajjis* under surveillance.

In any case, the *hajjis* travelling from the Balkans did not play an essential role in Western policies of prevention up to the late 1870s. Neither did they in Ottoman public health. The network of Ottoman sanitary offices, responsible for quarantines and control of maritime traffic, actually left large spaces uncovered. The few medical doctors in the Ottoman Empire were concentrated in the larger cities or were field surgeons serving in the army who did not visit the villages where the bulk of the Balkan Muslim population lived. Both the rural town and village Muslim populations in the region relied on folk healers, the so-called *hekimins*. Only the elites of Balkan Muslim society (mostly the governors of the provinces) had modern physicians at their personal service. These additional factors further explain the scarcity of information on the medical control of Muslim pilgrims from the Balkans. In the end, medical control of pilgrims, no matter what part of the Arab-Islamic world they came from, seemed to be limited to the Hejaz itself and to a handful of large Egyptian and Ottoman ports.

However, both the political situation in southeast Europe and the international sanitary policies addressing Muslim pilgrims would change by the end of the 1870s. With regard to the former, armed insurrections of the Christian population of the Balkans against Ottoman rule, a local war of the vassal states Serbia and Montenegro against the sultan and, finally, the Russo-Ottoman War of 1877–78 resulted in a tremendous defeat for the Ottoman Empire which drastically reduced its European provinces. In June 1878, the new political and territorial reordering of the Balkans was sanctioned by the European great powers at the Congress of Berlin stipulating the independence of Romania, Serbia and Montenegro from the Ottoman Empire, heralding the foundation of an autonomous Bulgarian principality, and the transfer of the administration of the province of Bosnia-Herzegovina from the Ottoman Empire to Austria-Hungary (Figure 6.1). Consequently, the local Muslim populations were bereft of their religious and secular ruler, which for centuries had protected and encouraged their existence in the European provinces of the Ottoman Empire. Change was particularly felt in the case of Bosnia-Herzegovina and Bulgaria, both home to considerable Muslim populations. In Bosnia, the new imperial Austro-Hungarian administration sought to patronise its Muslim subjects and to minimise the influence of the Ottoman Empire, with the sultan still formally the head of this province. In autonomous Bulgaria, which nevertheless remained an Ottoman vassal state, a more robust policy vis-à-vis Muslims was pursued instead.

Meanwhile, throughout this time and the following decades, international sanitary policies were evolving. After the 1866 conference in Constantinople, and in particular following the cholera epidemic of 1881–82 in Arabia and Hejaz, Muslim pilgrims passing the Egyptian port of Alexandria, the Suez Canal and/or the Red Sea would increasingly come under international sanitary control. The quarantine

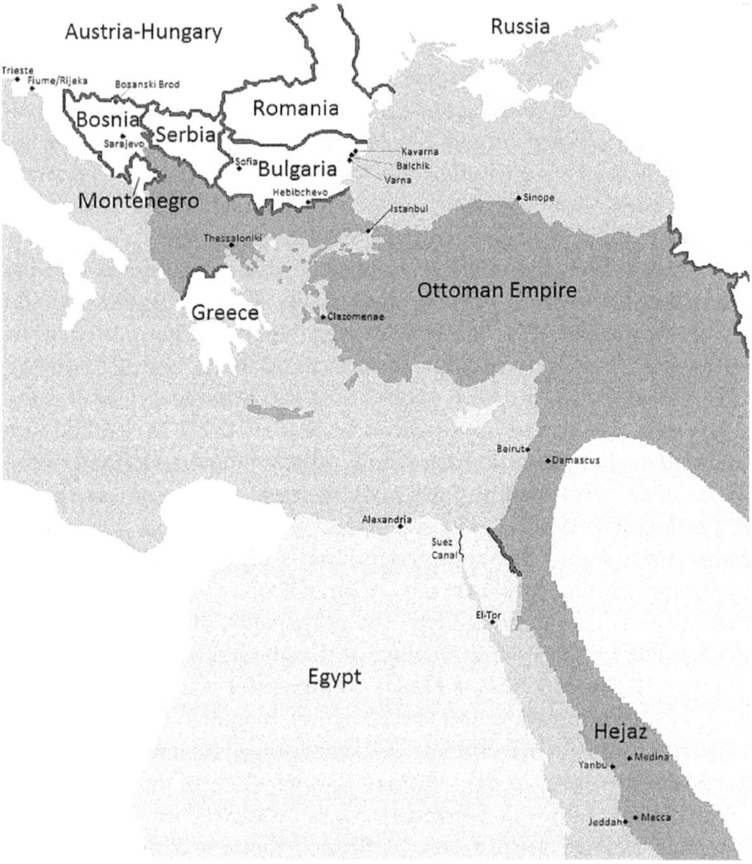

Figure 6.1 The Balkans and the Near East at the turn of the twentieth century.

stations of El Tor and Alexandria became the most important checkpoints for Ottoman and North African pilgrims. After a renewed outbreak of cholera in the Hejaz in 1890, European governments perceived the *hajjis* as an ever-greater threat to their countries. At the ISCs of Venice in 1892, Dresden in 1893, Paris in 1894 and Venice again in 1897, the 'Concert of Europe' agreed on a package of anti-epidemic measures (medical inspection, disinfection, quarantine, treatment of the diseased and deceased) to be applied to the *hajjis*.[16] The European powers dispatched permanent sanitary delegates to the Red Sea port of Jeddah, on the Hejaz coast, which was the principal gateway for pilgrims. On their return trip, the usual treatment for Ottoman and North African pilgrims in 1902 foresaw fifteen days of quarantine in El Tor under supervision of the Egyptian sanitary authorities, and thereafter five additional days of quarantine under Ottoman supervision – either in Beirut, in Lebanese Tripoli or in Clazomenae on the western coast of Anatolia. Those who did not return by sea, but joined the Holy Caravan on its way back through the Syrian Desert, had to undergo quarantine before passing the gates of Damascus.[17] But this was not the entire story. Returning Balkan pilgrims could expect further sanitary treatment in Bulgaria, Serbia and Bosnia itself, depending on where they came from and which itineraries they chose – whether travelling by train through the Balkan states or by ship to Trieste or Fiume/Rijeka for the Bosnian pilgrims or by ship to the Black Sea port of Varna for the Bulgarian *hajjis*. We will now proceed to examine in some detail the local measures applied to Muslim pilgrims departing from or returning to Bosnia-Herzegovina and Bulgaria.

The control of the Muslim pilgrimage from Bosnia-Herzegovina since 1878

Thanks to a short but remarkable article written by two Bosnian authors, Sreten Bošković and Ajša Smailbegović, we have precise information about the Muslim pilgrims from Bosnia during the period under study.[18] Their annual number was officially between 50 and 130 persons who, by and large, opted for the railway overland route to Constantinople with only a small fraction taking the ships of the Austrian Lloyd at Trieste or Fiume. The Austro-Hungarian authorities were rather concerned about the possibility of Arab agitators coming to Bosnia for encouraging participation in the *Hajj*, or returning Bosnian *hajjis* importing plague or cholera. Over the course of the fifth cholera pandemic, which hit the Arabian Peninsula and Mecca in 1881–82, the Bosnian local government resolved that Bosnian Muslims should only leave for the *Hajj* with special passports and only in groups. Beginning in 1890, the local government designated a formal leader (*Reis-ul Hudžadž*) for every pilgrim party. This leader would be an authoritative person with good knowledge of the religious rituals, able to supervise the health of the pilgrims and, on their return, to report on the health risks that they had encountered. In the same year, the Austro-Hungarian authorities signed an agreement with the Austrian Lloyd regarding the transport of Bosnian *hajjis* to the Hejaz.[19]

Bošković and Smailbegović have calculated that the average death rate among Bosnian *hajjis* in the last two decades of the nineteenth century ranged between 30 and 40%. They point out, however, that cholera was not the only cause of death while travelling. Many pilgrims were middle-aged or older and suffered from previous chronic or geriatric diseases and simply succumbed during the troublesome passage on ships and the aforementioned inhospitable caravans through the Arabian desert. Dysentery (the so-called *hajjis'* diarrhoea) and heat stroke also claimed their share. Naturally, such diseases made the older pilgrims more susceptible to attacks of cholera.[20] In 1890, out of 104 Bosnian *hajjis* only 63 would return to their home country. That time it was definitely the cholera epidemic in the Hejaz region which was responsible for the loss of life. Egyptian (i.e. British) medical authorities were on high alert. On their return, aboard an Austrian Lloyd vessel, the *hajjis* had to stop at the quarantine camp on the Sinai Peninsula in El Tor. They were medically inspected, their luggage was disinfected and they had to stay in quarantine for twenty days. On their way through the Suez Canal their ship was not allowed to come ashore at any Egyptian port. Because some of the *hajjis* were from Anatolia, the ship disembarked in Smyrna. There – on order of the International Sanitary Board of Constantinople – the Bosnian *hajjis* again had to undergo medical inspection and their luggage was disinfected once more. From Smyrna the ship took its passage to the Austrian port of Trieste. In the Hospital of St Bartholomew the *hajjis* were again, for the third time, put under quarantine – this time the procedure would last seven days. Over this entire trip starting from the Arabian port of Jeddah, about twenty-eight pilgrims died.[21]

The following year, cholera was again rampant in the Hejaz. This time the Bosnian Government sent a doctor to escort the pilgrims on their return from Jeddah. Unfortunately, Dr Julije Macanec succumbed to typhus upon his arrival there, so the Bosnian authorities had to dispatch another physician, Justin Karlinski, the district doctor from Konjic, a town located 50 km southwest of Sarajevo. In total, there were thirty-six fatalities among the Bosnian *hajjis* in 1891, which accounted for a mortality rate of 35.3%.[22] From that moment, the Bosnian Government would always dispatch a medical doctor with the departing *hajjis*. In 1892, the mortality rate sank to 'only' 9.5%, but it jolted up to 49% the following year, when a new wave of cholera reached the Hejaz region. In 1894, the death rate again decreased to 13.2%, and in 1895 – due to a new invasion in the Hejaz – it again reached 35.5%. In 1896, a massive cholera epidemic that was raging in Egypt led the Bosnian Government and the international sanitary authorities to dissuade prospective pilgrims from the journey. Among the few people who nonetheless went on the *Hajj* (seventy-four men) the mortality rate was relatively low (16.2%); the reason for this being that the Hejaz region was not affected by the Egyptian outbreak.[23]

To make matters worse, 1897 saw the third pandemic of bubonic plague spreading out from India – where it had arrived from its original 1893 foci in China. Fears arose that the plague would be communicated to Europe via the returning *hajjis*. Consequently, the ISC held that year in Venice passed several regulations which foresaw intensified anti-epidemic measures at the quarantine stations of El Tor, Beirut and Clazomenae. Like France and Russia did with their colonial and state Muslim populations respectively, the Bosnian Government forbade its citizens to go on the *Hajj*. This resolution was also supported by the local Muslim authorities but, as a matter of fact, several hundred males who realised that it was impossible to obtain the special '*Hajj* passports', went to other countries and took Ottoman passports before travelling on to Mecca. More than 500 people evaded control in this manner. The Bosnian Government threatened them with prohibiting their return home and burning their personal belongings should plague be discovered. However, the Austro-Hungarian authorities finally complied with the wish of the pilgrims and sent a doctor to join the travellers who had left the country without formal organisation. Since there were cases of plague in the Hejaz, these pilgrims had to undergo twenty-one days of quarantine in Constantinople upon their return and suffer several hardships by the national sanitary authorities of Bulgaria and Serbia when they took the overland route home. Despite such dangerous circumstances, the mortality rate was only about 7%.[24]

In 1898 and 1899, the epidemiological situation in the Hejaz region was still considered to be dangerous. In compliance with international regulations, the Bosnian Government forbade the *Hajj* once again, but eventually had to give in, and even organised group travels with a leader and medical doctor.[25] During the spring of 1898, many pilgrims had again made their way to the Hejaz outside of the officially organised travel group, forcing the Bosnian authorities to warn the neighbouring provinces of the Habsburg Empire – Croatia and Dalmatia – not to allow the passage of returning Muslim pilgrims through their territories so long as they were not in possession of official documents issued by the Bosnian provincial government. In the event of infection, they had to undergo a quarantine of seven days with their luggage and clothing being disinfected.[26] The same harsh measures were repeated in 1899.[27] In 1900, the situation in Hejaz improved, such that the official restriction of the *Hajj* could be suspended. The mortality rate among Bosnian *hajjis* sank to about 2%.[28] The following year sanitary facilities and protective measures along the Bosnian border underwent a revision owing to the large number of returning *hajjis*. In the town of Bosanski Brod, located on the northern frontier, where the *hajjis* who had taken the overland route from Constantinople arrived, a new quarantine station was erected. In addition to a medical inspection and the disinfection of the pilgrims and their luggage, the head physician also carried out bacteriological tests. After their return home, the pilgrims were kept under observation for at least ten days. The only other option for *hajjis* re-entering the territory legally (and in possession of a special permit) from Ottoman territory was through the Montenegro–Bosnia border crossing of Metaljka, but here too they had to undergo the same treatment as in Bosanski Brod.[29] Additionally, Arabian agitators for the *Hajj* were placed under severe sanitary control, as were those *hajjis* who had not travelled with the official tour groups.[30]

The regulation of 1901 was still in force in 1910. However, after the opening of the Hejaz railway from Medina to Damascus in 1908, many pilgrims chose to return in small groups or even individually by train instead of joining the common group of the *Reis-ul Hudžadž* and contending with the quarantine of El Tor. Austro-Hungarian experts on the region – geographers and diplomats – considered the Hejaz railway a possible sanitary threat, since pilgrims who used it could easily evade Ottoman quarantines.[31] In the interim, Russia had joined India as a second permanent centre of cholera, a significant circumstance since the recently completed Trans-Caspian railway could transport pilgrims from Central Asia and China to the Black Sea within five to six days. Already, in 1908, pilgrims from the Caucasus had introduced cholera to the holy sites of Islam, and two years later Russian steamboats transported diseased pilgrims who had caught the epidemic in Sinope (on the Anatolian shore of the Black Sea).[32] In the aftermath, Bosnian sanitary authorities instructed the border guards of the province to make sure that all returning *hajjis* produced a certificate that they had undergone sanitary treatment in Bosanski Brod, in default of which they were not permitted entry and had to be immediately sent to the quarantine station of this town.[33] This was only the final wall of protection. At the twelfth ISC of Paris in early 1912 the Austro-Hungarian delegate – who had been medical chief of the provincial government of Bosnia-Herzegovina since 1901 – praised the efforts to put either the passengers of pilgrim ships arriving from the north (i.e. from Russia) under quarantine in El Tor or to erect a separate new quarantine station for them along the northern coast of the Red Sea, as the Ottoman sanitary authorities had promised to do.[34] In actuality, the Balkan Wars and the ensuing outbreak of the First World War ultimately prevented any such plans from being implemented.

Bulgaria and the issue of Muslim pilgrims

The Muslim population remaining in Bulgaria – those who had not taken flight during the Russo-Turkish War of 1877–78 or subsequently immigrated to the Ottoman Empire – consisted predominantly of Turks. They were met with reserve, and in Bulgarian eyes they bore the stigma of being part of the increasingly odious Ottoman legacy. With regard to the *Hajj*, apart from these native Muslim Turks, the Bulgarian authorities also had to deal with Bosnian Muslims who took the transit route from Constantinople to Bosnia on the transversal Balkan railway completed by the early 1880s – which later became famous as part of the so-called 'Orient Express'. We should add that until 1908 Bulgaria remained a tributary state of the Ottoman Empire and that as a consequence the system of quarantines operated according to Ottoman regulations. Hence, the Supreme International Sanitary Board of Constantinople could theoretically outline the quarantine policies of the Bulgarian principality. Nevertheless, this prerogative left ample room for its Bulgarian interpreters, leading to permanent conflicts between the sanitary institutions of the Ottoman Empire and Bulgaria. The first incident occurred in late March 1882 when the Bulgarian authorities of the port of Varna detected several cases of cholera among the disembarked pilgrims who were returning from the *Hajj*. They ordered that a military cordon encompass the lazaretto of Varna, but the International Sanitary Board of Constantinople denied the occurrence of cholera, while further contradictory news about the incident was received. In order to assess the state of affairs, the representatives of the European powers dispatched a medical commission to Varna.[35] By early May it was an official fact that twelve pilgrims on board the steamer *Aurora* which had arrived from Constantinople had been struck by cholera, five of them subsequently succumbing to the disease. The chief physician of Sofia, the Bulgarian capital, who had also declared that the epidemic was Asian cholera, ordered the luggage of pilgrims (which allegedly spread loathsome odours) to be burnt. The authorities prohibited Muslims who returned from the Hejaz from entering Bulgaria by land. All pilgrims arriving by sea had to undergo a fortnight of quarantine in the lazaretto of Varna as well as in those of the nearby ports of Balchik and Kavarna.[36]

This initial episode would have longlasting and severe consequences for the further treatment of Muslim pilgrims in Bulgaria. From here on the Bulgarian sanitary authorities would resort on several occasions to intensive radical disinfection measures and, with respect to pilgrims entering the country by land, to excessive use of terrestrial quarantines. The latter measure would receive public criticism during the eighth ISC of 1893 in Dresden, which formalised the system of medical inspection that Peter Baldwin has called neoquarantinist. According to this system, the achievements of bacteriology would allow replacement of quarantine measures with regular medical inspection of suspect persons at their homes.[37] However, such a procedure was not perceived as adequate by 'Oriental' countries, where quarantine measures against Muslim pilgrims had been intensified. Baldwin argues on good grounds that:

> the attempt to loosen quarantinist measures in the West, to shift from old-fashioned precautions to the revision system and more generally to neoquarantinism, depended in large part on Europe's ability to impose more drastic regulations on the Orient than it was – increasingly – willing to tolerate at home.[38]

There was no Bulgarian delegate present at the Dresden conference, but the ample use of terrestrial quarantines by Bulgaria was for the first time criticised by the Romanian delegate in that meeting. His objection was not made out of sympathy with the fate of Muslim pilgrims, however, but rather owed to demands for freer traffic and navigation along the Danube, which were being hampered by Bulgarian quarantines.[39] The Serbian delegate paid lip service to the general condemnation of terrestrial quarantines. He reminded the conference delegates that both Turkey and Bulgaria maintained an excessive system of quarantines. Therefore, as long as its two nearest neighbours did not change their strategy, Serbia felt likewise compelled to retain terrestrial quarantines.[40] This conduct may have arisen from the fact that the Muslim pilgrims from Bosnia had to cross Serbia on their way back home.

One year later, the Austro-Hungarian delegate at the first ISC in Paris mentioned the hardships of the Bosnian pilgrims on their return through the Balkans. In 1893, with cholera raging in the Hejaz region, they had become victims of harsh treatment from the Bulgarian and Serbian authorities. Quarantines in these two countries – certainly not the first ones endured by the *hajjis* on their long way back home – lasted about five and three days respectively. Although not lengthy, the fact that accommodation of the pilgrims during these interludes was not provided for, together with disinfection measures allegedly involving the dousing of travellers in acrid phenol, made the experience quite trying.[41] With that denunciation Austria-Hungary wanted to trigger Bulgaria's and Serbia's compliance with Western countries in a shared refusal of quarantinist measures in their territories, since Muslim pilgrims were previously subjected to them in El Tor, Alexandria, Beirut and Smyrna. In the Austro-Hungarian conception of geo-epidemiology, Serbia and Bulgaria were therefore expected to comply with the West and to renounce harsh preventive measures which fettered them to 'the Orient', because in terms of hygienic standards they were considered as states which had already passed the test of being part of 'the Occident'. Ironically, it was the Austrian rejection of Muslims as reminders of a painful and despised Ottoman past that induced those two countries to continue with old-fashioned quarantinism.

The official Bulgarian point of view would be finally presented at the tenth ISC in Venice in 1897, when the issue of plague entered the agenda. For the first time a Bulgarian delegate, the medical doctor

Marin Rusev (1864–1935), one of the most avid promoters of public health in that country, was appointed. Rusev made clear that his position with respect to the maintenance of terrestrial quarantines by his country was not up for negotiation, and this applied particularly to Muslim pilgrims for whom the revision system – medical inspection of suspect persons at their places of residence – was impracticable:

> We have 800,000 Muslims among us, many of whom will make the pilgrimage each year. Pilgrims from Bulgaria, like those of European Turkey, usually arrive at Jeddah, the port of Mecca, and in this port and on their way to Mecca they meet pilgrims from Bombay, i.e. from the contaminated regions. In this way, they can bring us the plague, as they did more than once with regard to other diseases, such as cholera. And I must add that in our country the Muslims live in villages far from the doctors who could monitor their health after their return from Mecca.[42]

Rusev declared that his government would continue to follow the suggestions of the Supreme International Sanitary Board of the Ottoman Empire with respect to sanitary measures to be taken in view of the pilgrimage, as long as the conference did not decide otherwise. But he also left no doubt that the Bulgarian Government would prefer a total ban or at least a restriction of the pilgrimage to Mecca.[43] He explained his strong support for the ample use of quarantines together with the mandatory and rigorous application of disinfection through the fact that Bulgaria had remained free of cholera in 1892–93, while the surrounding countries had beoame infected.[44] The Venice conference nonetheless passed a convention with regard to land borders, railway traffic and travellers which once more condemned the use of terrestrial quarantines. Rusev succeeded, however, in having an ambiguous clause incorporated which allowed the backdoor use of quarantines.[45] Consequently, when Bosnian Muslims returned from that year's *Hajj*, they were subjected to a severe quarantine of twenty-four hours and a disinfection of their luggage at Hebibchevo (today Lyubemets), on the Bulgarian border with the Ottoman Empire. On their way through Serbia, they were sent back to the Serbo–Bulgarian border crossing at Tsaribrod (today Dimitrovgrad) where they had to undergo another twenty-four hour quarantine before their transit through Serbia was allowed. And finally, as already mentioned, at the border crossing of Bosanski Brod they had to pass a final medical inspection with their luggage being disinfected once again (Figures 6.2 and 6.3).[46]

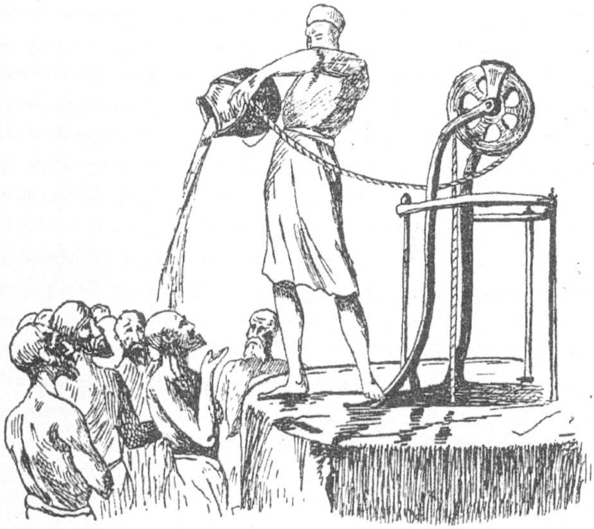

Фиг. VI.

Земземовски поливания отъ „Земземовския кладенецъ" при мусулманский пелеринажъ.

Figure 6.2 Muslim pilgrims experiencing the pouring of water from the Zamzam well.

In February 1903, Marin Rusev became head of the Bulgarian public health administration during a fluid and unstable period created by the presence of cholera and plague in the Red Sea region. As was already the case during the tenth ISC of 1897, Rusev remained categorical about quarantine and only one month after his promotion he tightened the regulations for the *hajjis*:

> 1) Mohammedans who depart for pilgrimage, on their return to Bulgaria, are allowed to enter only through [the ports of] Burgas, Varna, and [the terrestrial border crossing of] Hebibchevo; all other checkpoints are closed for them; 2) Mohammedan *hajjis* are only allowed to re-enter after strong medical examination and disinfection of their luggage and all their belongings, including [holy] water from the Zamzam Well [in Mecca]; for this end they are put under quarantine as long as is necessary to execute examination and disinfection; 3) Trains from Turkey carrying

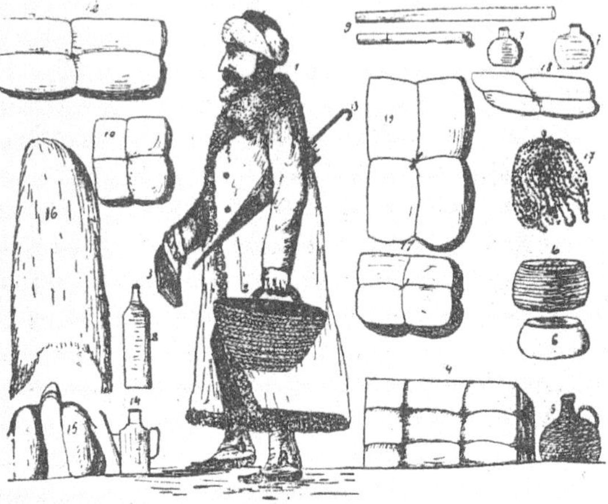

Фиг. V.

Типъ на мусулмански хаджия отъ България всрѣдъ своя типиченъ багажъ.

Figure 6.3 A typical Muslim pilgrim from Bulgaria with usual luggage.

> Mohammedan *hajjis* have to stop at the quarantine of Hebibchevo in order to drop the *hajjis* and their luggage; 4) Bosnian *hajjis* are only allowed when in transit, that is, they are not allowed to leave the train or to communicate in any way with the local population of the railway stations from which the train passes on its way through Bulgaria.[47]

And what is more, these measures were retained even after the plague in Egypt was officially brought under control, at least for the time being.[48] Consequently, during the eleventh ISC held some months later in Paris, the Ottoman Empire, Bulgaria and Greece were criticised by the Austro-Hungarian delegate for forming part of that block of countries – now already in a clear minority – which still upheld the principle of quarantinism thereby obstructing 'commercial transactions in the East'.[49] During the following years, the Bulgarian sanitary authorities somewhat eased their hitherto restrictive policy. In 1909, the Bulgarian 'Provisional Instructions for the Coastal Sanitary Service in Times of Cholera Risk' were enacted, taking a step toward the acceptance of the

1903 Paris ISC in questions such as the ample use of disinfection, though they still clung to the observation period of classical quarantine. Among the native *hajjis*, those who had not passed the quarantine in El Tor because they had used the Hejaz railway were treated with the utmost caution and had to undergo quarantine.[50]

Conclusions

This chapter has tried to show that the issue of Muslim pilgrims from the Balkans as possible vectors of cholera (and also of plague) came into the foreground only after the Congress of Berlin in 1878. Hitherto, it had not played any particular role in the general debates about how to protect Europe against 'Oriental' epidemics. This is surprising, because with the opening of the lower course of the Danube for international trade after the Crimean War, the protective character of the sanitary cordon at the Habsburg Military Frontier with the Ottoman Empire had been lost, and it was consequently abolished.[51] Only after Austria-Hungary began to administer the Ottoman province of Bosnia-Herzegovina in 1878 did the issue of medical control of Bosnian *hajjis* enter the agenda. Over the ensuing years, the newly founded principality of Bulgaria began to focus on its own *hajjis* as well as on Bosnian Muslim pilgrims crossing the country on their return home. At the time, Bulgaria was the only other region in the Balkans no longer under direct Ottoman control which nevertheless had a considerable Muslim population, if we leave aside the then small Muslim minorities of Montenegro (within its pre-1913 borders) and of the Romanian Dobruja. Serbia was in this period largely homogeneous from an ethnic-national point of view, a situation that would change after it took hold of the regions of Kosovo, Sandžak and Macedonia – with their considerable Muslim populations – after the Balkan Wars of 1912–13.

The treatment of Muslim pilgrims by the multi-ethnic and 'universal' Dual Monarchy and the 'parochial' Bulgarian nation-state seems to be different at first glance, though in practice it was very similar. The Austro-Hungarian authorities dealt with the Muslim pilgrims in an apparently benevolent way. They desired to win over a population which to a great extent still adhered to the social and political conventions of the pre-1878 order. This 'benevolence' had a patronising overtone, however. Epidemic control was introduced by organising pilgrimages under a leader and on a group basis. Control was further exerted by a medical doctor who accompanied the group on its return and by rigid measures of medical inspection, disinfection and quarantine, if advisable, on the return of the *hajjis*. As already said, it is still questionable whether these measures were experienced by all of the Bosnian *hajjis*, since there were always many who preferred to travel on their own. At the International Sanitary Conferences, Austria-Hungary advocated neoquarantinism and condemned the Bulgarian and Serbian adherence to old quarantinism, but at home – in the Bosnian quarantine facilities – it behaved not so differently from those countries. The ideological background underpinning this conduct shown by the Dual Monarchy – regardless of the reasonableness of the applied anti-epidemic measures – was one embedded in a sense of superiority of a Central European civilisation against the allegedly backward and fanatic Muslim population of Bosnia and Herzegovina. The reasons for Bulgaria's prolonged preservation of old quarantinism, enriched by the application of rigid disinfection are, in turn, manifold and not absolutely consistent. They were in part linked to Bulgarian dependence on Ottoman strategies with respect to the sanitary supervision of travellers and commodities, partly of a geo-epidemiological nature and finally attributable to an anti-Muslim attitude which was inscribed – as is the case of Serbian nationalism – in the Bulgarian national code (*Nationscode* in German). Bulgarian nationalism needed the local Muslims as a negative discursive figure which reminded of the perpetually reiterated oppression of the Bulgarian nation during the Ottoman period.[52] The Bulgarian case is only another example of how public health is always prone to serve an exclusive national cause.

It would be useful to discuss whether the case of the Balkan *hajjis* forms a variant of 'medical Orientalism', i.e. a specific attitude of containment of the Muslim world by the use of Western medicine. In this chapter, we have sought to demonstrate how practical measures reflected doctrinal changes with respect to the nature of cholera – namely the connection between contagionism and quarantines, miasma theory and the rejection of quarantines, bacteriology and neoquarantinism. The essence of 'medical Orientalism' was unequal power relations which are expressed in the fact that the old and rigid system of quarantine in the Orient was the precondition for the mild variant of neoquarantinism in Europe and therewith facilitated the prosperity of capitalist trade. But still, these theoretical combinations, put to practice, allowed for a degree of flexibility, this 'space' being subsequently used, for example, by the Austro-Hungarian authorities in an ambiguous way which could be described as 'nesting Orientalism'[53] in order to combine official neoquarantinism with tacit quarantinism at home. The Bulgarian case was much less complex, as authorities did not try to hide their intentions to subject native and Bosnian Muslim pilgrims to various hardships. But both examples show that the containment of Muslim pilgrims was not purely a sanitary/medical matter, but was also influenced by processes of cultural and political stigmatisation. In any case, the suspension of maritime traffic caused by the First World War in the Eastern Mediterranean, and the deep geo-political changes brought about by the conflict, relocated the nexus between the Muslim pilgrimage from the Balkans and the dissemination, not only of plague and cholera, but also of other epidemic diseases like typhus and smallpox, in a new context which falls outside the scope of this chapter.

Notes

1 Stefan Winkle, *Geißeln der Menschheit: Kulturgeschichte der Seuchen*, Düsseldorf, Artemis & Winkler, 2005, 3rd edn, 159–161, 1230; there is an entire chapter entitled 'Steamships and Cholera' in Francis E. Peters, *The Hajj: the Muslim Pilgrimage to Mecca and the holy places*, Princeton, NJ, Princeton University Press, 1996, 266–315; see also 'Health Maintenance and Disease Control on the Hajj' in Eric Tagliacozzo, *The Longest Journey: Southeast Asians and the Pilgrimage to Mecca*, Oxford and New York, Oxford University Press, 2013, 133–155.

2 Peter Baldwin, *Contagion and the State in Europe, 1830–1930*, New York, Cambridge University Press, 2005, 140, 228–231; Valeska Huber, 'The unification of the globe by disease? The International Sanitary Conferences on cholera, 1851–1894', *The Historical Journal* 49, 2, 453–476, 462–464.

3 N.N., 'Mecca Cholera Epidemic of 1831', in George C. Kohn (ed.), *The Wordsworth Encyclopedia of Plague and Pestilence*, Ware, Hertfordshire, Wordsworth Editions, 1998, 205–206.

4 'Asiatic Cholera Pandemics during the Life of John Snow: Asiatic Cholera Pandemic of 1846–63', www.ph.ucla.edu/epi/snow/pancholera3.htm (accessed 25 February 2016).

5 Cf. Mariko Ogawa, 'Uneasy bedfellows: science and politics in the refutation of Koch's bacterial theory of cholera', *Bulletin of the History of Medicine* 74, 4, 2000, 671–707.

6 Cf. Baldwin, *Contagion and the State*, 231–236; Cornelia Essner, 'Cholera der Mekkapilger und international Sanitätspolitik in Ägypten (1866–1928)', *Welt des Islams*, New Series 32, 1, 1992, 41–82; Daniel Brower, 'Russian roads to Mecca: religious tolerance and Muslim pilgrimage in the Russian Empire', *Slavic Review* 55, 3, 1996, 567–584; Michael Christopher Low, 'Empire and the Hajj: pilgrims, plagues, and pan-Islam under British surveillance, 1865–1908', *International Journal of Middle East Studies* 40, 2, 2008, 269–290. With respect to the Indian pilgrims, see Saurabh Mishra, 'Beyond the Bounds of Time? The Haj Pilgrimage from the Indian Subcontinent, 1865–1920', in Pati Biswamoy and Mark Harrison (eds), *The Social History of Health and Medicine in Colonial India*, London and New York, Routledge, 2009, 31–44; *Pilgrimage, Politics, and Pestilence The Haj from the Indian Subcontinent, 1860–1920*, New Dehli, OUP, 2011; T.M.P. Duggan, 'Western quarantine – excluding the other', *Mediterranean Journal of Humanities* 1, 2, 2011, 105–115; Luc Chantre, 'Le pèlerinage à la Mecque à l'époque coloniale (v 1866–1940): France-Grande-Bretagne-Italie', PhD thesis, University of Poitiers, 2012; 'Entre pandémie et panislamisme', *Archives de sciences sociales des religions* 3, 2013, 163–190; Valeska Huber, *Channelling Mobilities: Migration and Globalisation in the Suez Canal Region and Beyond, 1869–1914*, New York, Cambridge University Press, 2013; Elena I. Campbell, 'The "pilgrim question": regulating the Hajj in Late Imperial Russia', *Canadian Slavonic Papers* 56, 3–4, 2014, 239–268; Eric Tagliacozzo, 'Hajj in the Time of Cholera: Pilgrim Ships and Contagion from Southeast Asia to the Red Sea', in James L. Gelvin and Nile Green (eds), *Global Muslims in the Age of Steam and Print*, Berkley, Los Angeles and London, University of California Press, 2014, 103–120; Sylvia Chiffoleau, *Le voyage à La Mecque. Un pèlerinage mondial en terre d'Islam*. Paris, Belin, 2015; Michael Christopher Low, 'Ottoman infrastructures of the Saudi hydro-states: the technopolitics of pilgrimage and potable water in the Hijaz', *Comparative Studies in Society and History* 57, 4, 2015, 942–946, 957–960. In the last three chapters of her monograph on the impact of quarantines in the Ottoman Empire, Birsen Bulmuş also examines the role of Muslim pilgrims: Birsen Bulmuş, *Plague, Quarantines and Geopolitics in the Ottoman Empire*, Edinburgh, Edinburgh University Press, 2012.

7 Cf. Kemal H. Karpat, *Ottoman Population 1830–1914. Demographic and Social Characteristics*, Madison, Wisconsin, The University of Wisconsin Press, 1985, 55–58.

8 J[acob] E[duard] Polak, 'Itinerarien muselmanischer Pilger zu den wichtigsten Wallfahrtsorten, mit Bezugnahme auf Verbreitung von Cholera', *Mittheilungen der Kaiserlich-Königlichen Geographischen Gesellschaft* 10, 1868, 63–85, here 77–78.

9 Martin Dinges, 'Pest und Politik in der europäischen Neuzeit', in Mischa Meier (ed.), *Pest: Die Geschichte eines Menschheitstraumas*, Stuttgart, Klett-Cotta, 2005, 283–313, here 302–304 and 307–311.
10 [Karl Ludwig] Sigmund, 'Die Quarantäne-Reform, geschrieben nach einer Reise im Orient und in Egypten III', *Zeitschrift der K.K. Gesellschaft der Ärzte zu Wien* 6, 1, 1850, 165–178, here 166.
11 Daniel Panzac, *Population et santé dans l'Empire Ottoman (XVIIIe-XXe siècles)*, Istanbul, Isis, 1996, 77–85.
12 Marcel Chahrour, ' "A civilizing mission"? Austrian medicine and the reform of medical structures in the Ottoman Empire, 1838–1850', *Studies in History and Philosophy of Biological and Biomedical Sciences* 38, 2007, 687–705.
13 Erwin Ackerknecht, 'Anticontagionism between 1821 and 1867', *Bulletin of the History of Medicine* 22, 1948, 562–593.
14 Cf. Carl Ludwig Sigmund Ritter von Ilanor, *Die Quarantänereform und die Pestfrage. Beobachtungen und Anträge geschrieben nach einer im Auftrage der k. k. österreichischen Staatsverwaltung unternommenen Bereisung der Donauländer, des Orients und Egyptens*, Vienna, Braumüller, 1850.
15 Nermin Ersoy, Yuksel Gungor and Aslihan Akpinar, 'International Sanitary Conferences from the Ottoman perspective (1851–1938)', *Hygiea Internationalis* 10, 1, 2011, 53–79, here 59–61; Michael Christopher Low, 'The 1866 International Sanitary Conference through Ottoman Eyes: The Mechanics of Quarantine and Sanitary Reform in the Muslim Holy Land, 1866–1882', www2.iisg.nl/esshc/programme.asp?selyear=10&pap=8627 (accessed 31 August 2017).
16 Baldwin, *Contagion and the State*, 231–232; Ersoy et al., 'International Sanitary Conferences', 65–68; Huber, 'The unification of the globe', 467–476.
17 'Massnahmen zur Verhütung der Einschleppung der Cholera aus dem Hedjaz', *Das österreichische Sanitätswesen* 14, 16, 17 April 1902, 188.
18 Bošković and Smailbegović, 'Zdravstveno obezbjeđenje'.
19 Ibid., 75–76.
20 Ibid., 76, 81.
21 Ibid., 76–77.
22 Ibid., 'Bosnische Mekka-Pilger', *Wiener Abendpost* 202, 4 September 1891, 3.
23 Bošković and Smailbegović, 'Zdravstveno obezbjeđenje', 77–79.
24 Ibid., 79–80.
25 Ibid., 80–81.
26 'Oprezne mjere protí unosu kuge', *Liečnički viestnik* 21, 8, 1899, 267–269.
27 Bošković and Smailbegović, 'Zdravstveno obezbjeđenje', 81.
28 Ibid., 80–81.

29 'Sanitätspolizeiliche Behandlung der heimkehrenden bosnisch-hercegovinischen Mekkapilger in Bosnien', *Das österreichische Sanitätswesen* 13, 23, 6 June 1901, 254–256; 'Massregeln zur Verhütung der Einschleppung der Cholera durch zurückkehrende bosnisch-hercegovinische Mekkapilger', *Das österreichische Sanitätswesen* 14, 17, 14 May 1902, 203.
30 Bošković and Smailbegović, 'Zdravstveno obezbjeđenje', 81.
31 Alois Musil, 'Die Gefahren der Hedschasbahn', *Neue Freie Presse* 16232, 28 October, 1909, 21–23; E[manuel] A. Ziffer, 'Die mohammedanische Eisenbahn (Hedschasbahn)', *Zeitschrift des Österreichischen Ingenieur- und Architekten-Vereines* 62, 9, 1910, 133–140; Austrian State Archives, Allgemeines Verwaltungsarchiv, Ministerium des Innern, Sanitätsakten, Sign. 35, box 3105, Konstantinopel, 3 November 1911, no. 46913/8 in no. 7487/S.
32 Austrian State Archives, Allgemeines Verwaltungsarchiv, Ministerium des Innern, Sanitätsakten Sign. 35, box 3105, Vienna, 17 May 1911, no. 3611/S, G[eza] Kobler, 'Exposé, betreffend die bei der im Mai l.J. in Paris stattfindenden Sanitätskonferenz zu verhandelnden Fragen, insbesondere in Bezug auf den Pilgerverkehr'; cf. Campbell, 'The "pilgrim" question', 250–258.[Typesetter – please reverse highlighted speechmarks]
33 Austrian State Archives, Allgemeines Verwaltungsarchiv, Ministerium des Innern, Sanitätsakten Sign. 26/5, box 2645, Sarajevo, 21 October 1910, no. 4909/10.
34 *Conférence sanitaire internationale de Paris: 7 novembre 1911–17 janvier 1912, procès-verbaux*, Paris, Imprimerie nationale, 1912, 266.
35 'Sophia, 27. März', *Neue Freie Presse* 6316, 28 March 1882, 7; 'Bukarest, 31. März', *Die Presse* 35, 90, 1 April 882, 4; 'Cholera', *Die Presse. Erstes Abendblatt* 25, 101, 13 April 1882, 14; 'Notizen', *Wiener Medizinische Wochenschrift* 32, 15, 15 April 1882, 442.
36 'Varna, 5. Mai', *Die Presse* 35, 130, 12 May 1882, 3.
37 Baldwin, *Contagion and the State*, 179.
38 Ibid., 227.
39 *Procès-Verbaux de la Conférence Sanitaire Internationale de de Dresde, 11 mars–15 avril 1893*, Dresde, B.G. Teubner, 1893, 305.
40 Ibid., 107, 245.
41 *Conférence sanitaire internationale de Paris, 7 février–3 avril 1894: procès-verbaux*, Paris, Imprimerie nationale, 1894, 72; cf. Bošković/Smailbegović, 'Zdravstveno obezbjeđenje', 77.
42 *Conférence sanitaire internationale de Venise, 16 février-19 mars 1897: procès-verbaux*, Rome, Forzani et cie, imprimeurs du Sénat, 1897, 92.
43 Ibid., 92–93.
44 Ibid., 334.

45 Ibid., 447.
46 Bošković/Smailbegović, 'Zdravstveno obezbjeđenje', 80.
47 'Zapovedi', *Izvestiya na Grazdanskata sanitarna direktsiya* 1, 2, 1903, 1.
48 'Dnevnik no. 28 ot 15 Avgust 1903 god.', *Izvestiya na Grazdanskata sanitarna direktsiya* 1, 4, 1903, 6.
49 *Conférence sanitaire internationale de Paris, 10 octobre–3 décembre 1903: procès-verbaux*, Paris, Imprimerie nationale, 1904, 68–69.
50 Hr[isto] Doktorov, *Izlozhenie varhu Karantinata sluzhba v Varnenski Karantinen rayon*, Varna, Pechatnitsa 'Vzaimnost', 1911, 31, 37–41.
51 Erna Lesky, 'Die österreichische Pestfront and der k.k. Militärgrenze', *Saeculum* 8, 1957, 82–106; Gunther E. Rothenberg, 'The Austrian sanitary cordon and the control of the bubonic plague: 1710–1871', *Journal of the History of Medicine and Allied Sciences* 28, 1973, 15–23.
52 Mary Neuburger, *The Orient Within: Muslim Minorities and the Negotiation of Nationhood in Modern Bulgaria*, Ithaca, NY, Cornell University Press, 2004; cf. for Serbia, Dietmar Müller, *Staatsbürger auf Widerruf: Juden und Muslime als Alteritätspartner im rumänischen und serbischen Nationscode. Ethnonationale Staatsbürgerschaftskonzepte 1878–1941*, Wiesbaden, Harrassowitz, 2005 (Balkanologische Veröffentlichungen 41).
53 Milica Bakić-Hayden, 'Nesting orientalisms: the case of former Yugoslavia', *Slavic Review* 54, 4, 1995, 917–931.

7

Contagion controversies on cholera and yellow fever in mid nineteenth-century Spain: the case of Nicasio Landa

Jon Arrizabalaga and Juan Carlos García-Reyes

Introduction

In contrast to Edwin Ackerknecht's[1] long-prevailing dualistic views – miasmatism versus contagionism – on the causes and prevention of infectious diseases in nineteenth-century Europe, historians like Christopher Hamlin[2] and Peter Baldwin[3] have more recently emphasised the diversity and contingency of the links between aetiological knowledge of, and prevention practices against, these conditions in different countries at the time. Thus, no wonder quarantine techniques were rather widespread everywhere even during the heyday of environmentalism. In this regard, the period between the late eighteenth and late nineteenth centuries might be characterised as one of transition as a result of international commercial pressures and the new diplomatic context – particularly after the peace of 1815 – from the quarantine's old regime to a more systematic and liberal sanitary regime, cholera epidemics having been the major health challenge. The new regime applied the reform of quarantine regulations in many European countries, and led to the gradual construction of an international sanitary system, mainly through the International Sanitary Conferences.[4]

This chapter will examine contagion and quarantine controversies in mid nineteenth-century Spain through the views and practices of a remarkable physician of epidemics and reformist army medical officer, namely Nicasio Landa (1830–91).[5] Trained in the early 1850s, he is especially renowned, after 1863–64, as an early campaigner of the

International Red Cross movement in Spain and as a relentless promoter of the cause of war humanitarianism in both national and international medical and legal forums. Yet, the professional activities related to the causes and prevention of epidemics which he mostly undertook in the early stage of his career – between 1854 and 1864 – make him a suggestive case study to illustrate the controversies on contagion and quarantine in Spain and Europe at the time. These were mostly focused on cholera and yellow fever, regarding epidemics involving civil or military populations, in either metropolitan Spain (both the Peninsula and the Canary Islands) or in Morocco during the Spanish–Moroccan War of 1859–60. Always attentive to novel scientific ideas abroad – not only from French and German sources but also from British and North-American ones – Landa developed his own views and practices from his experiences as a physician of epidemics and a medical officer on campaign.

The quarantine regime in nineteenth-century Spain

The growing preception from the 1780s that politics, commerce and medicine were closely intertwined made merchants and humanitarian reformers on both sides of the Atlantic question quarantine as a 'relic of a less enlightened and brutal age'.[6] These circumstances led to the replacement in Britain of the Quarantine Act of 1753 by a new one in 1825 that, without abolishing the quarantine regime, brought some liberalisation to it.[7] Two years before, the Bourbon Restoration regime, whose defence of quarantine in France was implacable during the 1820s, had used a sanitary cordon to crush a liberal experiment in Spain – the so-called liberal Triennium (1820–23).[8]

Not incidentally, in 1822 the Spanish Parliament had developed a scheme for the introduction of a public health code of regulations – the *Código sanitario para la Monarquía española* (Health Code for the Spanish Monarchy). This liberal project that aimed to set permanent and systematic sanitary regulations, collected the quarantine measures implemented against the risk of 'exotic contagia', and divided them into those applicable to both the coastal or maritime and the terrestrial regimes.[9] While inland containment measures were based on military *cordons sanitaires* manned by the infantry or the cavalry or, in their absence, by the 'national militia' or 'armed civilians', the maritime littoral ones were put under the charge of *Juntas de Sanidad* (health boards) that were given the authority to set isolation or quarantine periods for ships, travellers or goods 'under suspicion'. Different periods of quarantine were established depending on whether the bill of health ('tainted', 'suspect', 'foul' and so on) involved passengers and cargo, or merely the latter. In the same way, goods susceptible to contagion, and therefore subjected to special attention, were distinguished from others, in principle, as 'free from suspicion'.

The 1822 Health Code never came into force because the Absolutist Monarchy was restored in 1823. During the subsequent quarter of a century, Spain remained rather active in the European debates about an international regulation of quarantine, usually opposing its relaxation.[10] And those physicians who paid attention to the health and epidemiological issue of cholera – like Manuel González de Sámano (c. 1832–c. 1860), Manuel Codorniu Ferreras (1788–1857) and Mateo Seoane Sobral (1791–1870) – looked for an ordered regulation of the quarantine system. Specifically, Seoane, who had figured prominently among the drafters of the 1822 project, held a new idea of public health, not limited to the setting up of temporal measures during epidemics but aiming at the organisation of a whole, permanent public health service, which would restructure the 'healthcare professions'.[11]

During the 1850s, a movement for health and social reforms took place in Spain – as in other European countries – with the active involvement of numerous physicians. Coinciding with this reformist period, during the so-called Progressive Biennium (1854–56), a new *Ley de Sanidad* (Health Law) that reflected the liberal spirit of the 1822 project was enacted.[12] To a great measure this law was motivated by the 1853–56 cholera epidemic which seriously affected various regions in Spain; actually the text paid great attention to the containment of this epidemic by quarantine.[13] Yet, in contrast to the more restrictive 1822 project, the 1855 law reduced and rationalised the periods spent in maritime quarantine,[14] abolished the terrestrial quarantines and assigned the regulation of *cordons sanitaires* not to local or provincial *Juntas*, but to the national government.[15] No wonder the new quarantine regulations in this law were rather influenced by the conventions agreed at the Paris ISC of 1851 – as Quim Bonastra has also pointed out in his Chapter 1 within this volume.[16]

After its enactment, quarantine measures provided for by the 1855 law were barely implemented despite the fact that a large part of the medical establishment supporting such measures continued lobbying for them during the subsequent years. This lobby mostly constituted physicians with great influence by virtue of their access to the royal court and/or their membership of the newly founded *Real Academia de Medicina* at Madrid (RAMM), among whom were Juan Drumen (1798–1863), Francisco Méndez Álvaro (1806–83) and Matías Nieto Serrano (1813–1902). At this point, Méndez Álvaro's work came to be seen as particularly remarkable after he was elected member of the *Congreso de los Diputados* (Spanish Parliament) in 1864, where he proposed a new health law whose main attention would be focused on reorganising the quarantine system. The recommendations regarding quarantines and sanitary administration that were given in the Constantinople ISC of 1866 served as bases for the Spanish decrees of 1866 and 1867 – modifying the 1855 law – which aimed to redefine maritime sanitary policy.[17] Marked by a greater propensity to believe in the contagiousness of cholera – the collective disease that caused most serious concern at the time – the introduced changes reinforced the barriers to prevent cholera from entering Spain, multiplying the number of lazarettos of observation in order to favour the flow of goods through a greater number of ports at a moment of profound economic crisis. As Quim Bonastra has also argued, this did not lead to a better articulation of the quarantine system, but the converse.[18]

Landa's views on cholera in peninsular Spain and Morocco (1854–60)

In 1854, just graduated as a physician at the Universidad Central of Madrid, Nicasio Landa looked after the victims of cholera in the south of his native Navarre on the occasion of a severe epidemic affecting Spain at the time. In this early professional 'baptism of fire' he worked along with his father Rufino Landa (1801–62), a surgeon-physician and hygienist who had already been involved in the fight against the previous cholera epidemic of 1833–35. Two years after having been awarded his doctorate at the same university, Landa joined the *Cuerpo de Sanidad Militar* (Army Health Service) which, like those of most European armies, was going through a period of reform. He and other young medical officers actively committed themselves to the collective aim of improving the Spanish military health services by applying scientific and technological advancements in order for the army to be able to meet the new challenges of modern warfare. For this purpose, in December 1858, a group of medical officers including Landa launched a collective editorial project, the *Memorial de Sanidad del Ejército y Armada*, the first Spanish journal specialising in military medicine. In August 1859, Landa published there his earliest work on cholera.[19]

After recalling that the epidemic outbreak he had faced with his father in a Navarrese town – Oteiza de la Solana – did not show a 'frontier' dissemination process, Landa questioned the dominant theory which defended the 'exotic origin' of the disease,[20] and expressed his conviction that cholera followed neither the course of rivers, nor any other 'topographic arteries', namely, ways, valleys, or mountain chains.[21] He claimed to have converted to his father's view that 'the traveller of the Ganges neither travels nor comes from Asia, but it is always a son of the country where it appears', and that the 'set of cosmic circumstances' under the influence of which cholera develops, 'can have and has its place at any point of the globe'.[22] For him, cholera was 'a native disease' – not derived from 'miasmas or bodies of exotic origin dissolved in the air' – that appeared when a 'certain set of cosmic circumstances' was given; and its propagation was neither by 'contagion ... nor even by infection according to the current meaning given to this word'. Although he recognised that these circumstances had not yet been cleared up, he considered that the conditions 'of atmospheric electricity first, and of heat and humidity then', might most probably play a key role in them.[23] Thus, when investigating the 'cause producing cholera' he emphasised the importance of the precedent or accompanying 'meteorologic circumstances', mostly those relative to 'electric tension'. He also recommended registering the 'composition of the air' and the 'hour of the invasions'. By then, Landa was already insisting on the need to study 'the facts' in an impartial way, and not 'on behalf of a certain system', in order to 'avoid the misfortune for humankind and the humiliation for science'.

In late 1859, when Landa and his colleagues were mobilised for the Spanish–Moroccan War, the publication of the *Memorial* was definitively interrupted. The military campaign caused a high number of victims on both sides, though fewer than those provoked by the epidemic outbreaks of cholera – a feature supported by the available statistics about the conflict that was emphasised by Landa and others.[24] Most contemporary physicians conceded that cholera was an endemic condition in northern Africa. Yet, Landa and his colleagues, like Fernando Weyler Laviña (1808–79) or Antonio Población Fernández (1822–1903), did not agree with this traditional view. Población and Weyler claimed that this and other epidemics, like dysentery and diarrhoea, were intimately associated with the stationing of the regiments, and insisted that cholera had been brought by the Spanish troops from the Iberian Peninsula to northern Africa.[25]

In coincidence with Weyler and Población, Landa claimed that any new landing of troops from Spain fuelled epidemic outbreaks. Moreover, he confirmed a complete lack of foresight by the Spanish military health services. This epidemiologic challenge had largely exceeded their resources and capacity of reaction.[26] Similarly, on the basis of his 'particular studies', Landa remained steadfast in his conviction that cholera was not 'contagious'. Well aware, however, of the scarce acceptance of this view in the medical world, he behaved in a professionally prudent way by ensuring that he always kept himself on guard in the face of any cholera 'symptom of propagation' during the healthcare tasks he performed in the hospital-ship wards where wounded soldiers crowded together. He also eventually felt relieved when the number of 'invaded' soldiers did not increase inside the ship.[27] Anyhow, by then Landa's professional experience with cholera had helped him to modify his original ideas on the origin of this disease with new knowledge which allowed him to explain the intensification of such epidemic outbreaks. For Landa, military station quarters – placed on the 'wrong' type of soils, in light of the geological theory to which he adhered to – coupled with the nutritional deficiencies and the overcrowding of the camps, were main causes which brought about the aggressive epidemic in Morocco.[28]

Two years later, Landa sent a report to the RAMM on the cholera epidemic of 1853–56 in Spain.[29] In this report, he related the varying intensity in the development of the disease in different geographical areas of the Peninsula, with the geological constitution of their soils. He confirmed the observation, already made in other European countries, that cholera developed with much less intensity in hipogenic or primordial (i.e. plutonic and chrystalline) soils than in others.

Then he proposed, allegedly 'for the first time', a gradation of chrystalline rocks that were refractory to the development of cholera, including granite (twenty times less intensity of cholera), gneiss (four times less), and limestones and schists (two times less).[30] Landa's *Memoria* drew from scientific sources that revealed his good knowledge of the state-of-the-art international literature on the matter, beginning with the investigations of the Bavarian physician, chemist and hygienist Max von Pettenkofer (1818–1901), father of the influential telluric theory according to which soil and subterranean waters were determinant elements in the propagation of cholera.[31] The apparent absence of Spanish translations of Pettemkofer's works in those days did not prevent him from reading them in their French, English or Italian translations.[32]

Other sources inspiring his telluric theorisations were originally francophone, such as the medical geography by the military physician Jean-Christian-Marc Boudin (1806–67),[33] and the studies by the physician and hygienist Alexandre Fourcault (1790–1853)[34] and by the geologist Nérée Boubée (1806–63)[35] on the relationships between geology and medicine on the occasion of the 1832–34 cholera epidemic in France. The severity of the disease in Paris in 1832 had led Fourcault and Boulée to take into consideration height as a variable among the geological conditions of soils determining a greater or lesser inclination in suffering from the disease. Landa also resorted to the works by the Belgian geologist André Hubert Dumont (1809–57)[36] and by two remarkable Spanish mining engineers – Guillermo Schulz (1805–77) and Joaquín Ezquerra del Bayo (1793–1859) – whose studies on mining soils were instrumental for his mapping of those soils prone to the propagation of cholera.

As recorded in the annual report of its activities, the RAMM did not acknowledge receipt of Landa's *Memoria* until 1862. The critical reception provided by the RAMM's Public Hygiene Section to his work (albeit recognising its worth) might explain why it remained unpublished, though this did not prevent Landa from being designated a corresponding member of the association.[37] Strikingly, the RAMM's report criticised not only the 'entirely unsecure' statistical data on which Landa's *Memoria* was based – although the source was the official report by the *Dirección General de Beneficencia y Sanidad* (General Health Inspection) – but also 'Boudin's, Boubée's, Fourcault's and Pettenkofer's inferences', all of which, they argued, lacked the 'best guarantees and foundations'.[38]

Landa and the epidemic of yellow fever in the Canary Islands (1862–63)

For centuries, the Canary Islands served as transit outposts in the communications between peninsular Spain and the colonial territories around the Caribbean, a region where yellow fever was endemic. As a result, the disease arrived to the islands from Cuba many times, the last three during the reign of Isabel II of Spain: 1838, 1846–47 and 1862–63.[39] The last epidemic between September 1862 and March 1863 affected the two largest islands of the archipelago, Gran Canaria and Tenerife. Landa, along with another colleague, was from February to mid August 1863 commissioned by the Spanish Government to visit Tenerife. Evidence of his viewpoint and actions were two letters he sent from the scene of the epidemic (dated in February and on 1 March)[40] and a speech he pronounced at the RAMM on 30 April.[41]

In his speech, Landa recognised that it was the first time that he had witnessed a yellow fever outbreak. He defined the disease as a 'great pathological phenomenon', 'lethal scourge' and 'pestilence' no less horrible than cholera, while describing in epic tone the devastation it had inflicted upon Santa Cruz de Tenerife, the island's capital, and its harbour. After having praised the 'abnegation of those honourable civil and military physicians' who had looked after the victims of yellow fever, and postponed for another occasion the unravelling of its 'ignored essence ... the conditions for its development, its probable cause, its fundamental lesions, [and] its curative treatment', he chose to focus on studying the origin of the epidemic. Landa justifies his decision with the assumption that such a question was not only the most controversial for science, and the most relevant for the 'health of peoples', but also the source on which authorities could build a solid basis for 'a public health regime able to answer to the advancements and complex needs of our times'.[42]

His analysis was drawn from the 'investigatory dossier' based on information gathered from witnesses, conducted in October 1862 by agreement with the Canary Islands' provincial health board. Landa used this to legitimise the 'arguments' which he formulated as propositions so that, he argued, they could 'be exempted from the blemish of being partial' and gain the impression of an 'almost official character'. He rejected point by point the theories that the epidemic 'germ' had been imported by sea from either the New World (Cuba) or the West African coast (Fernando Poo, Lagos or other areas in the region), respectively, by claiming that yellow fever's incubation period was much shorter than the sequence between the first cases in Santa Cruz and those in other towns on the island. After having ruled out both 'exotic' theories,[43] Landa favoured the 'hypothesis of the spontaneous development of the scourge', though he confessed that he felt unable to formulate 'a categorical statement instead of hesitant interrogations' on the origins of the epidemic. He finished his speech in this eloquent way:

> I have tried neither to have in this question preconceived inclinations, nor to give an *a priori* adhesion to anyone; lover of the truth, persuaded of how urgent it is for humankind to discover them [the origins of yellow fever], and convinced that my energies are not sufficient enough for such a big enterprise, I have believed as rightest to become the reporter of this important process, to bring you here all its pieces, and to submit it to the judgement of this supreme court of science.[44]

Landa's prudent and restrained interpretation of the origin of this yellow fever epidemic, whose 'exotic' nature he denied, was contested by the publication, in Tenerife in 1864, of two works rejecting his anti-contagionist theses. Written by two military subinspector physicians who were stationed there – Pedro Joaquín Vergara Díaz, on behalf of the provincial health board of the Canary Islands, and Francisco del Busto y Blanco, who inserted a chapter on the epidemic in his medical topography of the archipelago – both works located the most probable origin of the disease to a frigate from the Antilles that had docked at the port of Santa Cruz after spending eight days in Vigo's San Simón 'foul lazaretto'.[45]

The quarantine debate during the Spanish Medical Congress (1864)

In late September 1864, when the recent yellow fever outbreak at the Canary Islands was still alive in collective memory, a first *Congreso Médico Español* (Spanish Medical Congress) was held in Madrid. No wonder that one of its four monographic sessions was focused on quarantines and lazarettos.[46] The session began with the reading of a letter by Évariste Bertulus (1809–81) – a French military physician well accredited by his studies on epidemic diseases – who excused his absence from the congress due to his inescapable medical responsibilities at the Hôtel-Dieu of Marseille.[47] Bertulus praised the allegedly generalised support which 'Spanish physicians' gave to the 'maintenance of lazarettos and quarantines', and for claiming that these means were 'the sole reasonable and possible barrier against the invasion of great pestilential scourges'. For him, this feature made out of the Spanish physicians 'the last defenders of public health – so outrageously battered in our times', in contrast to French, Italian and English physicians' desertion. Bertolus evocated the vigour and eloquency of the Spanish hygienist Pedro Felipe Monlau (1808–71) when he had defended – as Spanish delegate to the first ISC in Paris in 1851, focused on maritime quarantines in the Mediterranean[48] – the 'healthy medical doctrines in a time when they were succumbing everywhere'. And he foresaw the day was soon to come when, once this question was definitely cleared up, public opinion would acknowledge that 'Spanish physicians' had been the 'wisest, most prudent, and most discerning' for not having been blinded by the dangers facing their country, by the 'love for money' and 'thirst for honours and properties', as well as for having 'known how to resist the torrents of new ideas'. After complaining about the 'scientific despotism' shown by Paris – which he defined as the 'great laboratory' where scientific 'systems', 'theories' and 'excentricities' originating from anywhere were celebrated to the detriment and exclusion of 'healthy medical doctrines' – Bertulus praised the favourable position taken by 'scientific and medical Spain', thanks to the fact that its 'men of science' were not obliged to 'fight against the lack of intellectual freedom [*ilotisme intellectuel*]', which he believed to be 'the most degrading among those afflicting humankind'.

Following the reading of Bertulus' letter, Antonio Fernández Carril (1823–91), an active general practitioner from Alhama de Aragón – an Aragonese town renowned for its thermal baths – delivered a report which was apparently intended as a general framework for the session.[49] His unequivocal defense of lazarettos and quarantines as an essential tool in the fight against those 'diseases imported from other countries', like cholera and yellow fever, was based on the assumption that their 'infection foci', either local, or larger in scope, produced the '*miasmas*, and these in turn, the *contagion*' from which it was necessary to be preserved. At the end of the report, Fernández Carril rejected the accusation that supporters of these measures were opposing the 'progressive movement of the age'. In this sense, he declared himself a fervent believer in the organisation of scientific congresses as he thought that the 'spirit of association' was the 'main agent' in the 'vanguard of universal progress'. Indeed, by invoking the Ciceronian principle *salus populi suprema lex est*, he underlined that nobody should get to the point of 'scorning the healthy precepts of public hygiene' in the name of 'free trade'.

Fernández Carril's report was followed by Nicasio Landa's paper about the nature of the miasma and by two other contributions, both of them openly aligned with the contagionist position. The first was a report by Jacinto Roger, a physician at Mahón lazaretto, on the quarantines against cholera and yellow fever implemented there since its opening in 1819. The other paper by José Varela de Montes, the dean of the medical faculty at Santiago de Compostela, underlined the importance of lazarettos and quarantines to prevent the importation of the three major exotic epidemics.[50] Roger sharply defended the need for quarantine measures to avoid the situation in which 'our coasts remained open to such mortiferous diseases'.[51] In contrast, Varela's defence – even in case of doubt – of quarantine and lazarettos against the importation of exotic diseases, did not prevent him from demanding a flexible and wise implementation of these measures, by restricting these practices specifically to those 'good maritime lazarettos located in convenient geographic positions' that took into account the comfort of those confined there, and avoided 'anti-humanitarian' conditions – to 'make quarantine laws the less onerous possible'. He also advocated new 'public health regulations' according to the 'maritime and terrestrial doctrine' with regard to 'the special conditions required of each exotic disease'.[52]

The subsequent debate, including more than a dozen rather lengthy interventions by different participants at the session, offers a representative panorama of the intensive confrontation then existing in Spain between contagionists and anticontagionists apropos the implementation of quarantine measures.[53] From the contagionist side of those defending quarantines and lazarettos, there were members of the RAMM such as its Perpetual Secretary, Matías Nieto Serrano, and the Professor of External Pathology in the Universidad Central (UC), José Calvo Martín (1814–1904); high public health servants to the royal court such as the first official of the *Consejo de Sanidad del Reino* (Royal Health Council), Ciriaco Ruiz Jiménez, and the subdelegate of medicine at the royal court, Santiago Iglesias; and Landa's colleague in the military health services, Antonio Población.[54] In contrast, on the anticontagionist side of those who opposed the maintenance of quarantine measures, one found professors of auxiliary medical disciplines – who were more open to the new experimental methods – such as those of natural history, Manuel M.J. de Galdo (1825–95), and chemistry, Ramón Torres Muñoz de Luna (1822–90); Teodoro Yáñez Font (c. 1830–1901), a disciple, as Landa himself, of Pedro Mata Fontanet (1811–77), who would succeed him in the chair of forensic medicine and toxicology at the Universidad Central; and, finally, Eduardo Sánchez Rubio (1833–1911), an active family doctor of the *Cuerpo facultativo de hospitalidad domiciliaria* (Home Care Medical Corps).[55]

Against bipolarisation: Landa's search for the nature of the 'miasma'

Landa rejected any irreducible bipolarity in the confrontation between contagionists and anti-contagionists – 'infectionists', as he preferred to call the latter. Showing professional and personal respect to all contenders, he claimed that the 'divergence' between the 'contradictory opinions' was itself evidence of the inaccuracy of their respective starting points. He called for a 'conciliation' between 'rival sides' by asking them to abandon the 'narrow spirit of faction', which he regarded as entirely alien to the 'spirit of science' since it led them to try to find in each epidemic 'less the absolute truth than the corroboration of their own doctrines' by means of 'the endless series, the eternal litany of contradictory facts, the ones not less certain and reliable than the others'. Landa also urged both sides not to succumb to the temptation of barricading themselves in a 'sectarian doctrinalism' and devoting themselves to 'a work of mutual demolition', but to direct their energy towards the unravelling of, by means of experimental research, the nature of the miasma, 'a *sui generis* entity, be it exotic, or native', in which, to the best of his knowledge, they all coincided in locating the 'cause and origin' of 'epidemic diseases'.[56]

Landa chose to begin his argument by quoting a passage from *Notes on Nursing* (London, 1859) where Florence Nightingale criticised nosological ontologism and defended the adjectival (not substantival) nature of infectious diseases that could allegedly be born spontaneously and transform their nature during their course.[57] He intended to establish, on this basis, 'a whole system of pathology' in accordance with the 'synthetic tendencies of modern science' and, more specifically, with the principle that 'nature tends to unity in its causes, and to infinity in its results' (while such tendencies appear to have a Comtean and/or Spencerian ascendant, the principle was explicitly associated to Pedro Mata, Landa's master). Therefore, by taking the British General Board of Health's *Report on Quarantine* (London, 1849) as a source of inspiration, he was inclined to consider all fevers (intermittent, typhoid, great endemic, eruptive, great epidemic and putrid) as 'varied manifestations of a single cause, very analogous if not the same', that were modified by 'the environment and the conditions under which it develops'.[58] And he located the cause of every fever in what was known as 'miasma', the 'essence' and 'nature' of which Landa claimed to be, at last, on the point of being elucidated thanks to the 'advancement of natural sciences':

> There are no more sterile hypotheses, nor cabinet lucubrations; there are exact observations, tangible and positive facts that have been studied thanks to the powerful instruments of physics.[59]

Landa illustrated his thesis by exposing some recent European and North American investigations on the question. First, he referred to the comparative studies about microphites and microzoaries present in the air of three different places in France – the marshy region of Sologne, the healthy area of Romainville and the Parisian *Jardin des Plantes* – published by François-Jules Lemaire (1814–66) in July 1864, barely two months before the congress.[60] By summing up the evolution of the 'world of microscopic organisms' that Lemaire had observed by microscope over fifteen days in drops of water vapour condensed at Sologne, Landa praised Darwin's principle of the 'struggle for existence' by applying it to these microorganisms.[61] And he associated these findings with the conclusive results presented by Louis Pasteur (1822–95) in Paris just five months before, in which the 'phenomena of organic decomposition' had been proved to be always due to the chemical action of bacteria.[62]

Landa proposed to identify miasma with these 'microscopic living beings' whose anatomy and functions were just being studied by other two French biologists, René Édouard Claparède (1832–71) and Félix-Archimède Pouchet (1800–72), respectively. To reinforce this hypothesis he resorted to different experiments and observations, having recently illustrated the action of microorganisms on 'animal economy'. On the one hand, he referred to the experiments through which Casimir-Joseph Davaine (1812–82) and Jules Signol (1824–1903) had proved in 1863 that carbuncle or anthrax could be transmitted to healthy rabbits by experimental inoculation of blood with 'infusoria' from sick lambs. Landa appears to have been punctually informed about them by means of the *Comptes Rendus de l'Académie des Sciences* of Paris.[63] On the other, he mentioned several observations and experiments in animals and humans made by physicians and surgeons during the American Civil War (1861–65) that linked the presence of spores, fungi or eggs of infusoria suspended in the air with intermittent fevers (W. Hammond), malaria (J.K. Mitchell), miasmatic fevers (J. Metcalfe) and 'camp measles' (J.H. Salisbury).[64] All these authors were more or less closely related to the U.S. Sanitary Commission whose activities Landa was following with greatest interest through its promptly received reports.[65] On these bases, he defended the 'essential unity of every popular disease', no matter how diverse were their 'morbid manifestations' depending on the distinct microorganisms – microphites ('mucedinea' and 'lycoperdon') and microzoaries ('bacteria', 'vibrio') – that could develop in them.

The question about the origin of these microorganisms led Landa to refer to the debate in the *Académie des Sciènces* of Paris that put an end to the lasting scientific controversy – from 1859 to 1864 – about the origin of microscopic life, in which the scientific coalition presided over by Pasteur proved that not even infusoria could be produced by spontaneous generation. Landa appears to have been well informed about the details of this debate since he reported the points of confrontation between the 'heterogenists' Pouchet, Nicolas Joly (1812–85) and Charles-Raymond Musset (1826–1892), and the 'panspermists' Louis Pasteur, J.J.M.C. Victor Coste (1807–73) and Édouard-Gérard Balbiani (1825–99), as well as the eventual 'conversion' into panspermism of some distinguished heterogenist biologists, such as Jean-Pierre Flourens (1794–1867), Edmond Frémy (1814–94) and Armand de Quatrefages (1810–92).[66]

Pleading for pragmatism and enlightened empiricism against the miasma

The observations and/or experiments showing that the miasma causing epidemic diseases was a 'microscopic organism' that could not grow out of spontaneous generation led Landa to infer that 'destroying the germ means destroying the scourge'. Thus, according to him, when it was definitely verified that 'the miasma is a microsporon' it would be possible: (1) to state that a 'distinct germ' corresponded to each 'popular disease', as had been already proven by Hammond for 'intermittent fever' and by Salisbury for measles; (2) to know in a precise way the diversity of its 'conditions of transmission' (e.g. within the 'hold of boats', the 'folds in the goods', the 'wings of the wind and of storm' and so on); and, in the end (3) to better understand the behaviour patterns of different epidemics. He exemplified these patterns through questions like the effects of some microorganisms on 'chronometric variations of atmosphere'; the variable ways of transmission (direct, indirect or mixed) for a single disease; and the reasons why a disease was sometimes exogenous, sometimes spontaneous, or why it appeared sometimes in an 'isolated place', and in others jumped from the coast to an island.[67]

In the end, for Landa this would definitely imply the 'absolute uselessness of those days of observation, during periods of quarantine' since he argued that the 'dried germs' could 'remain a long time inert' without losing their 'proliferation virtue'. Firmly convinced that scientific progress would soon allow 'a single, clear, and demonstrable theory' as well as 'a certain and infalible criterion' to solve any difficulty and antinomy in this matter, he was inclined to adopt a 'more conciliatory temper' until reaching a definite evidence. His firm commitment to pragmatism – 'not all that is beautiful in the absolute regions of theory is feasible in the conditional regions of practice' – and to governance – 'it is necessary to make concessions in order to rule well' – led Landa to formulate two pieces of practical advice. First, to maintain the 'sanitary precautions of empirism whereas we have no others to replace them', despite the fact that he claimed they should be informed by 'a more enlightened empirism'. Second, to mitigate 'useless rigours' resulting in 'discredit for science and authority' – something that he took advantage of for criticising the commercial protectionism then prevailing in Spain.[68]

As a guide for any sanitary regulations, Landa recommended following the agreement, then just signed between France and Italy, regulating quarantine measures in their Mediterranean ports for ships with foul bills of health due to yellow fever.[69] He considered this agreement as having achieved 'great progress' with respect to the Spanish legislation because, by applying different measures to travellers, goods and ships, it allowed harmonisation as much as possible between the 'interests of public health', the 'individual freedom of travellers' and the 'easiness of commercial transactions'. Among other advantages, Landa emphasised that these measures allowed free circulation of travellers whenever there were no cases of yellow fever during the voyage. They also introduced flexible criteria regarding the isolation periods for ships since they encouraged shipowners to incorporate the new technologies available for ventilation and hygiene so that ships could get pratique when their 'hygienic state' was 'satisfactory' or, if necessary, reduce to a few hours the previously much longer operation of 'disinfection from the miasma'.[70]

Conclusion

Nicasio Landa's opposition to the traditional quarantine model is an important example of his disapproval of the vitalist tendency that was hegemonic in the medical establishment of mid nineteenth-century Spain. Certainly, his ideas on this matter are associated with those of Pedro Mata, Professor of Forensic Medicine at the Universidad Central and supervisor of his doctoral dissertation entitled 'Considerations on the influence of civilisation on public health'.[71] The speech Mata pronounced at the RAMM in 1859 to vindicate positivism against vitalism in medicine had provoked unanimously tough responses during eighteen long sessions delivered by seven academics. These speeches were jointly published as a reply to Mata. Among these academics one finds Nieto Serrano and Calvo Martín, who five years later would defend contagionist views at the Spanish Medical Congress.[72]

Two decades after these debates on the causes and prevention of cholera and yellow fever in which Landa had been involved, the latter reasserted himself in his anti-quarantine position on two occasions, at a couple of scientific meetings. This was rather typical of the activities he developed during the last stage of his professional life. The first intervention took place on the occasion of a regional congress of medicine in Navarre – held at the town of Tafalla from 22 to 24 March 1886 – which was devoted to the impact left in the province by the 1884–85 cholera epidemic in Spain.[73] Landa, then a member of Navarre's provincial health board, was honoured with the presidency of the congress and submitted a report on the effects left by the 1885 cholera epidemic in the military district of Navarre – a report which unfortunately has been lost.[74] Yet, among the conclusions coming out of the congress were that on the one hand, cholera was an infectious epidemic, but not a contagious one, from 'some Asian regions', and produced by 'a telluric morbid germ' – the 'microbe of Koch' or 'Bacillus virgula' that was isolated in 1883. It was also concluded that its 'most probable' vehicle was the 'fluvial waters', though this required the concurrence of a 'telluric preparation' in order to become a 'pathogen'. On the other hand, it was underlined that the 'patient and systematic study of epidemics' was an equally (if not more) important means to get to know the 'etiology and pathogeny of cholera' as the microscope. A motion was almost unanimously approved discouraging the 'absolute confinement' of populations as an effective way to prevent cholera, for it was judged to be 'unrealistic and harmful', and 'ineffective' in preserving the community 'from the scourge', in addition to being a procedure that was 'expensive, humiliating and ruinous for agriculture, industry and commerce', and which made municipalities spend 'on illusory incommunication' substantial amounts of money instead of investing in their sanitation.[75] In the face of the threat of a new cholera epidemic in 1890 – a few months before he died – Landa still managed to impose his authority, albeit more tightly (eight against six votes) on the provincial health board of Navarre, with the support of its non-medical members, so that it adopted before a 'suspicious case' a mere 'medical inspection' instead of the more drastic confinement measures usually practised by physicians.[76]

His second intervention took place on the occasion of the eleventh congress of the *Institut de Droit International* (Lausanne, 28 September 1888). Proposing a project for an international sanitary convention to revise the 'current system of international sanitary policy' on bases which were 'irrefutable by experimental science', Landa summed up the different international law initiatives of the second half of the nineteenth century that had helped to suppress or attenuate the 'useless rigours of the quarantine regime [...] humiliating dispositions whose inefficiency modern science has admitted'. In accordance with the debates at contemporary International Sanitary Conferences,[77] his proposal suggested a substantial relaxation of the measures of sanitary police imposed on travellers arriving 'to a port or a border of any country' as well as on goods and ships. The regulation of those procedures that were considered most convenient 'according to the advice of science' to 'safeguard public health' would be left in the hands of each state. These procedures, that always needed to be published in advance and made available to the agencies of 'foreign trade', could be suspended or mitigated whenever ships had systems for 'constant ventilation or disinfection'; and compensation was foreseen for their owners (except in case of 'bad faith') when the sinking or destruction of ships or goods was mandated. Finally, no passerby could be subject to 'sanitary measures other than medical inspection'. On the contrary, immediate 'free circulation' should be given to each traveller without 'symptoms of a contagious or infectious disease' (even for those arriving 'under a foul bill of health'), though the 'medical inspector' could oblige them to take a bath and to allow 'their clothes to be disinfected'. Very significantly, Landa not only asked for hospital care to be provided for those 'sick people' that should always be subjected to 'all the considerations demanded by humanity', but he also demanded that states should renounce – by means of a treaty – the unnecessary rigours of quarantine measures, in the same way, he stressed, as was already being done in the face of the 'unnecessary rigours of war by means of the memorable Geneva Convention'.[78]

Notes

This chapter is an outcome of the research projects funded by the Dirección General de Investigación (Spanish Government), 'Military health services, war medicine and humanitarianism in nineteenth-century Spain' (HAR2011–24134) and 'Relief action and medical technologies in humanitarian emergencies, 1850–1950: agencies, agendas, spaces, representations' (HAR2015–67723P).

1 Erwin H. Ackerknecht, 'Anticontagionism between 1821 and 1867', *Bulletin of the History of Medicine* 22, 1948, 562–593.

2 Christopher Hamlin, *A Science of Impurity: Water Analysis in Nineteenth Century Britain*, Bristol, Adam Hilger, 1990; *Public Health and Social Justice*

in the Age of Chadwick: Britain, 1800–1854, Cambridge, Cambridge University Press, 1998; *Cholera: The Biography*, Oxford, Oxford University Press, 2009.

3 Peter Baldwin, *Contagion and the State in Europe, 1830–1930*, Cambridge, Cambridge University Press, 1999, 1–36.

4 For more information about this 'sanitary' period, see, among others, Mark Harrison, 'Disease, diplomacy and international commerce: the origins of international sanitary regulation in the nineteenth century', *Journal of Global History* 1, 2006, 197–217; Valeska Huber, 'The unification of the globe by disease? The International Sanitary Conferences on cholera, 1851–1894', *The Historical Journal* 49/2, 2006, 453–476.

5 For more information about Nicasio Landa, see José Carlos Sánchez-Vicente, 'El proyecto de manicomio agrícola de Nicasio Landa', *Gerónimo de Uztariz* 8, 1993, 123–135; José Javier Viñes, *El doctor Nicasio Landa, médico y escritor: Pamplona 1830–1891*, Pamplona, Gobierno de Navarra, 2001; *El doctor Nicasio Landa (1830–1891): cofundador de la Cruz Roja Española*, 2nd edn, Pamplona, Gobierno de Navarra – Cruz Roja de Navarra, 2014; Jon Arrizabalaga and Juan C. García-Reyes, 'Between a Humanitarian Ethos and Military Efficiency: The Early Days of the Spanish Red Cross, 1864–1876' in Wolfgang U. Eckart and Philipp Osten (eds), *Schlachtschrecken, Konventionen. Das Rote Kreuz und die Erfindung der Menschlichkeit im Kriege*, Freiburg, Centaurus Verlag, 2011, 49–65; Jon Arrizabalaga and Guillermo Sánchez-Martínez, 'Nicasio Landa, 1830–1891, le Comité de Genève et la première Croix-Rouge espagnole', in Valérie Lathion and Roger Durand (eds), *Humanitaire & médecine. 1. Les premiers pas de la Croix-Rouge 1854–1870*, Geneva, Genève Humanitaire, Centre de Recherches Historiques – Institut d'Histoire de la Médecine et de la Santé, 2013, 169–196.

6 Mark Harrison, *Contagion. How Commerce Has Spread Disease*, New Haven and London, Yale University Press, 2012, 50–79 (quotation on p. 50).

7 Ibid., 51, 62.

8 Ibid., 65–66.

9 'Proyecto de Código Sanitario para la Monarquía Española', transcribed in José María López Piñero, *Mateo Seoane y la introducción en España del sistema sanitario liberal*, Madrid, Ministerio de Sanidad, 1984, 49–122 (on quarantines, see articles nos 129–136, 79–80).

10 On some Spanish initiatives in this respect, see Francisco Javier Martínez, 'International or French? The early International Sanitary Conferences and France's struggle for hegemony in the mid-ninteenth century Mediterranean', *French History* 30/1, 2016, 82–85.

11 López Piñero, *Mateo Seoane*, 20.

12 'Ley de 28 de noviembre de 1855 disponiendo lo conveniente sobre el servicio general de sanidad', transcribed in López Piñero, *Mateo Seoane*, 219–235.
13 Quim Bonastra, 'La red de resguardo sanitario marítimo y la articulación del territorio costero español a mediados del ochocientos', *Scripta Nova. Revista Electrónica de Geografía y Ciencias Sociales*, 2012, 16/418 (18), www.ub.edu/geocrit/sn/sn-418/sn-418–18.htm (accessed 29 August 2017).
14 For the section regarding maritime quarantines, see articles nos 29–40 in López Piñero, *Mateo Seoane*, 223–225.
15 On the terrestrial quarantine system, see articles nos 57–59, in López Piñero, *Mateo Seoane*, 228.
16 Martínez, 'International or French?', 88–91.
17 Ibid., 95, 98.
18 Quim Bonastra, 'Del programa general a la solución de compromiso. Cuarentenas y territorio en la modificación de la ley de sanidad de 1866', in Quim Bonastra and Gerard Jori (eds), *Imaginar, organizar y controlar el territorio. Una visión geográfica de la construcción del Estado-nación*, Barcelona, Icaria, 2013, 123–165.
19 Nicasio Landa, 'Dos palabras acerca del origen del cólera-morbo [Pamplona, 21 agosto 1859]', *Memorial de Sanidad* 2, 19, 1859, 501–505. The article was fully reproduced in *La España Médica* 4, 199, 1859, 614–615.
20 'Ahora bien, este pueblo que según la teoría admitida debería ser fronterizo, se encuentra en medio de la provincia, se halla fuera de carretera, vive en el aislamiento, no había recibido viajeros ni mercancías, en fin, la presencia del cólera en el lugar de Oteiza era la refutación más completa de aquella teoría' (Landa, 'Dos palabras', 502).
21 Ibid., 503.
22 Ibid.
23 Ibid., 504–505.
24 Nicasio Landa, *La campaña de Marruecos: memorias de un médico militar*, Madrid, Imp. Álvarez, 1860, 62. On cholera in the Spanish–Moroccan War, see Joan Serrallonga i Urquidi, 'La guerra de África y el cólera (1859–60)', *Hispania: Revista española de historia* 58, 198, 1998, 233–260.
25 Fernando Weyler Laviña, *Apuntes topográficos sobre la parte del Imperio Marroquí que ha sido teatro de la última guerra con España*, Palma de Mallorca, Imp. de Pedro José Gelabert, 1860, 38; Antonio Población Fernández, *Historia médica de la guerra de África*, Madrid, Imp. M. Álvarez, 1860, 109–110. Cholera was also brought by French troops in a parallel campaign in eastern Morocco, as shown in F. Javier Martínez Antonio, *La otra guerra de África. Cólera y conflicto internacional en la olvidada expedición militar de*

Francia a Marruecos en 1859, Ceuta, Archivo General de Ceuta, 2010. The outbreak in Morocco was part of a larger western Mediterranean epidemic affecting Spain, Morocco and French Algeria.

26 'Sin duda no se había previsto esta calamidad, a pesar de ser bien sabido que es compañera inseparable de los ejércitos modernos, de que se había iniciado su desarrollo en el de observación: ello es que en Ceuta no había dispuesto otro hospital que el de los Reyes, y la única medida preventiva que se había adoptado era la de dotarle de un médico mayor y dos profesores más de su asignación en tiempo de paz. Ni se había acopiado en Ceuta utensilio y material de hospitales, ni contratado enfermeros, ni aun designado los edificios que a aquel uso pudieran destinarse; en suma la calamidad del cólera encontraba muy desprevenida a la Administración de nuestro ejército, que no había contado tal vez con que todo él fuere a desembarcar en un mismo puerto' (Landa, *La campaña de Marruecos*, 62–63).

27 'Aunque mis estudios particulares acerca del cólera me dan la convicción de que no es contagioso, como esta opinión se encuentra aún en minoría en el mundo médico, vigilaba yo sobre todo a los demás heridos, amontonados en aquellas salas, temeroso de percibir en ellos algún síntoma de la propagación de esta enfermedad, que en tal caso pudiera haber producido a bordo de aquel buque una catástrofe espantosa, a cuya sola idea se me erizaban los cabellos; pero felizmente no fue así, ni hubo más invadidos que los que ya lo estaban al entrar en el sollado' (Landa, *La campaña de Marruecos*, 157).

28 Landa's emphasis on the importance of soils is evidenced in *La campaña de Marruecos*, pages 41–42, 101, 104, 110, 125, 173. In order to illustrate the role played by the other two variables in the worsening of the epidemic, see Landa, *La campaña de Marruecos*, 68, 129 (on nutritional deficiencies and inadequate facilities); and 70, 77–78 (on overcrowding in hospitals and camps).

29 Nicasio Landa, *Memoria sobre la relación que ha existido entre la constitución geológica del terreno y el desarrollo del cólera-morbo en España*, Madrid, September 1861, transcribed in José Javier Viñes, *El doctor Nicasio Landa*, 2001, 227–243 and in 'El Dr. D. Nicasio Landa, médico oficial de epidemias en la de cólera de 1854–1855', *Anales del sistema sanitario de Navarra*, vol. 1, 2000, 93–102.

30 Landa, *Memoria*, in Viñes, *El doctor Nicasio Landa*, 2001, 240–242.

31 Pettenkofer's main works of the 1850s and the early 1860s were: *Untersuchungen und Beobachtungen über die Verbreitungsart der Cholera nebst Betrachtungen über Massregeln, derselben Einhalt zu tun*, Munich, Cotta, 1855; *Zur Frage Über die Verbreitungsart der Cholera: Entgegnungen und Erläuterungen*

zu Seiner Schrift 'Ueber die Verbreitungsart der Cholera', Munich, Cotta, 1855; *Die Cholera und die Bodenbeschaffenheit in der k. k. österreichischen Provinz Krain*, Munich, Christian Kaiser, 1861.

32 Another indirect source on Pettenkofer's work might have been González de Samano's unquoted *Memoria* on the cholera epidemic of 1854–55 in Spain: 'Para que los contagios se desarrollen en donde haya sido importado el germen, son precisas condiciones especiales de localidad. Los sitios movedizos y porosos son más a propósito, y las rocas gozan de inmunidad (Opinión casi universal entre nosotros apoyada en la de los profesores alemanes, a cuya cabeza podemos colocar a Mr. Pettenkofer)'. See Mariano González de Sámano, *Memoria histórica del Cólera-Morbo Asiático en España*, Madrid, Imp. Álvarez, 1858, vol. 1, 355.

33 Jean-Christian-Marc Boudin, *Essai de géographie médicale, ou Etudes sur les lois qui président à la distribution géographique des maladies, ainsi qu'à leurs raports topographiques entre elles, lois de coïncidence et d'antagonisme*, Paris, Germer-Baillière/ Labé, 1843.

34 Alexandre Fourcault, 'Influence des conditions géologiques et hydrologiques sur la marche du choléra en France', *Gazette Médicale de Paris* 4, 1849, 333–340, 357–360.

35 Nérée Boubée, *La géologie dans ses rapports avec l'agriculture et l'économie politique*, Paris, Bureau du Bulletin d'histoire naturelle de France, 1840; *La géologie dans ses rapports avec la médecine et l'hygiène publique: conditions géologiques des maladies épidémiques et endémiques en général et du cholera en particulier (Mémoire lue à l'Académie des Sciences de Paris le 18 juin 1849)*, Paris, Eloffe, 1849.

36 André H. Dumont, *Mémoire sur les terrains ardennais et rhénan de l'Ardenne, du Brabant et du Condroz*, Bruxelles, Académie Royale des Sciences, des Lettres et des Beaux-Arts de Belgique, 1847.

37 For the news that Landa's *Memoria* had been sent to the Academia in 1862, see *Discursos pronunciados en la inauguración de las sesiones de la Real Academia de Medicina de Madrid en el año de 1862*, Madrid, Imprenta de los señores Rojas, 1862, 13. Excerpts from the critical report of the RAMM that was signed by Juan Vilanueva y Piera as the secretary and rapporteur, and by Francisco Méndez Álvaro as dean are reproduced in Viñes, 'El Dr. D. Nicasio Landa', 90–91, 105–106. For Landa's designation as correspondent member, see Viñes, *El doctor Nicasio Landa*, 191.

38 Viñes, 'El Dr. D. Nicasio Landa', 90–91.

39 For a general view on the topic, see María José Betancor, *Epidemias y pleito insular. La fiebre amarilla en Las Palmas de Gran Canaria en el periodo isabelino*, Madrid, Ediciones del Cabildo de Gran Canaria-CSIC, 2002.

40 'Cartas del dr. Landa sobre la epidemia de Canarias', *La España Médica* 8, 376, 1863, 153; no. 381, 189.

41 Nicasio Landa, 'Investigaciones sobre el origen de la epidemia sufrida en Santa Cruz de Tenerife en 1862–1863'. This speach was published in June that year in the varia section of *La España médica, Iberia médica y crónica de los hospitales*, vol. 8, no. 393, 1863, 377–379; no. 394, p. 395; no. 395, 411–413; no. 396, 427–428; no. 397, 442–444; no. 399, 475–471; no. 400, 491–493; and in *El Pabellón médico: revista científica y profesional de medicina, cirujía y farmacia*, vol. 3, 1863, 260–261, 282–283, 293–296, 355–356, 402–403, 410–413.

42 '... y este [discurso] que ahora os prometo, trata de otra pestilencia no menos horrible, del cerbero que abre sus triples fauces en las costas americanas, del vampiro que sobre las cálidas ondas del golfo mejicano bebe la sangre de los europeos, del vómito negro que mi suerte ha querido que observara bajo el pico colosal del Teide' (*El Pabellón médico*, vol. 3, 1863, 260).

43 'Ya no hay en el sentido de la importación, otra hipótesis que examinar, ni otra teoría que discutir, ni otras sospechas que analizar' (*El Pabellón médico*, vol. 3, 1863, 413).

44 *El Pabellón médico*, vol. 3, 1863, 413.

45 Pedro Joaquín Vergara Díaz, *Ensayo histórico sobre la enfermedad que reinó epidémicamente en la ciudad de Santa Cruz de Tenerife*, Santa Cruz de Tenerife, Miguel Aranda, 1864; F. del Busto y Blanco, 'Fiebre amarilla padecida en Santa Cruz de Tenerife desde octubre de 1862 a marzo de 1863', in *Topografía médica de las Islas Canarias*, Sevilla, Imp. de La Andalucía, 1864, 213–236.

46 *Actas de las sesiones del Congreso Médico Español celebrado en Madrid. Setiembre de 1864*, Madrid, Imp. De José M. Ducazcal, 1865. The topics of the four monographic sections were 'importance of *lazarettos* and quarantines', 'surgical treatment of cancer', 'causes and means of avoiding or diminishing its [cancer's] havoc' and 'criterion of moral freedom in the perpetration of a crime'. For the contents of the congress session on lazarettos and quarantines (held on 26 September), see 218–331.

47 Évariste Bertulus, letter (Marseille, 15 September 1864), *Actas*, 218–220.

48 João Rangel de Almeida, 'The 1851 International Sanitary Conference and the Construction of an International Sphere of Public Health', PhD thesis, The University of Edinburgh, 2012.

49 Antonio Fernández Carril, 'La importancia de los lazaretos y cuarentenas', *Actas*, 221–233.

50 Jacinto Roger, 'Memoria de los sucesos ocurridos en el lazareto del puerto de Mahón, desde su apertura en el año 1817 hasta el presente' (*Actas*,

242–267); José Varela de Montes, 'Importancia de cuarentenas y lazaretos' (*Actas*, 268–271).

51 Roger, 'Memoria', 267.

52 Varela, 'Importancia', 271.

53 For this discussion that comprises over seventy pages of compressed text, see *Actas*, 272–334.

54 Matías Nieto Serrano (*Actas*, 279–281), Ciriaco Ruiz Jiménez (*Actas*, 298–307), José Calvo Martín (*Actas*, 314–323, 333–334), Antonio Población (*Actas*, 324–326) and Santiago Iglesias (*Actas*, 327–330).

55 Manuel María José de Galdó (*Actas*, 272–279), Ramón Torres Muñoz de Luna (*Actas*, 281–293), Yáñez (*Actas*, 294–297, 330–331), Eduardo Sánchez Rubio (*Actas*, 308–312). In the same year when the Congress' *Actas* were published, Torres Muñoz systematised his theses in the leaflet *El cólera morbo asiático considerado desde el punto de vista químico*, Madrid, Imp. Antonio Peñuelas, 1865.

56 Nicasio Landa, 'Sobre la naturaleza del miasma en las epidemias', *Actas*, 233–242 (233–235).

57 Ibid., 235–236.

58 Ibid., 236–237. For the context of this report on quarantine by the General Board of Health, see Harrison, *Contagion*, 99–101.

59 Ibid., 237.

60 Lemaire, 'Investigaciones sobre los microfitos y los microzoarios', *Revista de los progresos de las ciencias exactas, físicas y naturales* 15, 2, February 1865, 105–110 (originally published in *Comptes Rendus des Séances de l'Académie de Sciences* 59, 7, 1864, 317–321). The details collected by Landa had been presented by Lemaire in the session of 17 August 1864, and the summary of his intervention might have appeared in the *Comptes rendus* about two weeks after, in early September. On the other hand, Lemaire himself would present a small correction some days later, in the session of 22 August (59, 8, 1864, 380). There, he denied having had the purpose of teasing the chemists, as some had understood it, by claiming that, were the samples burned, what was important to collect and analyse was actually destroyed. He also added a bibliographic note reporting that in 1839 another researcher had departed from a similar assumption: 'reconnaissant l'insuffisance des analyses purement chimiques pour arriver à démontrer la nature des miasmes et des maladies contagieuses, [Chevreul] proposa une nouvelle méthode pour ces recherches. Le froid et le microscope sont conseillés. Je n'ai donc fait qu'imiter, sans le savoir, mon honoré maître. Je me ferai un devoir de rectifier ces passages de mon Mémoire'. Curiously, Landa used this correction in his reply to Ruiz Jiménez within the Spanish Medical Congress: 'no es la química la que nos dará la luz sobre este punto,

pero nos la dará muy esplendente el concurso de todas las ciencias naturales' (*Actas*, 308).

61 Landa, *Actas*, 237–238. Aparently, the phrase 'struggle for the existence' (*lucha por la existencia*), already in use at the end of the eighteenth century, does not come from any French translation of Darwin's *On The Origin of Species*, but from either the English original work or the English (or German) expositions of Darwin's theory: compare the phrases 'Struggle for life' and 'Struggle for existence' (Darwin, 3rd English edn) with 'Concurrence vitale' (Darwin, French translation by Clemence Royal, 1862, chap. III).

62 Pasteur had exposed the results of his experiments in the speech 'La génération spontanée', pronounced at a scientific soirée at La Sorbonne on 7 April 1864. On 23 April its contents were published in the *Revue des cours scientifiques* 1, 1863–1864, 257–265.

63 For an analysis of these experiments, see Jean Théodoridès, *Un grand médecin et biologiste: Casimir-Joseph Davaine (1812–1882)*, Oxford, Pergamon Press, 1968, 77–84.

64 William Hammond (1828–1900), *Treatise on Higiene with special reference to the military service*, Filadelfia, J.B. Lippincott, 1863; John K. Mitchell (1798–1858), *On the cryptogamous origin of malarious and epidemic fevers*, Filadelfia, Lea and Blanchard, 1849; John T. Metcalfe (1818–1902), *Report of a Committee of the associate members of the Sanitary Comission, on the subject of the nature and treatment of miasmatic fevers*, Nueva York, Baillière Brothers, 1862; James Henry Salisbury (1823–1905), *Remarks on fungi, with an account of experiments showing the influence of the fungi of wheat and rye straw on the human system, and some observations which point to them as the probable source of camp measles, and perhaps of measles generally* (n.p., julio 1862).

65 On the Sanitary Commission, see William Quentin Maxwell, *Lincoln's Firth Wheel. The Political History of the U.S. Sanitary Commission*, New York, Longmans, Green & Co., 1956. On Landa's interest for the Sanitary Commission, see Arrizabalaga and Sánchez-Martínez, 'Nicasio Landa, 1830–1891', 169–196 (at 183–184).

66 Landa, *Actas*, 239–240.

67 Ibid., 240–241.

68 ' … do not make the burden of sanitary protection so heavy as it is already that of commercial protection', See Landa, *Actas*, 241.

69 'Arrangement signé à Paris le 24 juin 1864, entre la France et l'Italie, pour régler les mesures de quarantaine dans les ports français et italiens de la Méditerranée', in M. de Clercq, *Recueil des Traités de la France… Tome neuvième 1864–1867*, Paris, Amyot, 1868, 43–44.

70 Landa, *Actas*, 242.
71 Nicasio Landa, *Consideraciones acerca de la influencia de la civilización en la salud pública*, Madrid, Imp. del Colegio de Sordo-Mudos, 1856.
72 Pedro Mata, *Hipócrates y las escuelas hipocráticas. Discurso pronunciado en la solemne apertura de las sesiones del año 1859 en la Real Academia de Medicina de Madrid*, Madrid, Imprenta de Manuel Rojas, 1859; Tomás Santero et al., *Defensa de Hipócrates, de las escuelas hipocráticas y del vitalismo*, Madrid, Imp. de Manuel de Rojas, 1859.
73 *El Congreso Médico-Regional de Navarra en 1886: memoria científico-descriptiva por la Comisión nombrada al efecto*, Pamplona, Imprenta Provincial, 1886; Pilar León, 'El Congreso médico-regional de Navarra (1886): un ejemplo de transmisión del conocimiento científico', *Anales del Sistema Sanitario de Navarra*, vol. 32, no. 2, 2009, 149–159; Pilar Sarrasqueta Sáenz, 'La epidemia de cólera de 1885 en Navarra y Tudela', PhD thesis, Universidad de Navarra, 2010.
74 'Memoria sobre la epidemia de 1885 en el Distrito militar de Navarra'. See *El Congreso Médico-Regional*, 14.
75 *El Congreso Médico-Regional*, 8, 19, 21, 23.
76 Junta de Sanidad de Navarra, act 111, 20 julio 1890, in José Javier Viñes, *La sanidad española en el siglo XIX a través de la Junta Provincial de Sanidad de Navarra (1870–1902)*, Pamplona, Gobierno de Navarra, 2006, 591–591.
77 Huber, 'The unification of the globe by disease?', particularly 471–476.
78 Nicasio Landa, 'Rapport sur police sanitaire internationale', *Annuaire de l'Institut de Droit International* 10, 1888–89, 251–256.

III

Power

8

Quarantine, sanitisation, colonialism and the construction of the 'contagious Arab' in the Mediterranean, 1830s–1900

John Chircop

Introduction

This chapter seeks to investigate quarantines – their set-up and sanitisation procedures – much as others have discussed other medical/hygienist institutions, in terms of their links with contemporary structures of power, mainly in connection with Western European colonial expansion in the southern and eastern littoral of the Mediterranean during the nineteenth century. As the growing volume of literature on the comparative history of colonial medicine demonstrates, Western biomedicine and sanitation were employed as 'tools of Empire' – to use Daniel Headrick's phrase[1] – as instruments to 'civilize' and control the 'indigenous body'.[2] Thus, it is increasingly being argued that the export of Western medicine and hygienist ventures – scientific discourse, practices – and hence the establishment of quarantine systems on the lazaretto model, was intimately embedded in and went hand in hand with informal colonial penetration and direct imperial acquisitions[3] of non-European lands, in the process corroborating Western European assertions of cultural–scientific superiority over 'native peoples'.[4]

Attentive to new insights emerging from recent literature, and engaging with the theoretical debates, this chapter focuses on the transfer of Western medical/hygienist theories and the related sanitary instruments and practices – in this case the quarantine lazaretto system – to various city ports in North Africa and the eastern Mediterranean during the nineteenth century. It consequently seeks to make evident the extent to which the conveyance of this Western sanitary technology and set of practices – presented to the local populations as beneficial instruments of modernity – facilitated colonial incursions in the political economies of these countries, most of which – apart from Morocco – were under Ottoman rule. In order to explore such issues, I shall focus on the several sanitary councils (also known as quarantine boards) created in the main regional ports. Although a thoroughly researched study still needs to be undertaken, this chapter uses the literature available to explore these sanitary councils as spaces of negotiation facilitating the transfer of contemporary epidemiological and medical knowledge – and the role they played in the construction of lazaretto establishments.

These sanitary councils have not received much scholarly attention in the historical literature, yet they were the earliest permanent sites of discussion on international sanitation – made up of resident European consuls, doctors and sanitary advisors in conversation with native physicians, public health and local state functionaries – and they preceded the first 1851 ISC by several years. By contrast, the history of the eleven ISCs until 1903 – also the subject of this chapter – has been dealt with by quite a number of scholars. Most studies shed light on the influence which these ISCs had on the shaping of interstate public health diplomacy[5] and how it came to exacerbate the 'South–North health divide'.[6] Other established scholarly works, such as Peter Baldwin's study of contagion and the state in Europe, make use of the ISC records to illustrate the strategies adopted by the modern European states to prevent the spread of epidemics as well as to investigate the intricate social and political consequences that these left on the evolution of their public health infrastructures.[7] For the purpose of this chapter, this historical literature helps to provide the wider contexts in which each ISC was convened, assisting in our understanding of the complex interests involved in the European countries' design and operation of the network of lazarettos in the Mediterranean and beyond.

By the time that the first ISC was convened, Western European trade, political hegemony and colonial projects were being bolstered by technological advances in transport and communication technology. Inducing an unprecedented acceleration in movement, they simultaneously spurred the rapid diffusion of epidemics by accelerating the transmission of disease from one regional corner to another and between continents, as happened with cholera in 1831–32. By exploring this wider context, and particularly indicating the various geo-strategic and colonial interests of the European powers in the Mediterranean region and how these were reflected in the proceedings of the ISCs, we can approach the operations of the lazarettos from a different perspective. This allows us to put at the centre of analysis the experiences of 'Arab' peoples themselves – often the focus of hygienist strategies including the lazarettos. By investigating the institutional architecture of these quarantine-lazarettos,[8] this study seeks to show their double role as preventive public health institutions but also, and more intriguingly, as devices for social control and colonisation. Focusing on specific quarantine practices – especially the disinfection of the body – which came to be rigorously conducted in these lazarettos, will make more visible the ways and the extent to which 'Muslim-Arabs', as local residents or/and as *hajjis* (pilgrims), were restrained, disinfected and put under surveillance: procedures which were also employed to reconstruct and publicly legitimise in contemporary discourse the stereotype[9] of the 'Muslim-Arab' as 'threatening 'contagious bodies' – these being essential features of the colonising process then underway.

Contraction of time and space: situating the International Sanitary Conferences

The first ISC was convened in Paris in 1851, at a time of rapid innovation in transport and communication technology – steamships, railways and the laying of the cable telegraph – which brought about an unprecedented shrinking of time and space. Intensification of speed was harnessed and used[10] by the European industrial powers, starting with Britain and France, to assist their colonial penetration of North Africa and the eastern Ottoman domains, which would eventually lead to their formal imperial acquisition.[11] This ushered in an era marked by velocity in human mobility, travel and exchange, by greater geographical interconnectivity[12] through which the various zones of the Mediterranean came to be incorporated in the emerging world economy.[13]

The complementary transition made from sail to steamships radically shortened travel time; for instance, the journey from Marseilles to Constantinople was reduced from six weeks to six days.[14] European steamships came to override traditional shipping routes, multiplying their interport linkages, criss-crossing from the west to the east of the region and beyond.[15] Actually, by 1846, British and French steamships had already forged direct and faster connections with the Black Sea and the Caspian Sea.[16] Subsequently, the opening of the Suez Canal in 1869 radically cut travel time further and condensed the spatial expanses between Europe, the East and India. The voyages from London to Bombay around the Cape of Good Hope, which covered 10,667 nautical miles, and to Hong Kong which travelled a distance of 13,180 nautical miles, were now being made across the Mediterranean and via the Suez Canal, cutting the nautical mileage to 6,274 and 9,799 miles respectively.[17] This continued to raise the volume of shipping and intensify the magnitude of human movement in all its forms:[18] from mass migration, particularly from southern Europe to the Maghreb and the Levant, to the rapid deployment of colonial troops to all corners of the region, to the numbers of Muslim pilgrims – markedly from British India – on their journey to Mecca.[19]

The increased speed of transport not only intensified human mobility and physical contact, it also accelerated the recurrence and transmission of contagious diseases within the region and from one continent to another.[20] Devastating epidemics – not least the plague – had of course been experienced before the nineteenth century,[21] but the speed and ferocity by which plague and, after 1831, cholera were now spreading caught European states unprepared, unable to effectively deal with and prevent them crossing their national frontiers. In the case of cholera, its spread was helped by the growth and speed of technologically-driven commerce, travel and colonial expansion, and the emergence of the ideology and practice of 'free trade'. Up until then, cholera had spread from India into Asia during the 1820s – coming to be known as the first cholera pandemic – but in 1831–32 the disease dispersed[22] in tentacle fashion, via the major travel routes on land, waterways and seas, passing through Russia and thence penetrating Europe, reaching Paris and London in 1832. Leaving a high mortality rate in its trail,[23] this epidemic raised alarm in the European states, creating a general sense of anxiety in their populations.

With the intention of discussing sanitary arrangements and of harmonising quarantine practices in the Mediterranean, the French Government in 1834 tried to convene an international conference, but without success.[24] Subsequently, cholera erupted time and again in epidemical waves, savaging Europe in 1848–49 (and then in 1854 and in the mid 1860s), following which the French Government, fretful about the vulnerability of its extensive national borders on the Mediterranean Sea to such diseases – made worse by its direct colonial contacts with Algeria – once again took the initiative to organise an International Sanitary Conference which this time was successfully convened in 1851.[25] Austria-Hungary, Great Britain, Spain, Portugal, Russia as well as Greece, Sardinia and Tuscany, the Papal states, the Kingdom of the Two Sicilies and the Ottoman Porte, besides France, sent delegates to Paris – from 23 July 1851 to 19 January 1852[26] – for the first international sanitary gathering, which put as its main objective the creation of an interstate mechanism to fight the increasingly rapid transmission of infectious disease[27] before it reached the European borders. European delegates sought to achieve this goal without giving away any of their shipping and commercial advantages or impeding their governments' expansionary designs in the Mediterranean.

However, for these envoys, both diplomats and doctors, the ultimate task of this conference was rendered difficult by the fact that in 1851, as J. Sheldon Watts argues, 'the old-style understanding of cholera was rendered obsolete',[28] as contagionism was being challenged by new miasmal–environmentalist theories, as discussed below. This meant that even though European representatives presented themselves as delegates of the most 'scientifically advanced' and 'civilised' countries, they could not but utter ambiguities, if not acknowledge outright ignorance, regarding the real causes and nature of cholera. In practical terms, they were unsure of how to effectively prevent any outbreaks or abate the accelerated spread of such trans-border pandemics. Moreover, as time passed, deepening conflicts among European nations made negotiations in the ISCs even more convoluted. As from the third ISC of 1866 in Constantinople, which was summoned against mounting rivalry between the European powers for control of the Mediterranean and particularly the Ottoman territories,[29] it became increasingly difficult for delegates to find common positions on various trans-border sanitary issues. The ensuing ISCs saw the European delegations expressing their different quarantine–sanitary views more firmly. The southern Europeans, who usually shared a pro-quarantine position, came under attack from the British representatives for both failing to thwart the spread of epidemics by their restrictive measures, and creating difficulties for commerce and travel.[30] Many of these incompatible positions reflected changing European geo-political concerns in the region, which need to be made clear.

Geo-politics of quarantine: the Mediterranean turned 'passageway' – laboratory

What comes out clearly from the proceedings of most of the ISCs[31] was that the Mediterranean came to be represented as a fluid carrier of contagious disease, and that this representation was framed in part by another representation of it as a a geo-strategic corridor (see Figure 8.1).[32] This means that a Western geo-political view emerged which encapsulated and reproduced deeply entrenched conceptions of the eastern and North African – mostly Ottoman-ruled – lands as disease-ridden and unhygienic, which were a dangerous source of contagious disease that threatened the rest of the Mediterranean and Europe.[33] Certainly the common representation of Egypt as a plague-nurturing terrain[34] and as a principal gateway of cholera from India fell within this Eurocentric view. Supported by an expanding volume of scientific knowledge gathered by European consuls, doctors and hygienists resident in the regional city ports, this geo-strategic perspective came to infuse the diplomatic sanitary discourse of the post-1866 ISCs and especially that of 1885 in Rome.[35] The last was convened as a result of the shocking death rate and social havoc caused by the 1883–87 cholera pandemic, which claimed some 20,000 lives in Spain alone in 1885, and sought to reach an agreement to strengthen the quarantine system by standardising regulations and practices of all lazarettos along the shores of the Mediterranean, the Suez Canal and the Red Sea, in direct communication with the Orient.

Coming around three years after the British acquisition of Egypt, the Rome conference, which was called by two of Britain's rival colonial powers – France and Germany – was marked by a concerted attack against the former for 'not taking seriously' its international obligations to tighten the quarantine system on the route from India to the Suez Canal and Egypt.[36] Such harsh criticism and antagonistic proceedings were these which, although delivered in the latest medico-hygienist parlance, were partly, indeed substantially, prompted by their aggressive rivalry over the Suez Canal area. In any case, similar geo-strategically motivated controversies between British envoys and other European delegates, especially the French, did direct the attention of the ISCs onto the Suez Canal as a shortcut which was accelerating the diffusion of 'Asiatic Cholera' into Europe (Figure 8.1). Hence the twenty-eight delegates attending the 1885 sanitary conference in Rome decided to appoint an independent sanitary board to regulate and oversee the quarantine procedures operated on all maritime vessels passing through the Suez Canal.[37] A similar sanitary board had been proposed by the French in the 1866 conference, but the British had opposed it. Now that they came to control Egypt, the British approved of such an initiative.

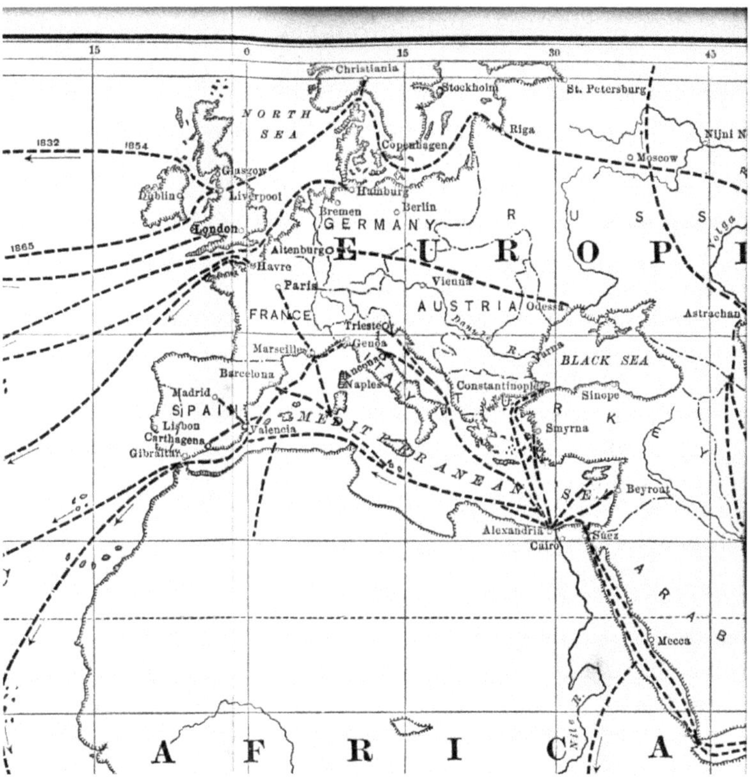

Figure 8.1 Chart of the Mediterranean as a main 'corridor' for the diffusion of cholera.

As a result, this zone came to be described as 'high risk' due to its direct links with the 'Orient', especially with the Hejaz and India that came to be marked red in the geo-epidemiological configuration of the world.[38]

The differences of opinion and positions taken on issues of quarantine among the European delegates at the ISCs were in various shades and measures articulated in two major medical theories – the microbial–contagionist and the miasmatic–environmentalist – which tended to divide the European medical body at the time.[39] On the one hand, the old contagionist medical school held the idea that cholera, like plague, and yellow fever were transmitted through physical contact with already infected human beings, animals and contaminated objects. In this view, the only instrument known to obstruct the spread of such contagious disease was quarantine – the physical segregation or spatial isolation of travellers, the fumigation of their clothes, personal belongings and merchandise – in maritime lazarettos and/or *cordon sanitaires* located on transit routes and access points on land.[40]

Contagionism as a medical philosophy was largely shared by the delegates of the southern European countries[41] – the Italian states, Greece and Spain, as well as Portugal. These, except for the latter, were all Mediterranean riparian states with extensive shipping interests and dense commercial networking with the Ottoman domains.[42] Experiencing rising vulnerability to rapidly transmitted disease, especially cholera, they favoured the maintenance of their quarantine institutions – in various degrees – as either inevitable or as a 'necessary evil'. Most of them pushed for the standardisation of quarantine regulations while trying to balance this with the least possible encumbrance on their shipping and travel activities. At a domestic level, the governments also feared that outbreaks of epidemics could instigate outbursts of popular rebellion,[43] and were therefore determined to maintain quarantine to keep disease out of their borders, to serve as a means of social control and to maintain public order. Quarantine stations and procedures also marked the crossing of a country's national frontiers and therefore helped to promote a collective feeling of national security. Hence it was feared that any act which could be perceived as intended to demolish lazarettos or quarantine stations could trigger social panic from sectors of the population and fuel political opposition.[44] This despite the fact that on numerous occasions it was quarantine itself – especially the cordoning of whole neighbourhoods or communities – which often created resentment and exacerbated social discontent in different countries,

All in all, the need to strengthen and regulate the increasing number of quarantine stations along the Mediterranean littoral with a uniform code of practice seemed to be the most pragmatic solution at hand for the governments in the region.[45] In truth many public health officials in Mediterranean Europe were not eager to experiment with sanitary measures that excluded the lazaretto institution, which, to their minds, was the only instrument that was proven to provide a realistic degree of protection against the infiltration of contagious disease through their national borders. These positions by and large usually conformed to those taken by the French delegations at the ISCs. Being a leading European power with an extensive Mediterranean coast and with huge trade, political and colonial interests in the region, France took an 'exemplary' pragmatic stand which held on to quarantine as a 'necessary evil', seeking to regulate and standardise its quarantine regulations and practices without hindering free-trade circulation. This even though some of the delegates themselves became increasingly sceptical of its worth in preventing epidemics.[46]

Elaborating on this solidly pragmatic platform, most of the European delegates attending the sanitary conferences granted that the lazaretto system, if regulated by them and extended to cover the southern and eastern rims of the Mediterranean, could develop a prophylactic barrier against the diffusion of plague, cholera and other contagious diseases before any of these reached the European borders. Quarantine continued to be operated even by the British in their Mediterranean domains where these were long-established practices. Being the most vociferous exponents of anti-quarantine policies internationally, the British were in a slow and piecemeal fashion relaxing, and by mid century rarely implementing, quarantine on their national territory.[47] On the other hand, by continuing to operate and actually consolidating the long-standing lazarettos in its network of colonial ports – which were known to be the strictest in the region[48] – Britain assured that its commercial ships were not denied pratique from other Mediterranean ports. Home-bound shipping from the East and North Africa underwent strict quarantine in one of its ports – usually either Malta or Gibraltar[49] or Corfu in the Ionian islands (up until 1864) – from where vessels carrying the British flag obtained a clean bill of health which enabled them to proceed directly to any regional/European port 'unhindered'.[50] In this way, the British sought to abide by their quarantine obligations – so deeply entrenched in Mediterranean shipping and port practices – while still adhering to an anticontagionist sanitary policy,[51] and without obstructing their international trade, shipping activities and travel. This pragmatism was lambasted as thoroughly inconsistent by uncompromising adherents of the miasmatic anticontagionist medical school, such as the editor of *The Boston Medical and Surgical Journal* who did not mince words to present Britain's quarantine practices in its Mediterranean ports as 'hyprocritical':

> England is as deeply in the mire as the Papal and Neapolitan governments, in regard to Malta and the Ionian Islands. How the minister of foreign affairs could play the hypocrite, without blushing to confusion, in sanctioning the movement of the General Board of Health, by sending a representative to Paris, is quite unaccountable.[52]

On the other hand, miasmatic environmentalism as a medical theory attributed the transmission of cholera and other contagious diseases to atmospheric pollution – foul air and climate – as well as contaminated water, decaying matter and putrescence which directly infected the body.[53] Propped up by accumulating scientific evidence, this miasmatic medical theory rejected quarantine measures as unwarranted and instead promoted regulated sanitation, cleanliness of the environment and personal hygiene.[54] Such anticontagionist philosophy was in harmony with Britain's 'free-trade' and 'open-sea' ideology. It was in Britain – more than in any other country – that the merchants' lobby, arguing that trade was bearing the brunt of quarantine restrictions, appealed to their government to abandon or at least radically prune such quarantine measures.[55] Antiquarantinism gained extensive influence in Britain due to the ties forged between prevailing trade, shipping and financial interests and the state's geo-strategic–imperial ventures around the globe.

In addition, because the aerial–miasmatic theory was environmentally based and hence solidly terrestrial, it came to be embroiled with the expansionary projects of the powerful colonial lobby. Identifying cholera and plague, together with diseases such as 'sleeping sickness' and schistosomiasis, as 'tropical diseases' and locating them in the 'hot climates' of extra-European lands, miasmatic theory was employed to assist colonial intervention in these territories as part of a self-proclaimed civilising mission imposed on indigenous people.[56] A case in point was the already mentioned contemporary association of plague with Egypt's climatic–environmental conditions – most emphatically with those 'endemically' found in the Nile Valley[57] – which in miasmatic terminology constituted the ideal ground for the eruption of contagious disease.[58] Keeping this contagion under control purportedly required the specialised assistance of Western sanitation and medical knowledge. From this miasmatic–environmentalist perspective, the principal cause of the outbreak and diffusion of cholera came to be linked with contaminated water in 'backward lands', as argued by the highly influential *British Medical Journal* in August 1893: 'the pollution of the wells at Mecca is the chief agent in the dissemination of cholera [...] water alone is the medium through which the pestilence spreads.'[59]

This quote exemplifies the political orientation which by the 1890s was taken by the miasmatic–environmentalists and which implicated them with British – and indeed European – imperial intervention in various parts of the globe.[60] Deeply influencing British medical thinking and public health practice, the aerial–miasmatic theory of epidemics was carried by the physicians and sanitarians who were despatched in the 'tropical colonies', that is, on the frontline of colonial expansion, and in our case in the East and North African territories.[61] In 1854–55, this medical philosophy had been given credit by John Snow's (1813–58) findings that cholera was – as later echoed in the above quotation – transmitted by drinking contaminated water.[62] Snow's discovery had been positively received by delegates attending the second ISC of 1859 which appointed an international board of physicians tasked with using data from these findings to investigate the link between atmospheric and environmental factors and the incubation and transmission of contagious disease in North Africa and the East. However, by 1884 Robert Koch (1843–1910) came out with a bacteriological explanation of cholera by identifying the cholera *comma bacillus*,[63] and came to emphasise the importance of quarantine in abating the proliferation of such epidemics. Koch's participation in the Rome conference spurred a rigorous scientifically informed discussion on the aetiology and transmission of cholera and the possible ways of preventing its diffusion, even though many medical specialists remained convinced that the *vibrio cholerae bacillus* was not the *cause* but the *product* of the disease. Yet again, Robert Koch's theory of the cholera microorganism was followed by another explanation provided by the German medic and hygienist Max von Pettenkofer (1818–1901), who argued that cholera could only be contagious under specific environmental conditions. Disagreeing with Koch's thesis that the *comma bacillus* was the only factor producing the disease,[64] Pettenkofer demonstrated that cholera showed contagious and miasmatic features. He proposed personal hygiene, home cleanliness and sanitary education to combat its diffusion.

In the imperialist climate generated during the last quarter of the nineteenth century, scientific–medical findings were appropriated by the colonial lobbies, which applied them to the idea of the civilising mission to provide the cultural, civil and moral justification for European intervention in non-European lands, most of which were under Ottoman control. Medical theories came to be more specifically employed in the colonial construction of the 'Arab Muslims' as potential carriers of contagion and their countries as 'disease-ridden' which required immediate sanitisation. In this colonising, Eurocentric discourse, the controversies initiated by the medical discoveries – which have historically proved essential for improvement in biomedicine[65] – were glossed over, while attention was directed onto the alleged 'contagious threat' coming from the Muslim *Hajj*.

The Mediterranean: Europe's imperial medical archive and 'prophylactic'

The urge to collect epidemiological information – through new medical specialisations such as medical topography – 'from source', and its processing and archiving in the metropolis (as in Paris and London), gained impetus following the first cholera epidemic in Europe. Physicians and sanitarians, many of whom were usually sent by their government or medical institutions to conduct research work on the spot, ended up advising local regimes and being involved in the design and implementation of public sanitary institutions. A number of these foreign resident doctors and sanitary advisors, merchants and consuls, conjointly with native physicians and state functionaries, were appointed by local authorities to sit on new sanitary councils – or boards of quarantine – created in the various ports of Turkey, Egypt, the Ottoman regencies and Morocco. As such these sanitary councils served as sites of negotiation between these European agents and their local counterparts, while charged with the construction and sharing of the management of lazarettos and other public health institutions in their resident city ports. It stands to reason that, therefore, these sanitary councils came to mirror the competing trade, political and colonial interests of each of their European members' nations, as much as echoing the varying claims made by native medics and public health officials.

On a sanitary level, these boards gave rise to dialogue – which nevertheless became ever more one-sided and dominated by Europeans – between the indigenous medical–sanitary traditions and the increasingly influential European medical theories and sanitary practices. On one occasion, Lord Ponsonby, acting as British ambassador to Constantinople, opposing the stricter quarantine regulations recently imposed, and drawing from miasmatic–environmental theories of epidemics, argued that quarantine was of no avail against the spread of contagious diseases. The ambassador further expressed his worries that despite the official assurances given by the Ottoman Capitulations, the new sanitary regulations empowered Turkish health officials to search the private homes of British subjects. In a letter to the Ottoman authorities in January 1839, Ponsonby declared himself strongly 'averse to these measures'.[66] Epidemics, he contended, could only be combated effectively 'by introducing cleanliness and ventilation in Constantinople', and not by restrictive quarantine. In a similar vein, anticontagionist miasmatic theories were frequently voiced by trade and shipping representatives within – and from outside – the sanitary councils, in support of appeals to abolish or at least reduce quarantine restrictions to the lowest possible. Frequently, merchants, supported by their consular representatives, many of whom were in business partnerships themselves,[67] came to be involved in the nationalistic agendas of their own governments. This complicated negotiations and hindered the taking of decisions and the carrying out of specific quarantine measures, regulations and procedures in their respective ports.

The first of such sanitary boards was set up in 1828 by Muhammad Ali (1805–48), the de facto ruler of an 'independent' Egypt – which came to occupy the Ottoman provinces of Syria and Cilicia (1831–40) – who was much influenced by Western European and especially French sanitary practices.[68] The 'quarantine board' set up in Alexandria was commissioned to establish a quarantine station to supervise its operations and to issue bills of health.[69] Also referred to as *Commission Consulaire de Santé* (Consular Commission for Health), this board included 'foreign' European doctors, sanitary technicians and consular representatives who rubbed shoulders with their Egyptian counterparts, giving it an international character. Apart from the one at Alexandria, other quarantine stations came to be built along the coast of Egyptian-ruled lands: one in Damietta, another one in Rosetta in 1831,[70] and four years later in Beirut to filter maritime traffic passing from Syrian ports.[71] In 1837, another sanitary board was founded with the task of creating a lazaretto to quarantine ships passing through the Bosporus.

By this time, the Ottoman Porte itself had taken the initiative to construct its own quarantine stations and thus extend the regional chain of lazarettos along the eastern rim of the Mediterranean and beyond the Bosporus. Actually, in 1836 the *Meclis-i Kebir-i Umur u Sihhiye* (Superior Council of Health) was founded at Constantinople, made up of eight Ottoman representatives and nine 'foreign' (European) physicians living in the city together with five representatives of foreign embassies.[72] As well as being handed the task of setting up a lazaretto, this Council was in charge of formulating 'modern' public health regulations and supervising their implementation in that city port. Presented as part of the *Tanzimat*[73] – the process of modernisation through the reorganisation of the Ottoman State – initiated by Sultan Mahmud II, supported by the Ottoman ruling elites, the new Superior Council of Health led to the building of quarantine establishments and infection hospitals in Turkey itself and in its neighbouring domains. By 1840, the Porte was able to pass a series of so-called quarantine 'organic regulations', which were compiled by the Council, to regulate all lazarettos under its control,[74] starting with that in Constantinople and including two stations located on the sea passages into Anatolia and Rumelia.

Concurrently with the setting up of sanitary boards and lazarettos in Turkey and its eastern possessions, other quarantine stations were being established in the North African ports, starting with that of Tunis in 1835.[75] Five years later, in 1840, the Sultan of Morocco formed a Sanitary Council which was to advise on the preventive measures to be applied against the importation of epidemics, including the need to construct a lazaretto which, together with the one in British-Gibraltar, would greatly assist the policing and filtering of the traffic flow through the western entry of the Mediterranean. Although varying in their lazaretto procedures and regulations, with some of the establishments considered operationally volatile, by the 1850s the principle of quarantining ships to prevent the spread of contagious diseases along the main routes came to be accepted by most Arab-Muslim governments in the Mediterranean.

During the fifteen years or so preceding the first ISC in 1851, these sanitary councils not only operated as negotiation sites of an international character, and as advisors and designers of quarantine establishments to the local administrations, but also served as information gathering centres. A large volume of the knowledge – of an epidemiological and sanitary nature – collected by these sanitary councils was to be tabled in the ISCs, in support of the many European delegates' proposals to standardise international quarantine regulations.[76] Most of this qualitative and quantitative data – packaged as scientific evidence – was despatched to, and processed in, European medical archives by consuls and physicians sitting on the several quarantine boards, as well as by explorers, colonial scientists and travelling scholars. These gathered all sorts of medical–sanitary knowledge, tabulated statistics, drew reports,[77] chartered disease-prone or 'ideal' breeding grounds of specific contagious disease and mapped regional–global epidemic routes. One eminent medical scientist was Robert Koch, who in 1883 went on an expedition in Egypt to investigate the aetiology of plague, sending back reports on a country which, as already noted, was considered a principal breeding ground of 'tropical disease'.[78] All in all, the scientific–medical investigations which researchers, physicians, medical topographers and others conducted in these territories were framed within, and reproduced, their own European medical and public health theories. Ostensibly objective and ideologically neutral, these theories of epidemics were frequently swathed in racial and ethnic presumptions of Western 'civilised superiority' over the non-European natives – in this case 'the Arabs'. This, of course, illustrates the extent to which European medical science was infused by the 'imperial spirit of the era'.[79] Having been collated and methodically organised in European medical archives, this knowledge was, as Thomas Richards argues, 'enlisted into the service of the Empire', and together with other emerging fields of expertise – like biology and geography – came 'to function as an extension of the imperial project'.[80]

Along with their gathering and despatching of information, as well as their direct involvement in the setting-up and administration of lazarettos, European consuls, traders and physicians came to take over a rising share of responsibilities over the domestic public health, which had previously lain in native and Ottoman hands. This in turn significantly boosted their influence on sectors of the local ruling elites and the state authorities. By supervising and administering quarantine procedures, they gained increasing control of entries and exits of these countries' coastal borders. Such transfer of decision-making power from local to 'foreign' hands reflected and sustained the ongoing informal colonial penetration,[81] which would eventually lead to the subjugation of these countries to Western European supremacy.[82] What happened in Tunisia can be taken as a case in point. Protesting against the restrictions imposed by the local authorities on vessels entering port to stop cholera, but which also disrupted British and European commercial activities,[83] resident foreign consuls and merchants solicited to be involved in any other decisions regarding quarantine arrangements in the regency. Consequently, a number of them were called by the Bey to form a new sanitary council in charge of formulating quarantine regulations.[84] This, of course, provided them with greater power leverage.[85] Decisions taken in the Tunis sanitary council and on the other sanitary boards in North Africa would in the long term have deep politico-economic effects – which were similar to the impact left by the Ottoman Capitulations – facilitating colonial infiltration and hastening the collapse of the Ottoman Empire.[86]

Actually, the regulations and codes of procedure adopted by the sanitary councils for local lazarettos, which were then elaborated and standardised by the ISCs and applied to the quarantine stations,[87] privileged trade vessels flying European flags and their merchandise over those from Egypt and the Ottoman ports.[88] The hierarchical classification of persons, merchandise and ships adopted in these lazarettos – indicating the intensity of disinfection and the required duration of quarantine according to their specific degree of 'contagiousness' – was determined by their declared 'origins'.[89] By and large, inward ships originating from 'Arab' ports and carrying indigenous products were marked as 'highly infective' and had to pass through stricter and lengthier quarantine procedures. Such classification encoded an essentialist bipolarity in which European 'white bodies' as well as their merchandise and vessels were unambiguously associated with outright cleanliness, while 'Muslim'/'Arab'/'Ottoman' bodies, products and ships were considered in various degrees as contagious. A standard scheme of classification was – through the work of the sanitary councils and the ISCs – transferred and structured in the regulations and operations of North African and Levantine lazarettos. Taking the Beirut lazaretto as example, a three-tier classification was adopted here: 'healthy European'; 'suspect Egyptian, Syrian and Greek'; and 'contaminated Ottoman'.[90] In the southern European lazarettos – such as British-controlled Gibraltar, Malta and Corfu[91] – quarantine procedures were carried out according to a scale of 'contagiousness' (or 'contamination') which listed ships, products and persons from Egypt and Ottoman ports as 'highly susceptible epidemic carriers', having to endure the strictest segregation and the most meticulous disinfection procedures in 'normal circumstances'.[92] This contrasted with the 'lighter treatment' and shorter quarantine duration awaiting British and other northwestern European crews, travellers, their vessels and their merchandise, especially those arriving directly from European ports.

Constructing the 'threatening' 'contagious' Arab

The setting up of lazarettos and quarantine systems in Ottoman and other city ports around the Mediterranean was presented as an act of European 'enlightenment' or of colonial 'benevolence', and considered by the native elites as instruments of 'modernisation' for their countries. As with the sanitary councils, the quarantine lazarettos functioned also as sites for European–'native' talks, negotiation and collaboration. In due course, however, they came to assert Western self-proclaimed scientific–medical superiority over the Arab populations who, it was claimed, if left to their natural inclinations would spend their 'barbaric existence' in foul, disease-ridden conditions.[93] Such contemptuous, inherently racist, attitudes and discourse against 'native Arabs' were expressed, visualised and circulated by the popular press and other genres of literature in Europe, and seeped into political and diplomatic parlance. Hence the condescending treatment of Arabs and Muslims in general, and of the Ottoman Porte in particular, as observed in the proceedings of the ISCs. A *British Medical Journal* article published a couple of months before the start of the 1894 ISC held in Paris illustrates such self-proclaimed European supremacy in no uncertain terms:

> The problem, indeed, is full of complexity […] It must not be forgotten, however, that in this Meccan business the Porte is the central figure, and that whatever any conference may decide will be of but small avail so long as the sultan remains passive. For any real progress we must look to the self-interest of the Mohammedans themselves.[94]

A narrative went that 'Arabs' – often disparagingly referred to as 'Mohammedians', as in the above quote – were so incompetent that they were unable to progress in the field of hygiene and sanitisation which, it was believed, contrasted with their cultural traditions, customs and way of life. 'Arabs' were stereotyped as lazy, dirty,[95] disease-carrying, disordered bodies, and as such comprised an enduring negative and 'threatening' image in colonial ideology and the European collective imagination.[96] Often modelled on the imagined figure of the *fellahin* as prototype, Arabs were depicted as slow moving, leading unproductive lives, overwhelmed by an enervating climate, and thus unadaptable to the accelerated rhythm of an ordered life,[97] considered to be a principal feature of 'modernity' characterising Western civilisation. In the different genres of European literature produced at the time, Arab countries and their predominantly Muslim populations were imagined, as Edward Said puts it, as a 'decrepit carcass awaiting his [European] restorative efforts'. The Oriental Arab had, according to this narrative, fallen 'into a savage state', with a 'civilization, religion and manners […] so low, barbaric, and antithetical as to merit reconquest'.[98]

This portrayal of the Arabs as unhygienic and disease-carrying bodies was superimposed on, and meshed with, the politically constructed representation of the Turkish Empire and the Porte itself as the 'Sick Man of Europe'.[99] This well-known label has historically been attributed to Tsar Nicholas I just before the outbreak of the Crimean War in 1853, when referring to the inability of the Sublime Porte to hold together its vast domains. 'We have a sick man on our hands, a man who is seriously sick,'[100] the Tsar was reported to have stated by G.H. Seymour, British ambassador at St Petersburg, in his correspondence to Lord Russell.[101] The image quickly percolated into political–diplomatic discourse during the course of the long debate on the Eastern Question. Recurring waves of so called 'Oriental', 'Asiatic' and 'Arabic' pestilential epidemics of cholera and plague – which devastated continental Europe, Britain and America during this same period – seemed to affirm these negative conceptions of the Arabs and of the Sublime Porte. For the remaining crises-laden period of the Eastern Question, that ran from the Crimean War to the First World War, the image of the 'Sick Man' characterised as infective, decrepit, terminally ill, continued to be used to represent the weak political state of the Sublime Porte and its crumbling empire in European literature and journals.[102] This portrayal intermeshed with the personification of cholera and plague as essentially 'Arab', which in turn reproduced the perception of the 'Arab-Muslim[s]' as threatening bodies (both in terms of contagious disease and political instability) that needed to be restrained and kept out of the European borders.

In real terms, in as much as the Porte was visualised as politically moribund – a 'very sick man' – it was kept on 'life support' by the Concert of Europe[103] (the alliance between the European Powers between 1814–1914), while the task of protecting the European borders from epidemics emanating from this 'insalubrious' body was given to the ISCs. With the Turkish state perceived as being unable to hold together its vast domains, and hopelessly incapable of implementing political and sanitary 'reforms', it lay with the 'enlightened' Europeans – as part of their self-proclaimed civilising mission – to intervene with their hygienist instruments, to do so. As *The British Medical Journal* put it:

> Since Turkey refuses to put her house in order, it is clearly the duty of the civilized world to take such steps as may be necessary to compel her to do so [...] From every point of view the Turkish authorities are to blame; and it is almost incredible that Europe should allow a state of things to exist which is manifestly fraught with peril to the commonweal.[104]

The use of hygienist interventionism – based on modern scientific sanitary–medical knowledge and technology – to drive the wider project of civilising the allegedly 'backward' Arabs,[105] gained impetus in the 1870s, with the creation of medical specialisms such as 'tropical medicine' – which dealt with diseases such as malaria, schistosomiasis and plague – in the chief European medical institutions. These were being utilised, as Roy Porter put it, in 'the spirit of the era of imperialism [by the great powers] battling to settle the "Less Civilized" parts of the globe'.[106] Such hygienist strategies were shaped by a Eurocentric bipolar vista – which posed the 'civilised Western Europeans' against the 'uncivilised Arabs' – that seeped into mainstream political discourse and articulated much of the proceedings of the ISCs from 1851 to 1894. With the opening of the Suez Canal in 1869, the principle destination of worship for Muslims – Mecca – was brought much closer in travel time to Europe. As much as it emerged as a highly strategic 'open nerve' in the European powers' – especially the British – global lines of communication,[107] the Suez Canal also came to be marked as a main passageway accelerating the diffusion of cholera into Europe. This prompted the European states to set up an interborder sanitary mechanism for the vigilance and filtering of traffic passing through the Canal and into the Mediterranean body of seas. Most sanitarians agreed that this objective could only be achieved by consolidating and standardising all quarantine stations into a prophylactic network covering the Mediterranean littoral, the Red Sea and beyond. Driven by this hygienist objective, from the late 1860s lazaretto establishments took on a sharper biopolitical *modus operandi*: physically restraining, segregating, clinically observing and disinfecting 'Arab Muslims' and other 'alien' bodies perceived as potentially contagious and 'threatening', before these could 'infect' the traffic flows on the major travel routes and lifelines of communication across the Mediterranean into Europe.

Quarantine measures on 'Arab-Muslim' bodies on the move were actually intensified following the outbreak of an epidemic during the *Hajj* of 1865.[108] This prompted European doctors, hygienists and politicians to point specifically to the Hejaz as a major incubation ground – a '*cholera nidus*' – and conveyor of this contagious disease into Europe.[109] In truth, this cholera epidemic came – as it did earlier – to be transmitted from India to Mecca, killing 30,000 solely at the Hejaz; it then savagely spread into Anatolia from where it penetrated Europe taking a heavy toll of 200,000 persons in the major cities that it hit. From then onwards, in the sanitary discourse and practice which came to dominate public health institutions around Europe, particularly in France, Muslim pilgrims came to be labelled as liable vectors of pestilential diseases. The French Government, alarmed by the growing numbers of pilgrims returning from Mecca to North Africa,[110] with whom there was uninterrupted intercourse – especially through Algeria under their colonial administration – took the initiative to call a third ISC in 1866.[111]

Mirroring the strong political–hygienist intentions behind its convening, this third ISC was organised in Constantinople, the seat of the Ottoman Porte that ruled over and was accountable for the Hejaz. While India was indicated straightaway as the 'home of cholera', with the Indian Government being advised to impose strict quarantine on pilgrims, the focus of attention shifted to the *Hajj*, the Hejaz and Mecca itself as European delegates pressed for a plan to regulate the clustering of pilgrims there and to sanitise this territory.[112] One main proponent of this hygienist strategy was the French delegate Dr Sulpice-Antoine Fauvel (1813–84), who bid the Ottoman Porte to dispatch a sanitary commission to the Hejaz to thoroughly investigate the real state of public health and of the pilgrims amassing there.[113] Demanding that the Porte take tangible action in 'its own domains' reflected the disparaging treatment the latter was receiving from most of the European delegates. These shared the belief that Turkey was incapable of taking seriously its international responsibilities of surveillance and sanitisation of the Hejaz, in addition to overseeing and disciplining the pilgrimages.

The identification of 'contagiousness' with Muslim pilgrims overcrowding Mecca[114] was further sustained by the repeated epidemic outbreaks reported in this area and which led to the convening of other ISCs. Hence, for instance, the 1872 cholera that erupted in the Hejaz and rapidly diffused into Egypt, where it took some 60,000 lives in three months before spreading further into Europe and reaching America, raised alarm in most governments and led to the calling of the fourth ISC in Vienna in July 1874. This conference was marked by 'scientifically informed' talks between envoys to find the most practical course to incisively intervene to filter all traffic – mainly, though not only, through lazarettos – passing from the Suez Canal zone and the Hejaz.[115] Nevertheless, it took until 1893 – with the eighth ISC in Dresden – for delegates to reach an agreement to secure a regulated standardisation of procedures in all lazaretto stations around the Mediterranean and on the major routes to Mecca. Subsequently, the Ottoman authorities, overseen by European hygienists, were obliged to rigorously enforce specific quarantine practices – including disinfection procedures on pilgrims – and execute social discipline in the Hejaz and all ports of embarkation en route to and from Mecca. Strict hygienist measures on individual Muslim bodies at these ports were further intensified by the eleventh ISC held in Paris in 1903, which was convened a year after another cholera epidemic had erupted during the *Hajj*.[116] This conference appointed a sanitary commission made up of foremost hygienists to supervise the carrying out of sanitary procedures and other preventive measures on location as well as distribute medicine in a concerted way:

> to regulate the pilgrim traffic in the Red Sea and Persian Gulf, with the view of preventing the importation of cholera to Mecca, and its dissemination thence along the track of the returning *hajjis*.[117]

One enduring effect left by this series of ISCs was the marking of the chief trajectories of the Muslim pilgrimage to Mecca as 'infective routes' of cholera into Europe and, by association, of the Arab-Muslims as vectors of such epidemics. This corroborated the deeply rooted stereotyped image of the 'Muslim-Arab' pilgrim which, as argued above, had been in circulation through Orientalist literature[118] – mainly in travellers' accounts, but also in works on medical topography and other 'scientific' narratives – which depicted the Hejaz as 'barren and retarded.'[119] Echoing this growing aversion towards Muslims in Europe was the French hygienist Adrien Proust (1834–1903), when in 1873 he wrote that Europeans were 'every year, at the mercy of the pilgrimage to Mecca.'[120] By this he was conveying the state of mind of most other European sanitarians, doctors and diplomats who held Mecca and the *Hajj* accountable for the breeding and transmission of the scourge of cholera in Europe. The article published in the authoritative *The British Medical Journal* on the 26 August 1893 is typical of this widely spread feeling in Europe:

> As long as the Hedjaz remains a closed book to the hygienic world, so long shall we be in danger [...] It is intolerable in the nineteenth century that fanaticism should be allowed to close the doors to all humanising influences throughout a vast territory [...] Is it not time that life in Paris and London were protected against the Old Coprophagan, the dirt-eating Death that abides at Mecca? Self-preservation is the first law of Nature. The Hadji must permit the setting of his house in order, or the Haj must not go on.[121]

By this time, the prophylactic chain of lazarettos stretching along the northern and southern Mediterranean coasts and the Suez Canal had been extended to the Red Sea and Persian Gulf to cover the length of the main passageways to Mecca. By 1885, two quarantine stations were set up in Jeddah and Yambo, while others had already been built on Perim Island in 1866 and on Kamaran Island in 1881. In this Kamaran establishment, for example, all disembarking Muslim pilgrims were treated 'as infected' and passed through a meticulous disinfection of their bodies, with their clothes and all other personal belongings being systematically 'fumigated'.[122] These painstaking and lengthy sanitary procedures became increasingly burdensome to, and negatively perceived by, the Muslim pilgrims and other travellers. All strict hygienist measures practised at the ports of departure for Mecca – particularly those decided upon at the 1894 Paris ISC – stretched the quarantine period for 'pilgrimage boats' from five to ten days, and thus led to substantial delays in the *Hajj*, creating wide-ranging disgruntlement.

In addition, the policing of the principal pilgrimage routes to Mecca[123] was tightened by procedures which responded to the general perceptions and fears of the 'Muslim-Arabs'.[124] In the chief ports of embarkation, the latter were to pass through a filtering process which selected those who could proceed on their pilgrimage according to their socio-economic status. This was based on the logic that wealthy pilgrims would be better equipped to travel in 'hygienic conditions' and to thus avoid contracting and transmitting disease. Still, selectivity according to one's wealth or social status went against Islamic teaching, which advocated opportunities for every 'able bodied Muslim', poor or wealthy, to accomplish the *Hajj* once in a lifetime.[125] The option thus left for the poor, who did not possess the officially demanded means to travel rapidly to the Ka'ba in Mecca and back, was the traditional and much slower journey on land and across the desert. In a way this long voyage served as an incubation period for any contagious disease to appear, with pilgrims who contracted cholera or plague usually falling ill and/or dying before their arrival. Then again, in all the quarantine stations, Muslim pilgrims had to undergo rigorous disinfection, including undressing 'in open space' – a practice which was felt to be debasing, particularly when it involved Muslim women.[126] Such routine sanitary procedures came to vindicate the fixed European identification of all 'Muslims'/'Arabs' as menacing bodies, needing to be socially disciplined, disinfected and subdued into 'modernity'.

Conclusion

By the second half of the nineteenth century, quarantine came to be deeply implicated with European colonial expansion in the Mediterranean basin. The numerous lazarettos which were established on the North African and the Eastern coasts of the region were designed by Europeans, and then operated on the Western sanitary quarantine model, with the guidelines, regulations and procedures set by the International Sanitary Conferences and expedited by European consuls, physicians and sanitary officials/hygienists on the spot. Many of these European agents had also served on – and actually patronised – the handful of boards of health (or quarantine boards) earlier established in some of these same ports and consequently came to act as advisors and administrators of the lazarettos which they had assisted to set up.

The ensuing network of lazarettos accompanied, and actually gave impetus to, the creeping economic penetration and ascending political hegemony of the European powers which gradually started to give way, in various degrees, to formal colonial rule – a process which hastened the disintegration of an already weak Ottoman Empire. Against such a complicated geo-political scenario, intensified by hostile intra-European imperial rivalry, the lazarettos, acclaimed as vital public health institutions, came to function as powerful instruments which vetted the bulk of the shipping traffic and led to the consolidation of new imperial steamship and communication routes. Concurrently, lazarettos served as nodal colonial sites, abetting the European powers' imperial expansion in multiple ways and means, including the use of elaborate institutional procedures and reconfiguring of a discourse (using modern medical–sanitary phraseology) and practices which endorsed the colonial subjection of 'native' Arabs as an 'inferior race'.

Most lazarettos located on the southern and eastern coasts of the Middle Sea and – following the opening of the Suez Canal in 1869 – on the major maritime routes to the Orient/India, fell directly under European surveillance and control. These came increasingly to be regulated and driven to operate on prefixed sanitary regulations and standardised practices issued and imposed by the series of international conventions and sanitary commissions ensuing from the ISCs. This chapter argues that with the construction of such a network of lazarettos, spread along the major seaways crossing the Mediterranean to India and the 'Orient', the European powers were assured of a frontline prophylactic barrier against the diffusion of contagious disease – especially cholera – into Europe. Narrowing down analysis on the actual quarantine procedures used in these lazarettos it has been shown how, through these fixed regulations and a selective code of practice, maritime quarantine favoured and facilitated European shipping, trade and travel, as much as it hindered 'Arab', 'Ottoman' mercantile ships, travellers and crews arriving from North African and Levantine ports. Standing quarantine rules compelled non-European vessels and travellers to undergo stricter and much lengthier detention, isolation and hygienist procedures. This proved to be a thoroughly discriminatory treatment which further intensified the unequal trade relations in the region in as much as it consolidated the European states' rising control over international maritime traffic and commerce.

This chapter has also explored the use of Western medical theories – articulated in pro- anti- or middle-of-the-way quarantinist positions – examining how these came to be entangled in the colonial discourse of the civilising mission, which nourished a racist sense of supremacy over purportedly 'inferior' Arabs. New and older medical/hygienist theories came to validate lazaretto practices based on a fixed hierarchy of classification which labelled as 'highly contagious' (or 'highly susceptible to epidemic disease') Arab and Ottoman vessels, merchandise, but most importantly persons. In practice this meant that these people had to undergo highly restrictive, heavily protracted and rigorous hygienist measures including the much-detested ritual of undressing and disinfection/fumigation. As such the lazaretto exercised strong biopolitical restrictions on Arab bodies, not only deterring their movement but elaborating, and continuously reproducing, the stereotyped image of the 'dirty' and 'contagious' Muslim-Arab – especially those on the annual *Hajj* to Mecca – as a 'threat' to public health, social order and Western civilisation.

Notes

1 Daniel R. Headrick, *The Tools of Empire: Technology and European Imperialism in the Nineteenth Century*, New York, Oxford University Press, 1981, 148–149.

2 Barbara Bush, *Imperialism and Postcolonialism*, Harlow, Pearson Educ. Ltd., 2006; J.N. Hays, *The Burdens of Disease. Epidemics and Human Response in Western History*, New Jersey-London, Rutgers University

Press, 2009, 179–186; John and Jean Comaroff, *Ethnography and the Historical Imagination*, Boulder Colorado, Westview Press, 1992, 215–235; John Chircop, 'Pax Britannica and "Free Trade and Open Seas": shifting British informal colonialism in North Africa, 1800–1860s', *Mediterranean Review* 8, 1, 2015, 29–57.

3 For the relationship between formal and informal empire building, see Bernard Porter, *The Lion's Share. A Short History of British Imperialism, 1850–1983*, London and New York, Longman, 1994, 8–12.

4 David Arnold, 'Introduction: Disease, Medicine and Empire', in D. Arnold (ed.), *Imperial Medicine and Indigenous Societies*, Manchester, Manchester University Press, 1988, 7–8; Pratik Chakrabarti, *Medicine & Empire 1600–1960*, London, Palgrave Macmillan, 2014, 57 and *passim*.

5 Norman Howard Jones, *The Scientific Background of the International Sanitary Conferences, 1851–1839*, Geneva, WHO, 1975; Mark Harrison, 'Disease, diplomacy and international commerce: the origins of international sanitary regulations in the nineteenth century', *Journal of Global History* 1, 2006, 197–217.

6 Aginam Obijiofor, 'The nineteenth century colonial fingerprints on public health diplomacy: a postcolonial view', *Law, Social Justice and Global Development* (2003) 1, 7–8; David F. Fidler, 'The globalization of public health: the first 100 years of international health diplomacy', *Bulletin of the World Health Organization* 79/9, 2001, 842; Valeska Huber, 'The unification of the globe by disease? The International Sanitary Conferences and cholera 1851–1894', *The Historical Journal* 49, 2006, 453–476.

7 Peter Baldwin, *Contagion and the State in Europe, 1830–1930*, Cambridge, Cambridge University Press, 2005.

8 In Foucaultian terms, lazarettos can be seen as 'enclosed functional sites' (Michel Foucault, *Discipline and Punish: The Birth of the Prison*, Middlesex, Penguin, 1991, 143–144).

9 For the deeply rooted negative stereotyping of the 'Arab' and the 'Turk' in the European imagination, see Ann Thompson, *Barbary and Enlightenment. European Attitudes towards the Maghreb in the 18th Century*, Leiden, E.J. Brill, 1987.

10 Headrick, *The Tools of Empire*.

11 France had already occupied Algeria in 1830 and in 1881 Tunisia. Britain gained Cyprus in 1878 and Egypt in 1882 – apart from its control of Gibraltar (from 1705), Malta as from 1800, and the Ionian Islands from 1814 to 1864.

12 Huber, 'The unification of the globe by disease?', 453–476.

13 On the integration of the various ports of the Mediterranean in the world economic system, see R. Kasaba, C. Keyder and F. Tabak,

'Eastern Mediterranean port cities and their bourgeoisies: merchants, political projects and nation states', *F. Braudel Review* X, 1, 1986, 121–135.

14 Yrio Kaukiainen, 'Shrinking the world: improvements in the speed of information transmission, c. 1820–1870', *European Review of Economic History* 5, 2001, 17–18, 26–29.

15 See David Haworth and Stephen Haworth, *The Story of the P & O. The Peninsular and Oriental Steam Navigation Company*, London, Weidenfeld & Nicolson, 1986, 32–36.

16 J.M. Wagdoff, *The Evolution of Middle Eastern Landscapes. An Outline to A.D., 1840*, Kent, Croom Helm, 2001, p. 235; Kaukiainen, 'Shrinking the world', 1–28. See also E.J. Hobsbawm, *The Age of Capital, 1848–1875*, London, Weidenfeld & Nicolson, 1985, 69–76.

17 *The Peninsular & Oriental Pocket Book*, London, 1879.

18 H.E. Fletcher, 'The Suez and world shipping in 1869–1914', *The Journal of Economic History* XVIII, 1958, 550–559 (559).

19 Obijiofor, 'The nineteenth century colonial fingerprints on public health diplomacy', 4–8; Saurabh Mishra, *Pilgrimage, Politics and Pestilence. The Haj from the Indian Subcontinent 1860–1920*, Oxford and New Delhi, Oxford University Press, 2011, 15–51.

20 Baldwin, *Contagion and the State in Europe*, 99–104.

21 Jean Noel Biraben, *Les hommes et la peste en France et dans les pays européens et méditerranéens*, vol.1, Paris, Mouton, 1976.

22 Mishra, *Pilgrimage, Politics and Pestilence.*

23 Roy Porter, *Blood and Guts. A Short History of Medicine*, London, Penguin Books, 2002, 15.

24 Krista Maglen, 'Politics of quarantine in the 19th century', *JAMA* 290, 21, 2003, 2873.

25 Francisco Javier Martínez, 'International or French? The Early International Sanitary Conferences and France's struggle for hegemony in the mid-nineteenth century Mediterranean', *French History* 36, 1, 2016, 77–98.

26 *Procès-Verbaux de la conférence sanitaire internationale ouverte à Paris le 27 Juillet 1851*, Paris, Impr. nationale, 1852, 1–2.

27 Jones, *The Scientific Background*, p. 10.

28 J. Sheldon Watts, 'From rapid change to stasis: official responses to cholera in British-ruled India and Egypt: 1860 to c.1921', *Journal of World History* 12, 2, 2001, 452–463.

29 M.E. Chamberlain, *The Scramble for Africa*, New York, Longman, 1995, 3–16.

30 Fidler, 'The globalization of public health', 843.

31 See, for instance, the *Procès-Verbaux de la Conférence Sanitaire', 1852 – Séance du 31 Octobre 1851*, 4–6; *Report of the International Sanitary conference of a commission from that Body, to which were referred the Questions Relative to the Origin, Endemicity, Transmissibility and Propagation of Asiatic Cholera*, Boston, Mass., 1866; *Conférence Sanitaire Internationale de Paris, 7 février–3 avril 1894; Procès-verbaux*, Paris, Imp. nationale, 1894.

32 On the political construction of the *Inland Sea* as a geo-strategic 'corridor', see C.B. Fawcett, 'The Life Line of the British Empire', in W.H. Weigart, V. Stefansson and R.E.H. Harrison (eds), *New Compass of the World. A Symposium of Political Geography*, New York, MacMillan, 1949, 238–248; John Chircop, 'The British Imperial network in the Mediterranean 1800–1870. A Study of Regional Fragmentation and Imperial Integration', unpublished PhD thesis, University of Essex, 1997, 233–235. See also the cartographic representation of cholera's epidemical routes in, for instance, Alfred Stille, *Cholera: Its Origins, History, Causation, Symptoms, Lesions, Prevention and Treatment*, Lea Brothers & Co., Philadelphia, 1885.

33 Walter Francois, *Une histoire culturelle XVI–XXI siècle*, Paris, Seuil, 2008, 144.

34 Laverne Kuhnke, *Lives at Risk: Public Health in Nineteenth-Century Egypt*, Berkeley, University of California Press, 1990, 65–67.

35 Mariko Ogawa, 'Uneasy bedfellows: science and politics in the refutation of Koch's bacterial theory of cholera', *Bulletin of History of Medicine* 74, 2000, 697–698.

36 Maglen, 'Politics of quarantine in the 19th century', 2873.

37 Baldwin, *Contagion and the State in Europe*, 206, 229–231.

38 See Mishra, *Pilgrimage, Politics and Pestilence, passim*.

39 On the great historical controversy between 'Contagionists' and the 'Miasmatics', see Peter Wright and Andrew Treacher (eds), *The Problem of Medical Knowledge: Examining the Social Construction of Medicine*, Edinburgh, Edinburgh University Press, 1982; Baldwin, *Contagion and the State in Europe*, 10–36; Margaret Pelling, *Cholera, Fever and English Medicine, 1825–1865*, Oxford, Oxford University Press, 1978; see also the seminal article by Erwin H. Ackerknecht, 'Anticontagionism between 1821 and 1867', *Bulletin of the History of Medicine* 22, 5, 1948, 562–593.

40 Ray Porter, *Health Civilization and the State: A History of Public Health from Ancient to Modern Times*, London, Routledge, 1999; P. Ziegler and C. Platt, *The Black Death*, London, Penguin, 1998.

41 Juan B.H. Jimenez, 'Actas de las Conferencias Sanitarias Internacionales (1851–1938)', *Revista Española de Salud Pública* 79, 3, 2005, 339–349.

42 Baldwin, *Contagion and the State in Europe*, 201.

43 R.J. Evans, 'Epidemics and revolutions: cholera in nineteenth century Europe', *Past and Present* 120, 1988, 123–146 (120).

44 Giorgio Cosmacini, *Le Spade di Democle. Paure e Malatie nella Storia,* Roma-Bari, Laterza, 2006, 123.
45 Baldwin, *Contagion and the State in Europe,* 201.
46 See speech by François Melier, French delegate at the 1851 Conference, 27 September 1851 in *Procès-Verbaux de la Conférence Sanitaire, 1852 – Séance du 31 Octobre 1851.*
47 Katrina Tower, 'Medicine and politics: the abolition of English quarantine 1872–1898', *Social History of Medicine* XV, 3, 2002, 413–428.
48 G. Bussolini, *Delle Istituzioni di Sanita Marittima nel Bacino del Mediterraneo,* Trieste, 1881, 95; *Handbook for Travellers in Greece describing the Ionian Islands, the Kingdom of Greece, the Islands of the Aegean,* London, John Murray, 1854, 10–15.
49 For Gibraltar, see 'Proclamation relating to Performance of Quarantine in Gibraltar – 22 June 1836', *Orders in Council, Ordinances and Proclamations relating to Gibraltar,* London, HMSO, 1839; Chircop, 'The British Imperial Network in the Mediterranean', 233.
50 'Quarantine laws and regulations – House of Commons Debates – 23 December 1844', *Hansard,* vol. 76, cc.1292–1293.
51 Tower, 'Medicine and politics', 413–418.
52 'Quarantine congress', *The Boston Medical and Surgical Journal,* Boston, 13 August 1851, 1.
53 Research in miasmatic–aerial aetiology produced a large volume of medical literature – mainly as 'medical topography' – with quite a proportion of it dealing with 'tropical diseases' in the colonies.
54 James C. Riley, *Rising Life Expectancy: A Global History,* New York and Cambridge, Cambridge University Press, 2001.
55 Baldwin, *Contagion and the State in Europe,* 201, 203–207.
56 See Philip D. Curtin, *Death by Migration: Europe's Encounter with the Tropical World in the Nineteenth Century,* Cambridge, Cambridge University Press, 1989.
57 Roy Porter, 'Medical Science', R. Porter (ed.), *The Cambridge History of Medicine,* Cambridge, Cambridge University Press, 2006, 136–175.
58 *Report on Quarantine London, 1848,* 8–9; Kuhnke, *Lives at Risk,* 65–67.
59 *The British Medical Journal,* 26 August 1893.
60 See Bush, *Imperialism and Postcolonialism,* 206; Comaroff, *Ethnography and the Historical Imagination,* 216–217.
61 In these territories where 'the periodical return of epidemic disease appears to afford further corroboration of the connection between this class of diseases and particular atmospheric conditions' (*Report on Quarantine and the whole class of epidemic disease,* London, HMSO, 1849, 8–9).
62 Cf. [Snow John], *Snow On Cholera being a reprint of two papers,* London, Milford Oxford University Press, 1936.

63 It must be noted that the *cholera bacillus* was already identified by Filippo Pacini in 1854, but was not accepted in the dominant medical climate of the time (William Coleman, 'Koch's comma bacillus: the first year', *Bulletin of the History of Medicine* 61, 1987, 315–342; also Cosmacini, *Le Spade di Democle*, 118.)
64 Roy Porter, *The Greatest Benefit to Mankind. Medical History from Antiquity to the Present*, London, Fontana Press, 1999, 436–437.
65 Baldwin, *Contagion and the State in Europe*, 231–233.
66 Philip Manel, *Constantinople. City of the World's Desire, 1453–1925*, London, Penguin Books, 1997, 256; Daniel Panzac, *La Peste dans l'empire Ottoman 1700–1850*, Louvain, Peeters, 1985, 476, 482.
67 As in the case of Tunisia: Nancy E. Gallagher, *Medicine and Power in Tunisia 1780–1900*, Cambridge, Cambridge University Press, 2002. See also D.C.M. Platt, *The Cinderella Service: British Consuls since 1825*, Connecticut, Archon Books, 1971.
68 See Panagiotis Krokidas and Athanasios Gekas, 'Public health in Crete under the rule of Mehmed Ali in the 1830s', *Egypt monde Arabe* 4, 2007, 35–54.
69 Panzac, *La Peste dans l'empire Ottoman*, 413–423.
70 Cf. Kuhnke, *Lives at Risk*, 2.
71 The Sanitary Board in Beirut was founded in 1834 and included the French, Greek, Danish, Spanish and Austrian consuls. It was followed by the establishment of a lazaretto in the same port where all Syria-bound ships were to stop for quarantine. Toufoul Abou-Hodeib, 'Quarantine and trade: the case of Beirut, 1831–1840', *International Journal of Maritime History* XIX, 2, 2007, 223, 230.
72 This Council was made up of 'local members': the president, the interpreter, two Muslim officials and four physicians trained in European universities. The foreign representatives came from Austria, Belgium, France, England, Greece, Russia, Sardinia and Italy.
73 On the Tanzimat as a modernising process initiated 'from within', see Dietrich Jung with Wolfgang Piccoli, *Turkey at The Crossroads. Ottoman Legacies and a Greater Middle East*, London, Zed Books, 2001, 38–40.
74 '*Per l'Impero è in vigor il regolamento organico 24 maggio 1840, compilato dal Consiglio di Sanità, per le provenienze di mare tanto a Constantinopoli che per gli altri scali dell' impero stesso*', Brussolini, 1881, 57–58.
75 Nancy E. Gallagher, 'Contagion and quarantine in Tunis and Cairo, 1800–1870', *Maghreb Review* 7, 1982, 108–111.
76 *Procès-Verbaux de la Conférence Sanitaire – 1851, passim.*
77 For instance: *Report on Quarantine*, London, 1849, 6–9 on Egypt.

78 Coleman, 'Koch's comma bacillus: the first year', 314–341; Kuhnke, *Lives at Risk*, 65–67.
79 Bush, *Imperialism and Postcolonialism*, 149, 163.
80 Thomas Richards, *The Imperial Archive. Knowledge and the Fantasy of Empire*, London and New York, Verso, 1993, 6.
81 P.J. Cain and G. Hopkins, *British Imperialism. Innovation and Expansion*, London and New York, Longman, 1993, 7–9, 235–238; Jurgen Osterhammel, *Colonialism. A Theoretical View*, Princeton, Markus Wiener Publishers, 1999, 18–20.
82 A.L. Macfie, *The Eastern Question 1774–1923*, London and New York, Longman, 46–47.
83 Gallagher, *Medicine and Power in Tunisia*, 40.
84 Ibid., 42.
85 For an analysis of the mounting European influence on the Tunisian ruling elites, see F. Robert Hunt, 'The comparative history of Tunisia and Egypt in the nineteenth century: a re-examination', *Arab Historical Review for Ottoman Studies* 7/8, 1993, 59–70.
86 L.S. Stavrianos, *Global Rift. The Third World Comes of Age*, New York, Quill, 1981, 129–131.
87 On the classification of persons, goods and ships according to specific scales of 'contagiousness' or 'infectiveness', see No.1 *Au Procès-Verbaux de la Séance du 21 Octobre 1851*, Annex No.1.
88 Bussolini, *Delle Istituzioni di Sanita Marittima*, 269–70.
89 Annex no. 1., *Proces-Verbaux de la séance du Octobre 1851*.
90 Abou-Hodeib, 'Quarantine and trade', 233, 236.
91 [Dr De Valcourt – letter to editor], *The British Medical Journal*, 26 August 1893.
92 John Davy, *Notes and Observations on the Ionian Islands and Malta; With Some Remarks on Constantinople*, vol.1, London, Smith Elder, 1842, 341; Chircop, 'The British Imperial Network in the Mediterranean', 148–150.
93 Bush, *Imperialism and Postcolonialism*, 162–163.
94 'A further International Sanitary Conference', *The British Medical Journal*, 27 January 1894.
95 According to Forbes: 'the Arabs among whom a garment is never changed or washed, until it drops in pieces from their bodies'. Frederick Forbes, *Thesis on the nature and history of Plague as observed in the North Eastern Provinces of India*, London, W.H. Allen & Co., MDCCCXL, 46.
96 Alatas Syed Hussein, *The Myth of the Lazy Native. A Study of the image of the Malays, Filippinos and Javanese from the 16th to the 20th Century and its Function in the Ideology of Colonial Capitalism*, London, Frank Cass, 1977.

97 See Patrice Bourdelais, *Les epidemies terrassées: une histoire de pays riches*, Paris, Le Martiniere, 2003, 122.

98 Edward Said, *Orientalism. Western Conceptions of the Orient*, Middlesex, Penguin, 1995, 171–172.

99 M.E. Chamberlain, *Pax Brittanica? British Foreign Policy 1789–1914*, London and New York, Longman, 1995, 90, 138–140.

100 This was later taken on and elaborated by European historians to become an established term in the historiography of the Ottoman Empire until very recently (Salto Rasha, 'The Not So Sick Man of Europe', *Al-Abram weekly – books supplement*, 15/25 August 2004, http://weekly.ahram.org (accessed 18 August 2017).

101 Lawrence Guymer, *Curing the Sick Man. Sir Henry Butwer and the Ottoman Empire, 1858–1865*, Netherlands, Republic of Letters, 2011.

102 Andrew Wheatecraft, *The Ottomans. Dissolving Images*, London, Penguin, 1995, 205.

103 Paul W. Shroeder, 'International Politics, Peace, and War, 1815–1914' in T.C.W. Blanning (ed.), *The Nineteenth Century. Europe 1789–1914*, Oxford, Oxford University Press, 2000, 158–209.

104 'Mecca and the cholera', *British Medical Journal*, 26 August 1893.

105 Comaroff, *Ethnography and the Historical Imagination*, 215–217.

106 Porter, 'Medical science', 163.

107 James Morris refers to the Suez Canal as 'an exposed nerve in the anatomy of the [British] Empire' (James Morris, *Pax Britannica. The Climax of an Empire*, London, Faber and Faber, 1975, 58). See also C.B. Fawcett. 'The Life Line of the British Empire', in W.H. Weigart and V. Stefansson (eds), *New Compass of the World. A Symposium of Political Geography*, London, H.G. Harrap, 1949, 238–248.

108 It has been consecutively estimated that during the period 1807–73, between 30,000 and 160,000 pilgrims visited Mecca each year, with the number rising more and more owing to rapid transport from the Mediterranean to the Mecca and from the latter to India. This pilgrimage and the crowded ritual gathering were marked as main conduits of epidemics to Europe and worldwide, with some twenty epidemics believed to have originated in the Hejaz during the period 1831–1900.

109 More importantly, this seemed to be confirmed 'scientifically' with the discovery of a variant of the *comma bacillus* (identified in 1883 by Robert Koch), which was named El Tor – taking the name of a locality in the Sinai, where this variant was found among Egyptian Muslim pilgrims coming from Mecca (Cosmacini, *Le Spade di Democle*, 118). A lazaretto was actually built on El Tor.

110 Shelton Watts, 'From rapid change to stasis', 344–345. See also F.E. Peters, *The Hajj: The Muslim Pilgrimage to Mecca and the Holy Places*, Princeton, Princeton University Press, 1994, 301–302.

111 This 1866 ICS was attended by representatives – both diplomats and physicians – of eighteen states. Salih Efendi and Dr Bartoletti represented the Ottoman State. Others represented Austria, Belgium, Denmark, Egypt, England, France, Greece, Iran, Italy, the Netherlands, Portugal, Prussia, Russia, Spain, Sweden and Norway and the Vatican.
112 Mark Harrison, 'Quarantine, pilgrimage, and colonial trade', *The Indian Economic and Social History Review* 29, 1992, 117–44.
113 Ibid. On the preventive measures to be adopted at the Hejaz, see Firmin Duguet, *Le pèlerinage de la Mecque au point de vue religieux social et sanitaire. Pier le Docteur Duguet, Médecin Général, Inspecteur général du Conseil Sanitaire, maritime et quarantenaire d'Egypte. Avec une préface de Justin Godard*, Paris, Editions Reider, 1932.
114 Peters, *The Hajj*, 301–303.
115 *Procès-verbaux de la Conférence sanitaire internationale Ouverte à Vienne le 1 Juillet 1874*, Vienna, Impr. Royale, 1874.
116 With delegations from Austria-Hungary, Britain, Belgium, France, Denmark, Greece, Germany, Italy, the Netherlands, Persia, Russia, Spain, Sweden and Norway, Turkey and the USA.
117 'A further International Sanitary Conference', *The British Medical Journal.*
118 Thompson, *Barbary and Enlightenment, passim.*
119 Said, *Orientalism*, 235.
120 A. Proust, *Essai sur l'hygiène internationale: ses applications contre la peste, la fièvre jaune et le choléra asiatique*, Paris, Masson, 1873; *La défense de l'Europe contre la peste: et la conférence de Venise de 1897*, Paris, Masson, 1892.
121 *The British Medical Journal*, 26 August 1893.
122 Baldwin, *Contagion and the State in Europe*, 231.
123 For a later discussion on the rigour of quarantine procedures and environmental hygiene as well as the possible use of inoculation, see Duguet, *Le pèlerinage de la Mecque, passim.*
124 David Arnold, *Colonizing the Body: State Medicine and Epidemic Disease in Nineteenth-Century India*, Berkeley, University of California Press, 1993, 186–189.
125 Azim Nanji, *Dictionary of Islam*, London, Penguin, 2008, 61.
126 Huber, 'The unification of the globe by disease?', 469. But even previously, in 1838, in the newly established lazarettos such as that of Beirut, travellers were examined 'by a European doctor who inspected their mouths with a stick and scanned their bare bodies for signs of plague' (Charles G. Addison, *Damascus and Palmyra: A Journey to the East with a Sketch of the State and Prospects of Syria under Brahmin Pasha*, London, Carey & Hart, 1838, 98).

9

Epidemics, quarantine and state control in Portugal, 1750–1805

Laurinda Abreu

Introduction

On 15 May 1756, some two months after reports had arrived of an outbreak of plague in Algiers and just a few days after his own appointment as Secretary of State for Home Affairs, the most important government post in Portugal, Sebastião José de Carvalho e Melo, the future Marquis of Pombal, ordered Dom João de Lencastre, Colonel of the Naval Regiment, to proceed immediately to the fort of Paço d'Arcos (on the northern shore of the mouth of the Tagus, west of Lisbon) and there to adopt all necessary measures to prevent the plague from spreading to Portugal (Figure 9.1). All ships arriving from 'infected lands' were to be subjected to 'strict quarantine' and their cargoes transferred to the lazaretto at Trafaria (on the opposite shore of the Tagus) for inspection. That day saw a flurry of other missives on the same subject rushed off from the Royal Palace. The letter to the *Provedoria Mor da Saúde* (Health Authority) – a body answerable to the Lisbon City Council – ordered the chief health officer (who was appointed from the city aldermen) to join Dom João de Lencastre and place himself at his service. Six letters were sent out to the *estribeiro-mor* (chief equerry) of King José I (1750–77) with instructions to place the army on high alert and to provide troops to man the 'towers, forts and other naval locations'. The military authorities in the country's ports received orders to put in place the protection measures laid down in the *Regimento da Saúde* (Health Statute). The crown-appointed representatives of the central government in the port

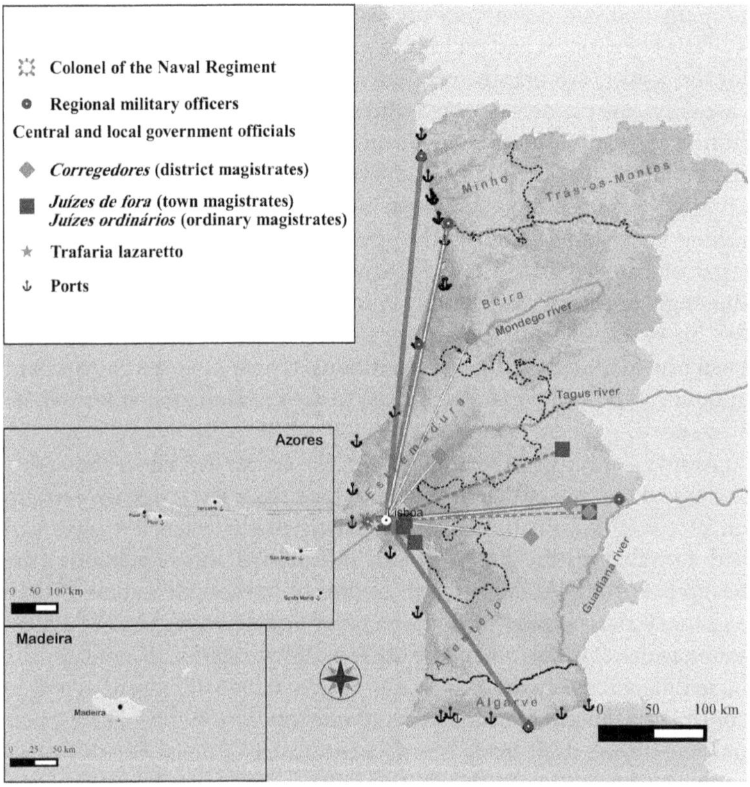

Figure 9.1 Plague in 1756 (path of communications).

towns – *corregedores* (district magistrates), *provedores* (administrators) and *juízes de fora* (town magistrates) – and the local town councils were told to cooperate with the army and to aid in implementing the control, prevention and isolation measures. It was only in the Atlantic archipelagos of the Azores and Madeira that vigilance was left entirely to the local authorities.

The following week, Carvalho e Melo and Dom Luís da Cunha Manuel, who had replaced him as Secretary of State for Foreign Affairs and War,[1] wrote to the Lisbon City Council again. In a dozen or so letters they criticised the chief health officer for not doing his job properly and laid down very precise instructions about repairing the Trafaria warehouses and building a new infirmary; recruiting labourers for the works; evicting the residents of houses around the lazaretto in case they were needed for quarantine purposes; preventing sick inmates from having any contact with the outside world; stopping vessels from the Barbary Coast from landing in Portugal; and quarantining all boats arriving 'from the Mediterranean or other ports in Italy', including fishing boats and warships.[2] The governors added that consuls in Portugal of France, Britain and Holland had already been informed of the ongoing operations, the fort commanders had been authorised to fire on vessels that dared to flout the royal decisions,[3] and they had been provided with additional munitions. On 30 June the government announced that all measures relating to the epidemic threat were to be suspended.[4]

At first glance, it would appear from the events described above that the crown had merely acted as it had done since the sixteenth century on receiving information that the plague might reach Portugal, and had activated all the public health institutions and regulations (the health boards, the Lisbon Health Authority, the Health Statute of 1526 and the Trafaria lazaretto) in the manner first developed by the Italian states, which Portugal and many other countries tended to emulate. The main difference between Portugal and other states with regard to plague control was the extent of government intervention. When plague broke out, the crown itself made the decision to set up local health boards (only in Lisbon was the health authority a permanent body) and laid down the measures that local communities were required to implement. This approach was part of the wider political project that saw public health as a matter of governance during the development of the Early Modern state. The project had begun in 1498 with the creation of the Lisbon *Misericórdia* – a crown-sponsored lay confraternity that had developed a standard model for dealing with poverty and hospital administration, which was soon copied throughout the country – and was strengthened in 1568 with the establishment of a kind of healthcare safety net designed to provide the poor with free medical assistance.[5] In this interpretation, there was nothing new in the way Carvalho e Melo pushed through the measures described above – known as the *Providências por ocasião do receio de peste em 1756* (Measures occasioned by the fear of plague in 1756)[6] – were it not for the political climate in Lisbon in the spring of 1756.

Epidemics used as tool for political survival

Sebastião José de Carvalho e Melo had been a not particularly notorious minister in King José's government before the terrible earthquake that struck Lisbon on 1 November 1755. He then seized the opportunity offered by the disaster to impose his authority and reform the state, sparing neither the Catholic Church nor the upper nobility in the process. So great were the changes he introduced that José Subtil has termed them a 'political earthquake'.[7] Public health, however, as pointed out elsewhere, was not one of his main areas of intervention, and he confined himself to protecting the *misericórdias* and securing state control over certain hospitals. He did not display any special concern about epidemics prior to 1756 (they had occurred in 1752, 1753 and 1754)[8] or even after that date (the country faced the threat of plague in 1758–61, 1764, 1767–68 and 1770)[9]. Yet, however serious the threat of plague might have been just months after the earthquake, and whatever public health concerns the Secretary of State might have had in mind, the 1756 Measures gain a whole new significance when examined in the light of the ongoing palace coup designed to strip Carvalho e Melo of his powers.

Seen purely in terms of epidemic control, the 1756 Measures were not innovative. As was the case in many other port cities throughout Europe, the line of defensive fortifications along the Portuguese coast acted as a *cordon sanitaire* that was relatively easy to bring into play. Protected by the early sixteenth-century Tower of Belém, the port of Belém near Lisbon and its westward extension in Paço d'Arcos, together with the lazaretto across the estuary in Trafaria, formed the physical space that materialised the Lisbon City Council's authority over public health matters. With every plague alarm, the crown ordered the chief health officer out to Paço d'Arcos to coordinate the country's protection measures. It should be noted that the administrative situation in Lisbon was very different from that in other towns in Portugal, which generally enjoyed considerable freedom. Since 1572, the chairman of the Lisbon City Council, a member of the country's aristocracy, and the aldermen had been appointed directly by the king[10] and were entitled to an annual stipend. As a result, the chief health officer ultimately was answerable to the monarch. Nevertheless, over time, the council had sought to assert its own authority and on many occasions entered into direct confrontation with the crown.

Although the substantial pay rise awarded on 23 March 1754[11] might seem to suggest otherwise, the absolutist process of centralising political power after the earthquake led the government to launch a number of attacks on the Lisbon City Council's financial privileges and client relations, particularly those associated with and/or dependent on the public health and hygiene portfolios.[12] Even before the 1756 Measures, the decree ordering the council to draw up a new statute for the pest-house and its staff[13] and the decision to take the lazaretto out of the council's hands so it could be used by the *Casa da Índia* (except during epidemics)[14] as a staging post for goods and prisoners bound for the East[15] accentuated the trend of forcing the city government to become institutionally dependent on the central government. The innovative aspect of the Measures lay in the governor's choice of the navy and not the chief health officer to organise ship quarantines: with a stroke of the pen, Carvalho e Melo flaunted his control over both the armed forces and the upper nobility as represented on the city council. The council's subordination was soon rewarded on 11 June with the reappointment of the chairman and aldermen,[16] followed by an order for special remuneration whenever the chief health officer moved out to Paço d'Arcos.[17] At the same time, the architects of the palace conspiracy were severely punished.[18]

It seems quite likely that two events – the publication in May 1756 of a tract by an anonymous writer entitled *Relaçaõ verdadeira da implacavel peste, que padece a cidade de Marrocos, Argel, e outras Africanas* [...][19] (True account of the implacable plague affecting the city of Marrakesh, Algiers and other African cities [...]), relating the horrors caused by the epidemic in the lands affected, and the presence of the royal family at a military exercise carried out by João de Lencastre's regiment as part of the 'convenient preventions to preserve this kingdom from contagion',[20] in the words of the *Gazeta de Lisboa* on 27 May that year[21] – may have been engineered by Carvalho e Melo to justify and legitimise his actions. The manner in which the crown dealt with epidemics reveals the importance of policies on poor relief and public health to the Early Modern state in Portugal, in that they helped the monarchy to strengthen its power over the towns and their elites.[22] Towards the end of this process, in 1756, in the midst of the chaos and disorder that followed the earthquake,[23] the news that the plague was spreading in the Mediterranean seems to have been used to ensure

Carvalho e Melo's political survival and to advance the reformist project he had begun the previous year. The symbolic, if not the physical, target of the disproportionate military strength deployed along the coast, especially in Lisbon itself, were certain members of the nobility who had always dominated politics at court and whom the governor was now preparing to subject to the royal yoke.

The epidemics of 1800: the first *cordons sanitaires*

Events at the dawn of the next century again suggest that epidemics were being managed politically for purposes that lay outside the field of public health per se. In the threats of plague and yellow fever that circulated between 1800 and 1804, the sea was still considered the main source of contagion, yet most of the measures taken related to the land border. On this occasion the leading role was played by one of Pombal's creations, the Intendancy-General of Police. In early 1780, only two decades after it was founded on 25 June 1760, the Intendancy-General of Police under its new intendant, Diogo Inácio de Pina Manique, began to take an active interest in the field of poor relief and public health, thereby coming to resemble other European police forces in its social aims. In Pina Manique's mercantilist plans for a populous, prosperous and educated country, which were heavily influenced by the values of the medical police as embraced by the German doctor Johann Peter Frank, it was the state's duty to care for the people's health and, therefore, to steer the actions of local government and healthcare professionals to this end. Of the many aspects of public health that the police addressed after 1780, epidemics (both on home soil and coming from abroad) were among those that had the greatest social and political impact. They were also the area in which the intendant soon met with most resistance – in this particular case from the towns and cities, which were reluctant to contribute financially to the proposed measures, and from medical practitioners, who were hardly enthusiastic about the requirement to provide the poor with free healthcare.

To combat 'epidemics of putrid fevers among the destitute'[24] – diseases usually resulting from the deplorable sanitary conditions in which the majority of the population lived – the Intendancy-General of Police reacted immediately to news of an outbreak by sending a small group of doctors and/or surgeons to the affected areas to provide care and to work with the local authorities in investigating the source of the outbreak and seeking the best way to resolve it. Where disease might be brought in by sea or by travellers crossing the border from Spain, situations that came under the Lisbon City Council's jurisdiction, as mentioned above, the role of the police was transformed during Pina Manique's term of office (1780–1805). At first it merely gathered and passed on information on the movement of diseases and their carriers – as was the case in 1783 when the plague hit Cadiz, Constantinople, Crimea, Bohemia, Poland, Danzig, Prussia and Pomerania, or in 1787 during the plague in Algiers.[25] By 1799,[26] however, when Morocco was considered 'plague-ridden' ('*empestado*'),[27] the intendant had become the crown's main advisor on such matters: not only was it his idea to send one cavalry detachment to Paço d'Arcos and another to Trafaria to strengthen the surveillance of people and vessels,[28] but the police were also increasingly involved in the inspection of vessels putting in to Tavira, Faro[29] and Lagos before being sent on to the lazaretto in Trafaria, the only place where quarantine measures were implemented.

It was also the intendant who on 19 September 1800 notified Dom Rodrigo de Sousa Coutinho, Secretary of State for the Navy and Overseas Territories, that Cadiz was in the grip of a yellow fever epidemic. His informant, the merchant Jacob Dahorman, had warned that the disease was highly contagious, and in fact it had caused the death of 2,616 people in two weeks (24 August–8 September).[30] Armed with a list of the ships then anchored in Cadiz harbour, Pina Manique stressed that although only one of them had Portugal as its stated destination the others could easily change course and put the country at risk. Seeing Cadiz in dire straits with the loss of between 7,400 and 8,500 inhabitants[31] (13–15% of its population) in less than five months, the government entrusted the organisation and implementation of epidemic control measures to the Intendancy-General of Police. At first it focused on the seaports and on setting up temporary lazarettos, but soon it turned its attention to establishing a land-based *cordon sanitaire*. Regular troops were stationed in Trás-os-Montes district in the north of the country to form the cordon there, whereas in the south the task fell to local, unpaid militias (*Ordenanças*).

With the authority to issue 'the most severe orders to prevent any kind of communication allowing such a disease to spread to the towns and villages of this kingdom', Pina Manique was given powers over the royal magistrates, the chief health officer and the military governors of the country's ports. He was also to liaise with the military governor of Alentejo to prepare quarantine for 'everything that might come from Andalusia and even from Spain'.[32] There is little in the archives that reveals what happened between late September and November 1800, while these inland cordons were being organised. It seems, however, that they merely consisted of men deployed along the Spanish border. The Health Statute provided for the use of troops during epidemics, but only in the port of Lisbon; vigilance elsewhere in the country remained in the hands of the health officers, although since 1695 they had had permission to bear arms.[33] No evidence has yet been found that troops had ever been used to protect the land frontier against epidemics prior to 1800.

As Gunther E. Rothenberg has pointed out,[34] quarantine measures were generally much more difficult to implement on land than at sea, and Portugal proved not to have any experience in the matter. Added to that was the state of friction between the intendant and the royal ministers, most of whom he accused of being negligent, irresponsible, lazy and corrupt. By the end of 1800 he was also criticising the head of the postal service[35] and the chief health officer,[36] making extremely damning remarks about the latter. Relations were likewise strained between the Intendancy-General of Police and the military hierarchy, which refused to supply the troops that the public health officers needed to enforce the maritime quarantine measures, as reported by the *juíz de fora* for Setúbal;[37] nor was it particularly happy about the intendant's increasing prominence.

On the ground, there were problems in abundance. The military governor of Trás-os-Montes, Manuel Jorge Gomes de Sepúlveda, expressed his perplexity at the contradictory instructions sent to him from Lisbon regarding the real purpose of the cordon. In the south, relations between the civil and military authorities were difficult[38] – the militia cordon was under the command of Field Marshal José Joaquim de Melo Lacerda assisted by the *corregedor* of Beja – and recruits were poorly trained. On 31 October, the *corregedor* of Elvas complained that 'a cordon without regular troops is always to be feared because it is susceptible to laxity [of manners]',[39] and the men who formed the cordon along the border of Alentejo were rough, illiterate (any written document presented to them as a health passport was accepted as such) and easily corruptible. Moreover, the family ties linking people on both sides of the border made it practically impossible to enforce the ban on communication between Portugal and Spain, as the *provedor* of Beja was at pains to point out (Figure 9.2).

Without underestimating the impact that fear of yellow fever, which was rife on the other side of the border, may have had on the

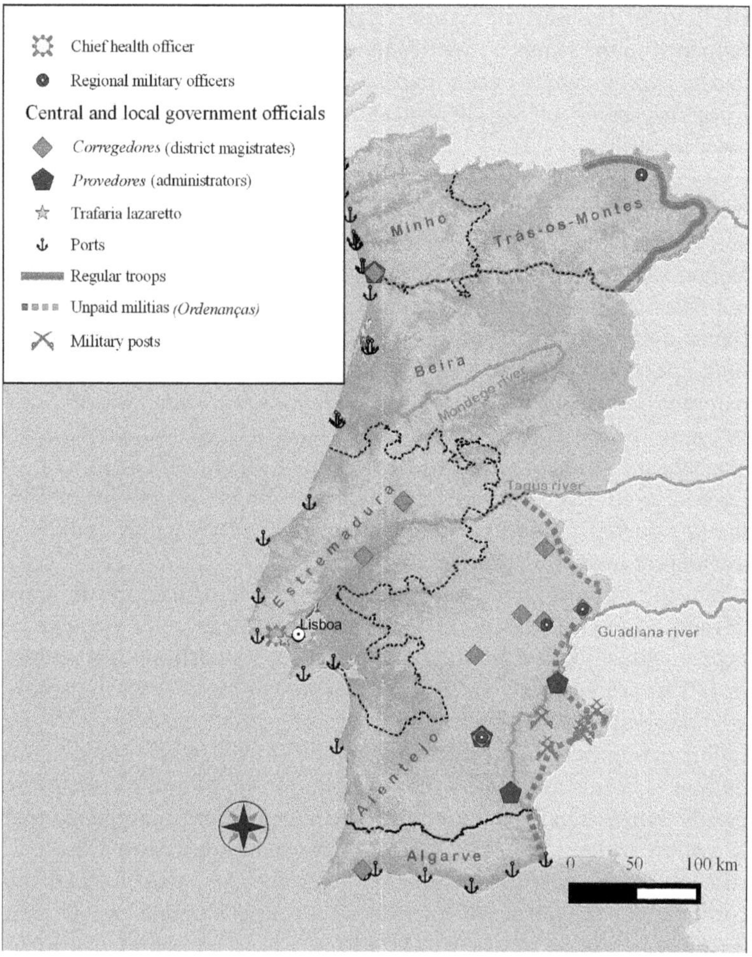

Figure 9.2 *Cordon sanitaire*, 1800.

government's decisions in 1800, it is difficult to avoid harking back to the political situation in the country. Only politics can help explain why, for example, the militia-manned *cordon sanitaire* was apparently lifted in November that year, even though across the border in Spain epidemics continued claiming victims until December 1801. Such a view is supported by the government's decision to waive quarantine for the British warships blockading Cadiz and by the letter sent by the *corregedor* and *provedor* of Porto district on 11 October 1800 informing the government that when monitoring the ports he had paid particular attention to ships from 'enemy and suspect nations, coming from said port of Cadiz or from those in Africa, or from North America'.[40] The fact is that Napoleon Bonaparte's return to France in October 1799 had once again raised tensions in Portugal in the context of the Continental Blockade. With war looming, Portugal sought military assistance from Lieutenant-General Ralph Abercromby, who was stationed in Gibraltar at the time; between 8 and 14 November 1800, Abercromby sent 2,222 British soldiers to Lisbon (out of the 12,000 requested). The country began to prepare for Spanish invasion and war, which eventually happened in May–June 1801.

In this situation, it appears from ongoing studies that the Portuguese authorities were dealing jointly with the dual threats of yellow fever and war. The difficulty in recruiting soldiers for the army and retaining them was well known. In 1796, with conflict on the horizon, the government had entrusted the police and its intendant with the task of extraordinary recruitment, thereby, in the view of Fernando Dores Costa, acknowledging the failure of the recruitment system based on the network of militias.[41] The task proved to be Herculean, despite the various tactics used by Pina Manique to overcome the people's resistance and circumvent the devices they used to avoid enlistment. The greatest opposition was encountered precisely in Alentejo, in contrast to the north, where the number of volunteers even earned an accolade from Pina Manique. These different attitudes may have underlain the decision to man the cordon in Alentejo with militias, perhaps playing on the fear of yellow fever to persuade men to join up. Once they had enlisted, the *cordon sanitaire* was probably transformed into a military cordon.[42]

This idea is supported by the geography of the cordon: if the epidemic was confined to Andalusia with its main focus in Cadiz, why emphasise the land border to the detriment of the seaports, where no special measures appear to have been taken apart from a tightening of ship inspections in the Algarve and Porto? And why extend the land cordon only as far north as the Tagus, leaving the whole border from the Tagus to the Douro open, and then deploy troops in Trás-os-Montes? The answer is to be found in Spain, which had been moving troops to the border area since 1797 and in 1800 was preparing for war, setting up field hospitals and supply depots in Galicia, Extremadura and Andalusia. It was precisely along the border with the last two regions that the Portuguese had ranged their *cordon sanitaire* of militias. Even so, and despite the many weaknesses exposed by the Portuguese army and made plain in its defeat in what came to be known as the War of the Oranges (1801),[43] the fact is that the country entered the new century having avoided the epidemics.

The role played by the press in this process should not be underestimated. It was used politically to keep the population alert by teaching it how to recognise signs of disease and what steps to take to avoid it. Equally important were the publishing houses, likewise encouraged by the government, which sponsored a number of translations of works publicising successful experiments in epidemic control in Smyrna,[44] Ragusa and Dalmatia.[45] A book published in Lisbon in 1800 describing how Marseille, Toulon and Moscow had defeated the plague became a best-seller, with nine editions appearing the following year.[46] A short pamphlet on lazarettos extracted from John Howard's well-known book *An Account of the Principal Lazarettos in Europe* [...][47] was published at government expense in November 1800. The purpose in this case was to justify the request of Prince Regent João (future King João VI) for a public loan of 40 million *réis*[48] in order to build a new lazaretto, which was announced in the same month and was promptly subscribed to by thirteen Lisbon merchants.[49]

Making the most of the favourable winds blowing from the Royal Palace, which had issued a statement praising his 'zeal and incomparable activity', Pina Manique attempted to ensure that the extraordinary powers he had been given on account of the epidemic[50] should be taken as a 'rule for the future' (a request that does not seem to have been granted, as will be seen below),[51] while also trying to persuade the crown to regulate the relationship between the police and the armed forces ('so that the police authority can act in agreement with the military').[52] In 1804, he was again chosen to lead the fight against the new threats of epidemics.

The 1804 yellow fever outbreak and the frontier cordon

The alarm sounded again in Portugal in the summer of 1804. There had been yellow fever in Cadiz and Malaga[53] for some years, but now it was spreading throughout Andalusia and coming perilously close to the Portuguese border. Portugal was in a particularly difficult economic situation, and the prince regent once again called on the Intendancy-General of Police to deal with the impending epidemic. Since 1802, the country had been trying to maintain its policy of neutrality in the Franco–British conflict, which enabled it to import goods from Britain and re-export them to France and Spain. The government was determined to defend the port of Lisbon, which acted as an 'economic lung for the warring countries',[54] and Pina Manique was ordered to implement immediately the measures 'that in previous years were put in place to the great benefit and security of public health.'[55] The intendant was vested with a wide range of policing powers and the authority to coordinate the royal magistrates,[56] which, together with his experience of enlisting troops[57] and organising the *cordon sanitaire* in 1800, placed him in a unique position to be able to address the imminent crisis. Having received his orders from the Royal Palace on 27 August, Pina Manique set to work on the very same day.

The first measures taken by the Intendancy-General of Police included organising temporary lazarettos in all seaports[58] so as to ease the concentration of quarantined vessels in Trafaria that the Health Statute required, and introducing stricter controls over fishermen, whom he described as 'ambitious' people who were all too eager to take the small rewards offered by vessels to tranship passengers.[59] The provincial governors of Alentejo and Algarve were sent instructions to 're-form the cordon of militias'[60] and the town councils were told to pay for the running of the lazarettos and to set up 'medical boards' that would assess travellers' state of health[61] and then, depending on the outcome, either issue them with health certificates[62] or quarantine them. In a letter to the royal ministers, Pina Manique stressed that the news from Malaga was still 'most disastrous and worthy of the greatest precautions for the sake of preserving public health.'[63] He placed the blame for the scale of the outbreak squarely on their Spanish counterparts for not having taken action promptly enough,[64] and put pressure on the government's representatives around the country to carry out his orders by threatening to have them arrested if they prevaricated. He appealed to the prince regent to allow him greater freedom of movement to ensure the success of his operations by granting him the same extraordinary powers that he had enjoyed in 1800.

The correspondence exchanged between the government and the Intendancy in the first weeks of October 1804 portrays particularly anxious times and reveals a veritable obsession with controlling people's movements regardless of social status[65] or country of origin,[66] and with inspecting premises that gave lodging to foreigners.[67] There was also concern for the sanitary conditions in which people lived, as they were advised to avoid domestic waste dumps, protect their goods and be wary of markets and slaughterhouses.[68] It proved difficult to organise the various different bodies and jurisdictions involved, not least because the orders issued sometimes conflicted with the legislation in force, particularly with regard to the quarantining of vessels.[69] As a result, everybody was seeking 'to arrogantly ascribe to himself the authority to order others about, overstepping the limits laid down by law', as the chief health officer complained on 24 October, referring to the dispute between the health officers of Portimão and Faro, their respective ministers of justice and the military governors.[70]

On 21 October 1804, the crown responded by setting up the *Junta de Inspecção sobre as Providencias para a Peste* (Plague Measures Inspection Board), primarily to deal with opposition within the armed forces.[71] The Board was to 'adopt all necessary measures using the means available to prevent the spread of the said plague to the kingdom', and was given the power to 'issue orders and [ensure] that they are obeyed by all institutions and persons in the kingdom'[72] and to mete out punishment if they were not. This was essentially a crisis cabinet made up of the chairman of the Lisbon City Council, the general of the infantry, the admiral and vice-admiral of the fleet and the Intendancy-General of Police. Everything suggests that this *Junta de Inspecção* was the embryo of what in 1813 became the *Junta da Saúde Pública* (Public Health Board). Apart from the intendant, none of the Board's members had apparently been informed that it was being established.[73] The same seems to have been true of the government's ministers, who on the same day were told of the purpose of the Board and that the monarch required each of them to collaborate with it insofar as it affected them 'without delay or hindrance'.[74] The Lisbon Council chairman was also told to place the senate assembly hall at the new institution's disposal,[75] pay for its expenses[76] and chair its meetings.[77] Copies of all documentation exchanged between the office of the Secretary of State for Affairs of the Kingdom and the Intendancy-General of Police and between the latter and the magistrates[78] were forwarded to the Board so it would have 'intelligence of its content in order to take account of the measures adopted'.[79]

By including the chief health officer and the heads of the army and navy on the Board, the prince regent aimed to remove the obstacles that the Intendancy-General had encountered in making the quarantine and *cordon sanitaire* system work.[80] This decision had an immediate impact on the chief health officer's performance. He swiftly produced a long and markedly self-justificatory description of all the work that had recently been carried out, which he presented on 26 October.[81] He subsequently updated this information at the end of every week,[82] with the addition of 'a true report [...] of the state of health of the city [Lisbon]' compiled from public health and epidemiological information from a number of sources.[83]

Pina Manique had ordered that the militia cordon[84] be re-formed, but the plans that Colonel José Carconte Lobo, the main architect of the *cordon sanitaire,* drew up and forwarded to all the division commanders on 11 October 1804 suggest that the intendant's words were not to be taken too literally. Although the experience gained in 1800 had been valuable, the 1804 cordon was, if not completely innovative, then certainly much more complete than the previous one. The model on which it was based is not known, but it is likely to have resulted from a combination of the expertise brought by the Prussian generals who were reorganising the Portuguese army[85] and the procedures followed in the *Cordão de Cautella Nova* (Cordon of New Precaution) organised by Madrid, to which the Lisbon Government had access.[86] According to the document entitled 'Recapitulation of the total force necessary for the organisation of a Cordon of Troops on the frontier from the Tagus beginning in Montalvão, to the Guadiana',[87] the cordon would require a total of 3,151 cavalry and infantry (including twelve different ranks) in eight military divisions, tasked with controlling the 'points of sale of tobacco' and the movement of people and correspondence, as well as protecting hospitals, lazarettos and boats on the River Guadiana.

The 'Instruction for the commanders of the divisions that form the frontier cordon'[88] laid down not only the places where the troops should be stationed but also the *misericórdia* hospitals that would take care of sick soldiers and the lazarettos to which infected travellers should be sent. It also provided specific information on how to set up and run a lazaretto and even on what treatment should be given. Particular attention was devoted to the relations between the troops and the local communities and officers of justice (Figure 9.3).

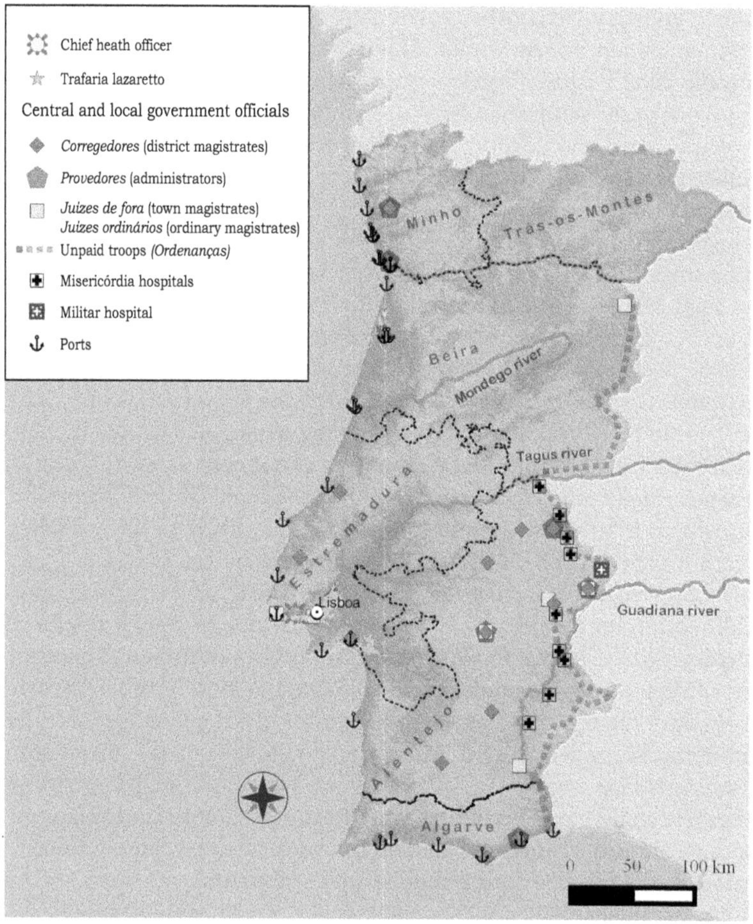

Figure 9.3 *Cordon sanitaire,* 1804.

Mapping this information reveals that the *cordon sanitaire* comprised three lines of protection: the first comprised the soldiers stationed along the border; a series of lazarettos some distance behind them formed the second; and the third was made up of the *misericórdia* hospitals at a much greater distance from the front line.

This time there was practically no connection between the *cordon sanitaire* and the line of fortifications, as there had been in 1800 (Figure 9.4). The troops now surrounded villages and blocked roads – from highways to rural lanes and byways – not to mention almost 200 small ports. The distances kept between units and the care taken in identifying the outermost limits of the towns and villages to be patrolled show that international criteria on the spacing of guard posts were being followed. In addition, cavalry detachments were sent to patrol the border constantly, and division commanders were required to perform random checks on their troops, who were relieved every 48 hours. On 22 November, the prince acknowledged everyone's efforts and gave thanks that the country had remained free of contagion;[89] two days later he ordered that the cordon be lifted. However, further outbreaks in Spain in December would delay the process, and it was only on 20 January 1805 that the Board ordered most of the troops back to barracks, transferring control of the military cordon to the district magistrates. It had not been possible to test whether the chief health officer had been right when, on 26 October 1804, he had criticised the flimsiness of the cordon, which, he claimed, would only 'be of service if the contagion does not come'.[90]

Conclusion

Public health and poor relief were areas in which the Portuguese crown asserted and demonstrated its power during the construction of the Early Modern state. Having been subject to government intervention since the late fifteenth century, hospital management, disease control, the regulation of the 'medical' professions and the distribution of poor relief and healthcare assistance came to reflect all the vicissitudes that influenced the exercise of political power. A study focusing on the late sixteenth century showed, purely with regard to epidemics, that populations were better protected under a strong government that was able to impose itself on the towns and force them to implement

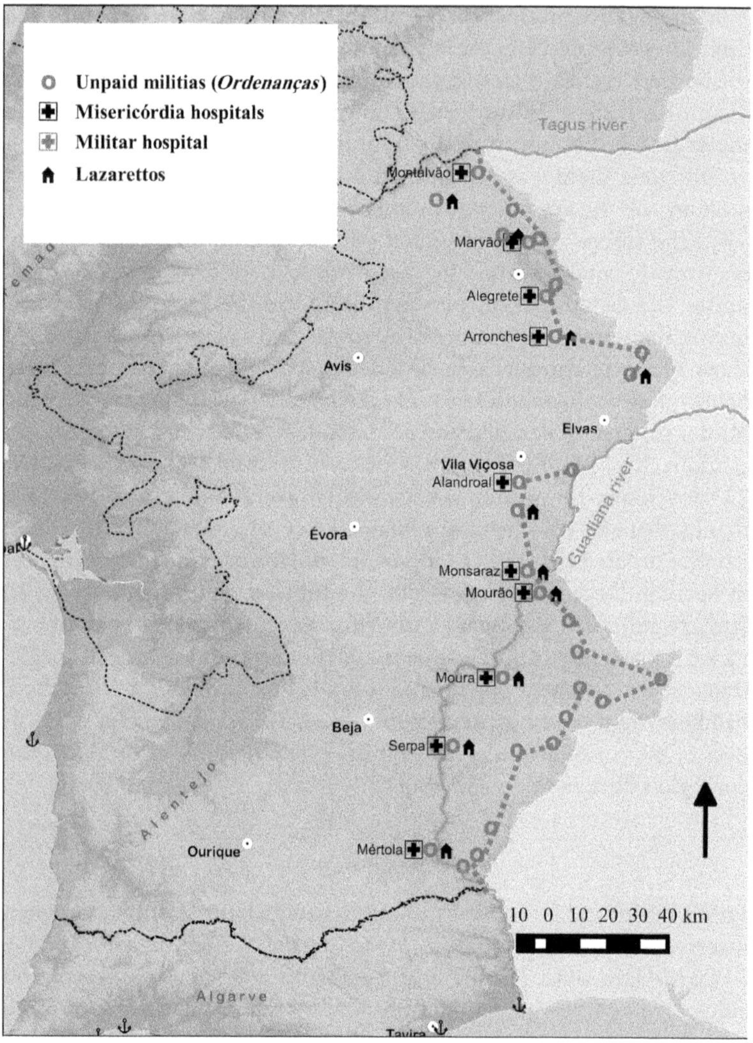

Figure 9.4 *Cordon sanitaire,* Alentejo 1804.

the crown's orders and sanitary measures. Conversely, whenever royal power appeared weaker, as it often did, the plague tended to spread uncontrolled while the towns waited for instructions or were forced to implement counterproductive measures. This pattern, which may also be examined as a barometer of the relations between central government and local communities, continued without major changes until the latter half of the eighteenth century, when new factors were added to the equation.

The possibility that the fear of epidemics and the introduction of public safety measures may have been exploited for purely political gain can be seen first in May 1756 and again in late 1800. In the first case, Sebastião José de Carvalho e Melo used a remote threat of plague – reported two months before in Algiers – to ensure his political survival. By controlling the navy and army, which he deployed along the Atlantic coast supposedly to protect the country from a peril that by then was threatening Naples, Carvalho e Melo displayed the extent of his power to those who were manoeuvring to oust him but ended up being banished from court themselves. In 1800, the situation was rather different, in that this time the government as a whole presented its actions as being a response to the yellow fever epidemic in Cadiz, when in fact the country's military defence was also at stake.

The notion that this first military *cordon sanitaire* to be established in Portugal had been planned more to police the border with Spain than to control the spread of the epidemic is supported by its geography. Even though the Mediterranean was the main source of contagion, the government decided to deploy troops along the country's northern border and to man the cordon in the south with militias. In both cases, men were deployed on the Portuguese side of the frontier to shadow the movements of the Spanish army, which was massing near the border in preparation for an invasion. A significant point in this interpretation is that the task of organising the cordon of militias was entrusted to Pina Manique, who was also responsible for recruiting soldiers for the army. This proved extremely difficult in Alentejo, where there was little appetite for enlisting in the army voluntarily. Everything suggests that this short-lived *cordon sanitaire*, which has left little trace, was immediately prepared for war.

The last case analysed in this chaper is from 1804. Although the political scene was still highly unstable – after the Portuguese defeat in the War of the Oranges the country feared French reprisals for refusing to close its ports to Britain, a choice that ultimately led to the Napoleonic invasions of 1807–11 – there is no sign that any political capital was made out of the genuine danger posed by the yellow fever epidemic that had spread throughout Andalusia and was threatening Portugal. The cordon established this time was significant in that it was a genuine *cordon sanitaire* (in contrast to the cordon of 1800, which had not gone beyond the stage of troop deployment) and marked the beginning of a new phase in the way the country dealt with epidemics. Ongoing research has revealed that it drew on the experience of recruitment gained in 1800 and closely followed the prevailing ideas in Europe[91] regarding the arrangement of military guard posts, the inspections to be performed by the municipal medical boards, and the roles planned for local hospitals and temporary lazarettos. Many of the difficulties encountered by the authorities in setting up the 1804 *cordon sanitaire* have now been elucidated, but one fact unarguable: the country escaped again the scourge of yellow fever, whereas, for example, the epidemic killed 36% of Malaga's population in that year.

Notes

I would like to thank Christopher Tribe for the translation of this chapter and to Luís Gonçalves for the figures.

Work developed in the framework of UID/HIS/00057/2013 (POCI-01–0145-FEDER-007702) – FCT, COMPETE, FEDER, Portugal2020.

1 Joaquim Joaquim Veríssimo Serrão, *História de Portugal [1750–1807]*, Lisboa, Verbo, 1982, 37.

2 This applied immediately to *Navio de Guerra La Gloria*, a British warship sailing from Algiers, Arquivo Nacional da Torre do Tombo (ANTT), *Ministério do Reino*, book 415, fl.11v.

3 ANTT, *Ministério do Reino*, book 415, fl. 5.

4 ANTT, *Ministério do Reino*, book 415, fls 13–15.

5 See L. Abreu, 'Assistance et santé publique dans la construction de l'État moderne: l'expérience portugaise', *Revue d'histoire moderne et contemporaine* 3, 2014, 67–97. 'A General Overview on the Poor Relief and Health Care "System"', in L. Abreu, *The Political and Social Dynamics of Poverty,*

Poor Relief and Health Care in Early-Modern Portugal, Oxford and New York, Routledge, 2016.

6 ANTT, *Ministério do Reino*, book 415, fl.1v.

7 J. Subtil, *O Terramoto Político (1755–1759) – Memória e Poder*, Lisboa, UAL, 2007.

8 Respectively, Eduardo Freire de Oliveira, *Elementos para a História do Município de Lisboa*, Lisboa, Typografia Universal, tome X, 1885–191, 326–327; Arquivo Municipal de Lisboa (AML) – Arquivo Histórico (AH), *Health Provision, Register of the chief health officer's rulings on the plague*, fls 11v–12v; de Oliveira, *Elementos para a História do Município de Lisboa*, 35–36.

9 The vast majority were from the Mediterranean: AML-AH, *Provisões régias*, 345–346; fls 14–21v.

10 Except for the city and guild attorneys, who joined the council in 1591.

11 de Oliveira, *Elementos para a História do Município de Lisboa*, tome XV, 500–522.

12 For example, by abolishing a number of posts created by the chief health officer.

13 de Oliveira, *Elementos para a História do Município de Lisboa*, tome XVI, 35.

14 de Oliveira, *Elementos para a História do Município de Lisboa*, tome XV, 188 and 213.

15 de Oliveira, *Elementos para a História do Município de Lisboa*, tome XVI, 294–295.

16 Ibid., 250.

17 Ibid.: payment was authorised in August 1756.

18 Serrão, *História de Portugal*, 35–36.

19 *Relaçaõ verdadeira da implacavel peste, que padece a cidade de Marrocos, Argel, e outras Africanas, e da grande trovoada, que a 15. de Março do prezente anno de 1756. experimentou a Berberia, Lisboa, 1756.*

20 'prevenções convenientes para preservar este reino de contagio'.

21 *Gazeta de Lisboa* no. 21, 1756-05-27, 177–178.

22 See L. Abreu, 'The city in times of plague: preventive and eradication measures against epidemic outbreaks in Évora between 1579 and 1637' *Popolazione Popolazione e Storia* 2, 2006, 109–125.

23 Subtil, *O Terramoto Político*, 112–113.

24 'epidemias de febres podres em gentes miseráveis'.

25 AML-AH, *Provisões Régias*, fls 19v–21v; fls 23–28; fls 29–30; fls 33–34v; fl. 36v; fls 39–43v; AML-AH, *Chancelaria Régia, Livro 1° de avisos de D. Maria I*, fls 111–112v.

26 Arquivo Histórico Ultramarino (AHU), *Reino*, box 417, bundle 9; box 177, bundles 2, 3 and 5.
27 AHU, *Reino*, box 177, bundle 2; AHU, *Reino*, box 177, bundle 3.
28 AHU, *Reino*, box 177, bundle 5.
29 AHU, *Reino*, box 417, bundle 29; box 31, bundle 29.
30 ANTT, *Intendência Geral da Polícia*, book 161, fls 278v–279.
31 J. Fellowes, *Reports of the pestilential disorder of Andalusia, which appeared at Cadiz in the years 1800, 1804, 1810, and 1813: with a detailed account of that fatal epidemic as it prevailed at Gibralter, during the autumnal months of 1804: also observations on the remitting and intermitting fever, made in the military hospitals at Colchester, after the return of the troops from the expedition to Zealand in 1809*, London, Printed for Longman, Hurst, Rees, Orme, and Brown, Paternoster-Row, 1815, 50.
32 AHU-Reino, box 31, bundle 30.
33 J.R.C. Sousa, *Systema, ou Collecção dos Regimentos Reaes*, Lisboa, Oficina de Simão Thaddeo Ferreira, 1785, IV volume, 349–350.
34 G.E. Rothenberg, 'The Austrian sanitary cordon and the control of the bubonic plague: 1710–1871', *Journal of the History of Medicine and Allied Sciences* 28, 1, 1983, 15–23.
35 The intendant accused him of only starting to purify correspondence after he had been severely reprimanded. ANTT, *Intendência Geral da Polícia*, book 6, fls 97–97v.
36 ANTT, *Intendência Geral da Polícia*, book 200, fls 215v–217.
37 AHU, *Reino*, box 238, bundle 4.
38 AHU, *Reino*, box 156, bundle 15.
39 'o cordão sem tropa de linha sempre é temível por susceptível à relaxação'.
40 'nação inimiga e suspeitosa, vinda do dito porto de Cádis, ou dos de África, ou da América Setentrional'. AHU, *Reino*, box 31, bundle 31.
41 F.D. Costa, 'O bom uso das paixões: caminhos militares na mudança do modo de governar', *Análise Social* XXXIII, 5, 1998, 969–1017.
42 This has long been common practice in many countries. Several examples can be found in K. Friedrich *Brandenburg-Prussia, 1466–1806: The Rise of a Composite State. Studies in European History Series*, Houndmills, Palgrave Macmillan, 2012.
43 R. Bebiano, 'Organização e papel do exército', in L. Torgal and J. Roque, João (coord.). *História de Portugal*, vol. V. Lisboa, Círculo dos Leitores, 1993, 252–263.
44 *Exposiçaõ de hum novo remedio curativo e preservativo da peste, presentemente usado com feliz sucesso no hospital de Santo Antonio de Esmyrna* (…) Lisboa, 1797.

45 *Methodo com que se Governa o Estado de Raguza e Dalmacia, quando nos confins se percebe algum ataque de peste ou outro mal contagioso* (…) Lisboa, 1800.
46 *Advertencias dos meios que os particulares podem usar para preservar-se da peste, conforme o que tem ensinado a experiencia principalmente na Peste de Marsalha em 1720, de Toulon em 1721 e de Moscou em 1771* (…), Lisboa, 1801.
47 *Historia dos principaes lazaretos da Europa* (…), Lisboa, 1800.
48 A.D. da Silva, *Collecção de Legislação Portugueza desde a última Compilação das Ordenações*, 1791–1801, Lisboa, Typografia Maigrense, 1828, 654–655. F.D. Costa, 'Capitalistas e serviços: empréstimos, contratos e mercês no final do século XVIII', *Análise Social* XXVII, 2–3, 1992, 441–460.
49 da Silva, *Collecção de Legislação Portugueza*, 657.
50 Or that the intendant had taken upon himself, as when he authorised innkeepers to arrest any strangers who appeared on their premises.
51 'regra para o futuro'. ANTT, *Intendência Geral da Polícia*, book 6, fls 97v–98.
52 'para a autoridade da polícia poder ir de acordo com o poder militar'. ANTT, *Intendência Geral da Polícia*, book 6, fls 99v–100v.
53 Málaga had lost some 7,000 inhabitants between August and December 1803.
54 J.H. Saraiva, *História de Portugal*, Lisboa, Alfa, 1993, 297.
55 '… que nos anos passados se puseram em observância com tanto proveito e segurança da saúde pública'. ANTT, *Ministério do Reino*, book 415, fl. 18.
56 For example, he was given direct access to the Lisbon Customs House, although he had been removed from its governing board the previous year.
57 F.D. Costa, 'O bom uso das paixões'.
58 ANTT, *Intendência Geral da Polícia*, Contas para as Secretarias, book 8, fl.16v.
59 ANTT, *Intendência Geral da Polícia*, book 162, fls 155–155v.
60 AHU, *Reino*, box 179, bundle 31.
61 ANTT, *Ministério do Reino*, book 415, fl. 18v.
62 ANTT, *Ministério do Reino*, book, 415, fls 19v–20.
63 '… a ser as mais desastrosas e dignas das maiores cautelas em favor da preservação da saúde pública'. ANTT, *Ministério do Reino*, book 415, fl. 18.
64 ANTT, *Intendência Geral da Polícia*, book 162, fls 172v–173v.
65 ANTT, *Ministério do Reino*, book 415, fls 18v–19; fls 20–20v.
66 Which included Ireland, Germany and Spain.

67 For example, the Prior General of the Carmelites was strongly censured for taking in an Irish friar.
68 ANTT, *Intendência Geral da Polícia,* book 162, fls 171v–172v.
69 As happened in Tavira, for instance.
70 '… com prepotência, arrogar cada um a si a autoridade de mandar aos outros, saindo fora dos limites descritos pela lei'. AML-AH, *Provimento da Saúde,* cód. no. 29, fls 14–17v.
71 ANTT, *Ministério do Reino,* book 415, fl. 21v.
72 '… tomar todas providências necessárias, usando os meios disponíveis de modo a evitar a propagação da dita peste para o reino […] promover ordens e de que estas sejam respeitadas por todas as instituições e pessoas do reino'.
73 ANTT, *Ministério do Reino,* book 415, fls 24–24v.
74 'sem demora nem embaraços'. ANTT, *Ministério do Reino,* book 415, fls 23v–24.
75 ANTT, *Ministério do Reino,* book 415, fl. 24v.
76 ANTT, *Ministério do Reino,* book 415, fl. 25.
77 AML-AH, *Provimento da Saúde,* bundle no. 3, fls 29–32v
78 ANTT, *Ministério do Reino,* book 415, fl. 22v.
79 '… inteligência do seu conteúdo para dar conta das providências tomadas'. ANTT, *Ministério do Reino,* book 415, fl. 22v.
80 It was at the Board's request that the prince regent ordered the Secretary of State for Foreign Affairs and War to supply the troops engaged in the cordon with tow in addition to their daily ration of bread, at the Royal Exchequer's expense.
81 In this he stressed the criticism he had had to face from the commanders of foreign vessels.
82 For the measures mentioned here that were taken in November 1804 alone: AML-AH, *Provimento da Saúde,* cód. no. 28, fls 1–8v.; fl. 29; fls 78–95v.; fls 98–101v.; fls 104–109v.; fls 112–113v.; fls 116–117v.; fls 136–163v; no. 29, fls 76–77v.; fls 96–97v.; fls 102–103v.; fls 124–133v.
83 'uma verídica notícia (…) do estado da saúde da cidade (de Lisboa)'. He enclosed fifteen copies of the measures he had taken and stated that 'other highly extraordinary' measures had also been adopted.
84 For the Barcelos section: AML-AH, *Provimento da Saúde,* file no. 10 of the papers for the province of Minho e Porto, fls 4–7v.
85 Probably based on the guidelines set out in the *Pest Contumaz Pate,* 1785.
86 ANTT, *Ministério do Reino,* book 415, fl. 26.
87 'Recapitulação da força total necessária para a organização de um Cordão de Tropas na fronteira desde o Tejo principiando em Montalvão, até ao Guadiana'.

88 'Instrução para os senhores comandantes das divisões que formam o cordão da raia'.

89 ANTT, *Ministério do Reino*, book 415, fl. 27.

90 '... serviria caso o contágio não chegue'.

91 On this topic, see A. Cliff and M. Smallman-Raynor, *Oxford Textbook of Infectious Disease Control: A Geographical Analysis from Medieval Quarantine to Global Eradication*, Oxford University Press, Oxford, 2013, 1–13.

10

Quarantine and British 'protection' of the Ionian Islands, 1815–64

Costas Tsiamis, Eleni Thalassinou, Effie Poulakou-Rebelakou and Angelos Hatzakis

> It is here a custom strictly observed not to suffer any to traffike or come ashore before they have a Pratticke from the Seniors of Health: which will not be granted until forty dayes after their arrival, especially if the ship come from Turkie, and bring not a certificate, that the place from whence they come is free from the infection. 'A Relation of a Journal Begun', Sir George Sandys (London 1610)

Introduction

This chapter seeks to present a case study of public health in a colonial context by focusing on the organisation of lazarettos in the British Protectorate of the Ionian Islands (1815–64). The British inherited these quarantine structures from the Venetians and, nothwithstanding their anticontagionist discourse, consolidated all quarantine facilities which they found. Quarantine was important not only for colonial rule on the Islands but also in terms of British seaborne power in the Mediterranean. By focusing on quarantine in the Ionian Islands we can come to understand better the links between local politics, medical theory and sanitary practice.

This, then, is a story of British sanitary policy writ small: how colonial policies towards quarantine played out at a local and regional level within those parts of the Mediterranean controlled by the British. It echoes a theme highlighted by others in this volume that, despite the domination of anticontagionist thought in Britain itself, Britain tended to promote quarantine measures in its Mediterranean possession, and indeed to strengthen them. It did this, we suggest, not only to counter the spread of cholera, plague and other contagious diseases, but also to police regional commerce and shipping, to allow its own ships to move smoothly through Mediterranean at a time when quarantine was widely practised across the region, and to manage local problems such as smuggling from the mainland of Greece, the arrival of Greek refugees from the Ottoman Empire and local resistance to British rule. Indeed, local perceptions that the quarantine system was not working fed into broader Ionian criticism of British rule, the most recent of a long line of conquerors that worked against Ionian independence or union with the rest of Greece.

Sanitary models in the Ionian Islands before the British

The Ionian Islands, traditionally called '*Επτάνησα*' (Seven Islands; from the Greek word *επτά* meaning seven), are a group of islands located off the West coast of Greece, in the Ionian Sea. The seven islands, from north to south, are Kerkyra (Corfu in Italian), Paxi, Lefkada (Santa Maura), Ithaca, Cephalonia, Zakynthos (Zante) and Kythira (Cerigo). Presently, Kythira belongs, from an administrative point of view, to the Prefecture of Athens (Figure 10.1). After the Fourth Crusade of 1202–04 that culminated in the sack of Constantinople, the Venetians significantly enlarged their possessions as they became the main beneficiaries of the partition of the Byzantine Empire. Following Corfu, the rest of the Ionian Islands would be conquered one by one by Venice and retained until the eighteenth century.[1] When the *Serenissima* was dissolved by Napoleon in 1797 the Ionian Islands fell under French domination, but after two years they became a Russian protectorate. In 1800 a short-lived independent state by the name of the Septinsular Republic was created – which went on until the French re-occupied the islands in 1807.[2]

Among these various powers that predated the British in the rule of the Ionian Islands, Venice was obviously the most influential, also in terms of the protection against epidemics. As is well known, during the second plague pandemic (Black Death, fourteeenth century) several Mediterranean states introduced quarantine measures to counter the spread of the outbreak. The first elementary quarantine for visitors from

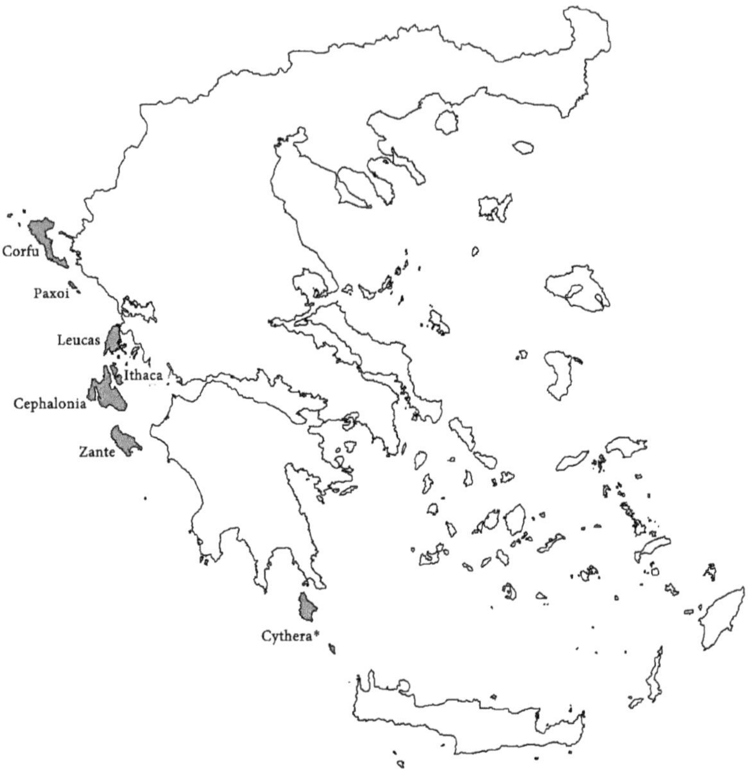

Figure 10.1 The Ionian Islands.

plague-affected areas was introduced in 1377 in the Republic of Ragusa (modern Dubrovnik, Croatia), a former Venetian colony on the Dalmatian coasts.[3] In the metropolitan territory of the Italian states, maritime quarantine was also pioneered by the Republic of Venice with the establishment of the first lazaretto on the island of *Santa Maria di Nazareth* in 1403,[4] in part to ensure the military, demographic and commercial stability of its possessions in the East. The geo-strategic position of its Greek possessions – used as a gateway in the maritime passage from the Levant to the West – forced the Venetians to translate metropolitan sanitary measures there.[5] Quarantine formed an integral part of a sanitary model based on the protection against a disease rather than its prevention or eradication. The Venetian model was characterised by a strict administrative hierarchy, heavy bureaucracy and a chaotic legislative system. In every Venetian territory, including the Ionian Islands, a *Proveditore alla Sanità* (Health Proveditor) was in charge of controlling a *Magistrato alla Sanità* (Health Magistrate) and a lazaretto.[6]

The following rulers of the islands, the French and the Russians, adopted the Venetian model but failed to reform it, in our opinion, due to the prevailing political instability. In the case of Imperial France, efforts to implement a massive, compulsory vaccination against smallpox, together with the subordination of the *Magistrato alla Sanità* to the *Commissaires de Police* (Police Inspectors) in case of epidemics, led to angry reactions by the local population. Of course, there were additional causes behind these reactions, such as the delay of the French in fulfilling their promise of creating an independent Greek state in the Ionian area and the gradual transformation of the islands into a French protectorate at the time. As far as quarantine was concerned, the French reformed the system with the State Order of the 1 June 1810 issued in Corfu, the capital of the Ionian Islands, by the Imperial Commissioner Mathieu Lesseps. The main articles of this official order regulated the location where ships were obliged to berth at the port of Corfu; the documentation required for issuing health certificates (article 2); the isolation procedures for the crews and merchandise (article 7); it also forbade the secret transportation of passengers and smuggling to the coasts of the island (article 11).[7]

Sanitary organisation under British 'protection'

With the end of the Napoleonic Wars, the Treaty of Paris (1815) handed the Ionian Islands to the British as a 'protectorate', the new possession being granted nominal independence.[8] According to the Ionian Constitution of 1817, drafted by the first High Commissioner, Lord Thomas Maitland (1815–24), the executive power was laid in the hands of a Senate and a Parliament took on legislative responsibilities. Despite this, in practice, the High Commissioner had the right to veto the Parliament's decisions. The Ionian Parliament comprised three parties: the Conservative Party (pro-British party), the Reform Party (promoting the independence of the islands) and the Radicals (promoting union of the islands with the Kingdom of Greece after the latter became independent from Ottoman rule).[9] In 1864, by means of the Protocol of London, the islands would be finally annexed to Greece as a 'present' made by the British to King George I, whom they themselves had sponsored as candidate for the throne.[10]

With the establishment of British rule, the new authorities adopted the old Venetian sanitary model albeit with a few administrative modifications. The first actions of the British included the codification of a chaotic Venetian sanitary legislation and attempts at reducing administrative bureaucracy. In accordance with Maitland's 1817 Constitution, the Venetian *Provedittore alla Sanità* was renamed General Resident of Health (Part 5, Article 1), and his election was to be decided by a written examination and a personal interview with the High Commissioner.[11] It is important to note that previously under Venetian rule, the *Proveditore alla Sanità* had been elected by local committees representing the local Greek population. Therefore, in most cases, they were not physicians but judges or notaries. Venetian archives provide us with reports on the difficulties faced by the public health services due to poorly trained health officers.[12]

Among the various administrative and legislative duties of the General Resident of Health were the management of epidemic crises and the supervision of the workings of the lazarettos. First, the General Resident of Health, in collaboration with the *Collegio Medico* of Corfu (a scientific association founded in 1802, whose members included the most prominent Greek physicians who had graduated from Italian universities, such as those in Bologna, Padova and Sienna), determined the duration of quarantine for each infectious disease in 1861.[13] Second, the General Resident of Health, just like his predecessor, the *Provedittore alla Sanità*, supervised lazarettos through his control of the *Magistrato alla Sanità* (the Health Magistrate of the islands). The *Priore* (President) and the *Protomedico* (Chief Doctor) of the Magistrate were in direct communication and collaborated with the chief and physicians of the lazaretto. Hence, the reports they transmitted to the General Resident were of great importance in cases of epidemic outbreaks.

Finally, the General Inspector of the Coast (established in 1820) – who was in turn under the direct command of the General Resident – was tasked with supervising compliance of quarantine by everyone. During the British presence on the islands, a new programme was launched, aimed at the reorganisation of the maritime sanitary

Table 10.1 Venetian and British lazarettos in the Ionian Islands

Island	Venetian era	British protection
Corfu	1588 (Sanitary Station) 1705 (Lazaretto)	1814 (renovation)
Cephalonia	1705 Lazaretto 1719 (renovation)	1841(renovation)
Zante	1690 Lazaretto	1854(renovation)
Santa Maura	1718 Lazaretto	1820 c. (New lazaretto)
Ithaca	1560 Lazaretto	1817(renovation)
Cerigo	Without Lazaretto	1817 (New lazaretto)
Paxi	Without Lazaretto	1820 c. (New lazaretto)

Source: Data from John Lascaratos, *The Prevention of Disease and the Establishment of a Social Welfare Policy in the Islands under British Protection, 1814–1864*. Table by the authors.

procedures and the renovation of the Venetian lazarettos or the building of new ones (Table 10.1). One of the major problems found with the Ionian lazarettos derived from the islands' location at the most active seismological zone of Greece. Many Venetian lazarettos had suffered heavy damage from high-magnitude earthquakes during the eighteenth century – these included that in Corfu in 1743 (7 degrees, Richter magnitude scale) and 1786 (6.5 R), and the enormous one of 1767 (7.2 Richter degrees) affecting Cephalonia, Zante and Santa Maura and leaving many victims.[14] During the period of British protection, dozens of strong earthquakes were recorded, the most noteworthy being those of Santa Maura in 1815 (6.3 R) and 1825 (6.7 R), Zante in 1820 (6.7 R) and 1840 (6.7 R) and Cephalonia in 1862 (6.6 R).

Lazarettos and seaborne infectious diseases

The port official responsible for the surveillance of every ship approaching the islands was a state appointed physician. These officers had the duty to control the ship's bill of health (the so-called *Fede di Sanità*), which confirmed that the port of departure was free from infectious diseases.[15] The certificates were signed by the British ambassadors or consuls in states such as the Ottoman Empire, Italy and the newly independent Greek territories.

Captains were required to answer the physician's questions regarding any cases of disease detected among the crew or the passengers, or any contacts made with other ships. In case of a suspect case or a declared patient, the crew was obliged to be hospitalised in the lazaretto. The Magistrate had the obligation to supply the isolated persons with new clothes. This while the blankets and coverlets of the sailors in the ship had to be cleaned and exposed to the sun. The duration of quarantine depended on the nature of the disease and the port of departure; hence, the forty-day quarantine was not compulsory for every disease. According to the instructions in force under British rule, the duration of the quarantine ranged from nine to forty days. For a vessel which came in contact with another ship while at sea (the ship having departed from a port where an epidemic had broken out), another twenty-four days of isolation were added. In 1861, the duration of quarantine was determined according to the particular disease detected, plus a compulsory isolation period for every ship departing from certain ports (having had or not an epidemic outbreak): twenty-four days for vessels coming from Albanian ports, ten days for those arriving from the Aegean Islands and seven days for arrivals from Constantinople. The period of quarantine isolation stretched over the actual incubation period of plague, cholera and yellow fever (Table 10.2).[16] This means that with quarantine the physicians had the time to detect a suspect case and communicate it to the authorities. (Figure 10.2)

During quarantine, crews were isolated, the cargo and their vessel were subject to clearance procedures consisting of fumigation by the *Sborratori*, a special corps of cleaners who were experts in disinfection. During cleansing, a yellow flag was raised signalling the ship's isolation. The isolated persons and the cargo were guarded by a squad of sanitary armed guards, the *Quardiani*. When the period of quarantine ended, the *Protomedico* of the Magistrate of Health would allow the ship to carry a clean sanitary certificate signed by the *Protomedico* – which enabled it to continue its commercial activities (*Pratigo*) – and a licence for free departure (*Fede di Partenza*) (Figure 10.3). The British authorities provided trilingual public documents (in Greek, English and Italian), but naval documents were exclusively delivered in Italian. The *Magistrato alla Sanità* was obliged to record all events by keeping a 'port

Table 10.2 Comparison between days of quarantine and the incubation period of plague, smallpox, cholera and yellow fever.

	Plague	Smallpox	Cholera	Yellow fever
Quarantine Duration (days)	40	12	9	40
Incubation period (days)	2–6 (bubonic) 1–3 (pneumonic)	12–14 (range 7–17)	2 hours–5 days	3–6

Sources: *Report of the Central Medical Society of Corfu to H. Drummont Wolff, Secretary of H.M. Lord High Commissioner, Corfu 24 March 1861*; J. Poland and D. Dennis, 'Diagnosis and Clinical Manifestations', in: D. Dennis et al. (eds), *Plague Manual: Epidemiology, Distribution, Surveillance and Control,* World Health Organisation, Geneva, 1999; W. Joklik, H. Willett, B. Amos and C. Wirfeut, *Zinsser's Microbiology,* Norwalk, Appleton Lange, 1999; J. Vainio and F. Cutts, *Yellow Fever,* World Health Organisation-Department of Emerging and other communicable Diseases Surveillance and Control, Geneva, 1998. Table by the authors.

diary', which was also written in Italian. During his term of office, High Commissioner Lord John Colborne of Seaton (1843–49), who was extremely popular among the local population, decided to start having all naval and port documents produced in Greek.

Lazarettos and endemic infectious diseases

Lazarettos were places of isolation not only for crews and passengers affected by 'exotic epidemics', but also for the natives of the Ionian Islands suffering from endemic infections. British physicians studied a wide range of local diseases. Following neo-Hippocratic medical concepts widespread at that time, they took into consideration many parameters and factors, such as the environment, climatic disturbances, humidity and the temperature fluctuations of the islands, the level of agricultural production, the professions of the inhabitants, even their diet and their daily social life. According to the data, the most frequent

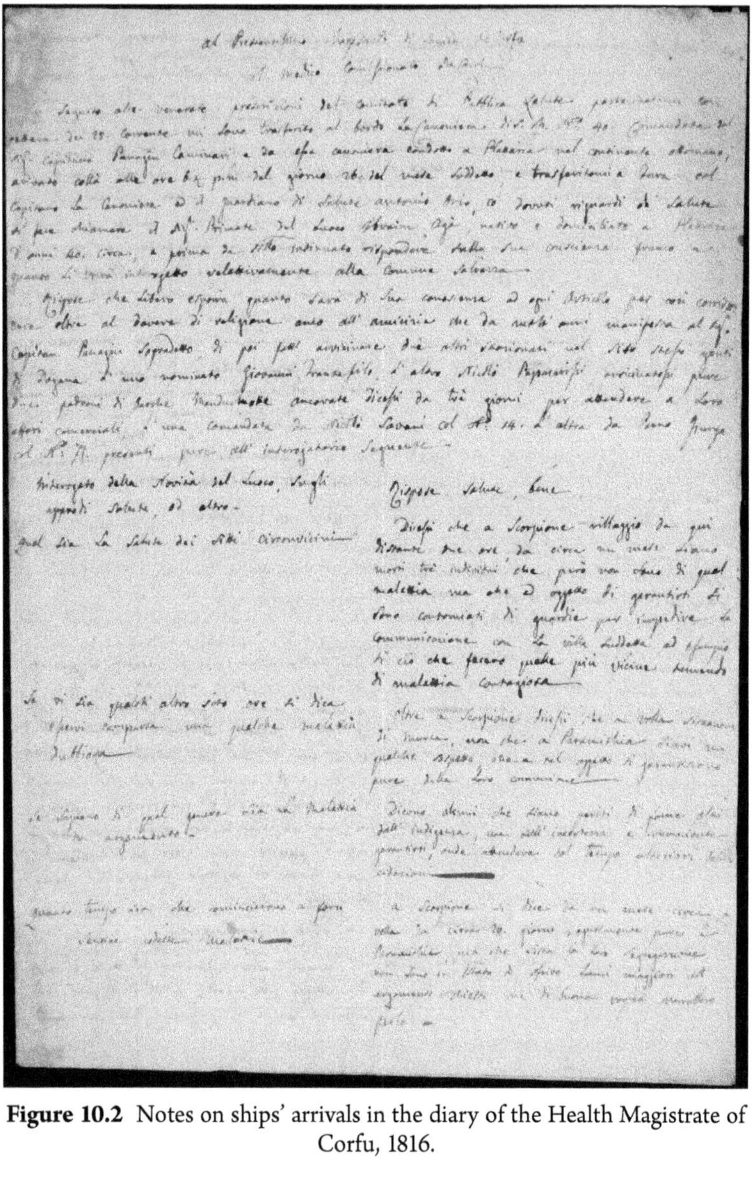

Figure 10.2 Notes on ships' arrivals in the diary of the Health Magistrate of Corfu, 1816.

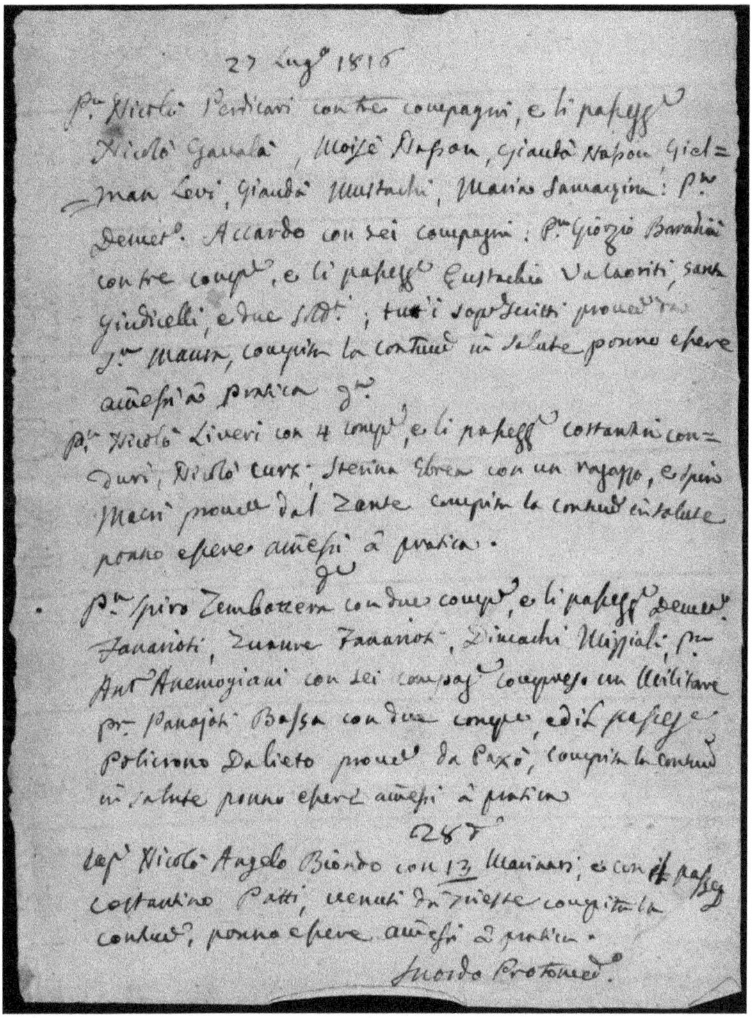
27 Lug.o 1816
P.n Nicolò Perdicari con tre compagni, e li passegg.i
Nicolò Gavalà, Moisè Nasson, Giacobbe Nasson, Giel=
=man Levi, Giacobbe Mustachi, Marino Samaragina: P.n
Demet.o Accardo con sei compagni: P.n Giorgio Baradà
con tre comp.i, e li passegg.i Eustachio Valaoriti, Santo
Giudicelli, e due sold.i; tutti i sopradetti provenienti
... mare, compita la contumacia in salute ponno essere
ammessi a pratica g.i
P.n Nicolò Liveri con 4 comp.i, e li passegg.i Costantin Con=
duri, Nicolò Curx, Stefano Ebreo con un ragazzo, e Spiro
Macri provenienti dal Zante compita la contum.a in salute
ponno essere ammessi a pratica.
g.i
P.n Spiro Zembazzera con due comp.i, e li passegg.i Demet.o
Fanarioti, Zuanne Fanarioti, Dimachi Missiali; P.n
Ant.o Anemogiani con sei compag.i compreso un Militare
P.n Panajoti Bassa con due compag.i, ed il passeg.e
Policrono Dalieto proven.ti da Paxò, compita la contum.a
in salute ponno essere ammessi a pratica
28 d.o
Cap.n Nicolò Angelo Biondo con 13 marinari, e con il passegg.
Costantino Patti, venuti da Trieste compita la
contum.a, ponno essere ammessi a pratica.
Giordo Protomed.o

Figure 10.3 *Fede de partenza* signed by the Protomedico of Zante for a ship travelling to Corfu, 1816.

infectious diseases in the Ionian region were malaria, dysentery and pneumonia.[17] The major endemic disease in the area was malaria and all kinds of 'fevers', as British and local physicians called them: *therma continua, amphimerina paludoza, tertian fever, quartian fever, malignant fever*.[18] Malaria did not justify isolation, but it was nevertheless a serious disease having great social, economic and military impacts. The records of British military hospitals in the Ionian Islands during the period 1822–29 show that malaria was the primary cause of death in the British garrisons.[19] During the period 1837–46, the total morbidity rate in garrisons due to malaria reached 22.47% (6,703 cases).[20] Malaria was a cause of hospitalisation and not a disease for isolation in the lazaretto.

Official instructions issued by the health authorities made it compulsory for persons who were found with a serious infectious disease (plague, smallpox, dysentery) in the main towns or in villages to be isolated and monitored in the lazaretto. In case of large-scale epidemics, the General Resident of Health could decide to expand the lazaretto quarantine and to establish temporary isolation facilities in churches, monasteries and special camps. According to archival records, no large-scale epidemics broke out in the Ionian Islands, in comparison to the Greek Kingdom and the other Greek lands under Ottoman rule, apart from the outbreaks of cholera in Cephalonia in 1850 (992 deaths) and of smallpox in Corfu in 1852 (365 deaths).[21] Other recorded epidemics, either originating on land or coming from the sea, were the outbreaks of plague (Corfu 1815 and Cephalonia 1816), cholera (Corfu 1855 and Zante 1856), smallpox (Cephalonia, Zante and Santa Maura 1837) and meningitis (Corfu 1843–44), though all these cases left minimal casualties (Figure 10.4).[22]

Some contemporary impressions of the Ionian lazarettos

According to the British sanitary legislation for the Ionian Islands, it seems that quarantines were strictly adhered to, even if their duration varied from time to time and was influenced by specific circumstances. The British authorities in particular were keen to demonstrate the rigour with which quarantine was applied, and that the High Commissioner himself could not escape it. Zante's newspaper *Ioniki* reports that: 'His Excellency, High Commissioner-General Lord Thomas Maitland, landed in our town after his quarantine.'[23] It seems that Lord

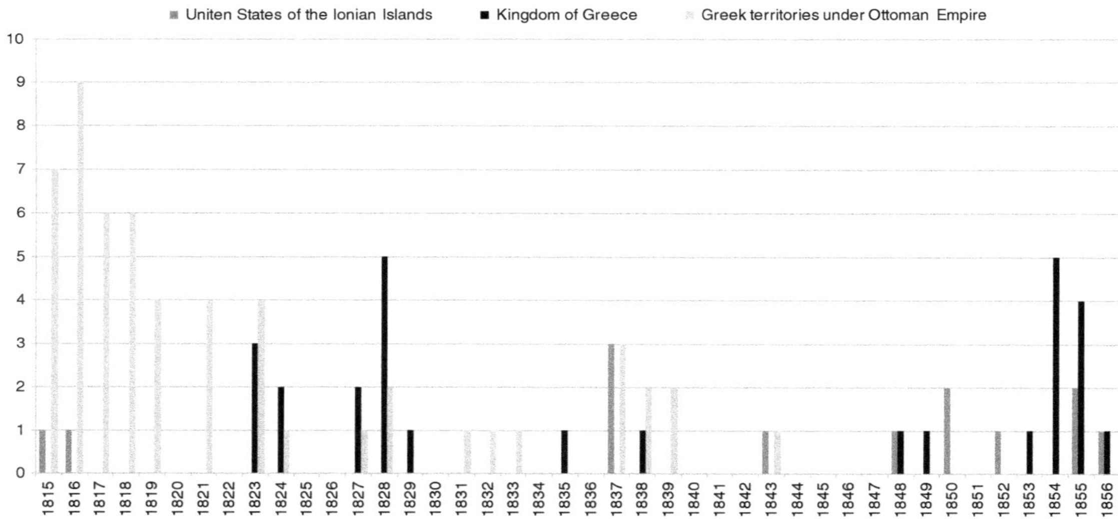

Figure 10.4 Epidemic outbreaks of various infectious diseases in the Ionian State, the Greek Kingdom and the Greek territories of the Ottoman Empire.

Maitland set a good example to the locals, demonstrating that no one was above the law in this case.

Travellers' diaries provide a more complex picture, with accounts of a rigorously enforced quarantine countered by examples of exceptions to the rule. Thus, the British traveller Hugh Williams wrote in 1820, seeming to support the image of a rigorously applied quarantine, albeit one that applied differently depending on where the ships came from:

> At present all persons coming from the Ionian Islands perform a quarantine of twenty-eight days. The recent plague at Corfu and Cephalonia seem to justify the measure. On the other hand, there is a quarantine of ten days on all vessels from the coast of Calabria, in consequence of the appearance of pestilence last year in the town of Noja.[24]

The point of rigorous enforcement may also have been supported by the tendency of both sailors and travellers to present lazarettos as prisons. Hence, according to Edward Giffard (1837):

> We had therefore what anywhere else would have been an agreeable society, but in this quarantine prison nothing can be agreeable, and the time crawled but heavily along, our chief occupation being to watch the boat which brought over our breakfast and dinner from the town …[25]

It was perhaps for this reason in part that there were frequent infringements of quarantines, and that passengers were not equally treated: while the poor were confined in lazarettos, the wealthy remained on the ships moored outside the ports, a privilege they obtained from the port authorities who many a time also reduced the duration spent in quarantine. The case of the American traveller Samuel Barrows shows the typical 'modification' of quarantine procedures for the wealthy or powerful on board a ship at the port of Corfu:

> Life at the Vido was a happy dream. We learned then, if never before, the true meaning of *dolce far niente* … A thousand happy memories will always cling to Vido: the hot afternoons that we spent listening to the military music floating across the water from the fortress; the cool evenings when the wandering musicians from Corfu serenaded us with mandolin and guitar …[26]

Some of the prominent passengers enjoyed another privileged procedure when they were 'hospitalised' in the residencies of British officers.[27] Another unusually alternative case of 'strict' quarantine was recorded in the travel diary of Hugh Williams, published in 1820. He revealed that:

> We landed at the health office, and a small adjoining house within the precincts of the office, and enclosed with palisades, was allotted for our residence during our days of quarantine. After our introduction to the Governor-General Sir Thomas Maitland, we were invited by his Excellency to dine with him, and an apartment was provided for us in the Palace. We remained there about 10 days, and nothing could exceed the kindness of Sir Thomas Maitland ...[28]

Beyond individual examples, the most serious violation of the quarantine procedure occurred in 1850 during a popular revolution against the British in Cephalonia. Under pressure of such an uprising, the British brought in several regiments from their nearby island colony of Malta in order to reinforce their troops in Cephalonia. It seems that some suspect cases of cholera were detected among their ranks. However, the British overrode their own quarantine procedures and, a few days after the regiments' landing, an outbreak of cholera struck the island. This epidemic was to become the deadliest sanitary episode during the whole period of the British Protectorate, causing 992 deaths among Cephalonia's inhabitants.[29] The case fatality rate of the 1,858 patients was high (53.3%) and the mortality of the population (8,966 citizens) was 11.1%.[30]

Economic, social and political impact of lazarettos

It should be clear by now that the implementation of the quarantine system was not always as rigourous as the British authorities suggested. Indeed, the British authorities attempts to impose quarantine were often challenged by shipowners and merchants concerned about the blockade of their products at the lazarettos; smugglers who brought contraband from distant shores; the clandestine arrivals of Greek rebels and their families from the mainland of Greece during the revolution against the Ottomans between 1821 and 1832; and the general opposition of the Ionian islanders to British rule. Finally, the British authorities themselves were often conflicted about quarantine, trying to reconcile two often opposing imperatives: preventing infectious diseases from crossing the borders and minimising the economic impact of disease-related restrictions on travel and trade.[31]

Such problems were exacerbated by the rapid 'globalisation' of Mediterranean trade – accelerated by the opening of the Suez Canal in 1869 – and by the increasing importance given to miasmatic medical theories, and the fact that persons and merchandise were regularly isolated and put under surveillance. The British authorities claimed that it was a priority to protect the islands against the short- and long-term impact of an infectious disease outbreak. However, in practice they tried to balance the protection of public health with the maintenance of economic activities, so that the detection of a person suspected of being infected did not always result in the blockade of a port or an island and the authorities often sought to facilitate commerce even among those subject to quarantine. For example, after the fumigation of merchandise, the Ionian sanitary authorities allowed quarantined merchants to carry out their trade exchanges with local merchants: negotiations between the two parties would take place in the lazaretto and under the supervision of the medical officers. Almost all the Ionian lazarettos had a place designated for such meetings. The native merchants would remain at a distance and in a separate space from their isolated colleagues. In this way, quarantined merchants enjoyed the opportunity to spend some of the 'wasted' time in isolation on negotiating and closing business deals.[32]

Blockading a port was always a critical issue for local and British trade. During such cases, the British introduced the system of so-called 'hygienic convoys'. This meant that a flotilla of vessels from an island put under quarantine carried out commercial exchanges in open sea, under the supervision of a sanitary magistrate. The procedure was almost identical to that being done at other ports. Merchants from the other islands were obliged to carry their ships' certificates and to be visited by physicians. Upon their return to the blockaded island, if any suspect patients were detected, the sanitary ship would raise a yellow flag in order to alert the Magistrate and the lazaretto personnel.[33] With these hygienic convoys, the British managed to avoid economic collapse and above all secured the necessary food supplies for the local population of the island being quarantined. However, when the blockade was prolonged, strong reactions became unavoidable. This phenomenon was in part the result of pressing interests in resuming economic activities as soon as possible. After a period without patients or deaths in the lazaretto, the local communities would always emphatically demand the resumption of trade. The decision to end a blockade rested on the High Commissioner. During certain outbreaks, such as in the cases of plague in Leukimmi in Corfu (1815), cholera in Corfu (1855) and Zante (1856), the High Commissioners ordered the opening of the ports a month after the last case of disease had been recorded.[34] Such delays often caused public tensions and clashes between local inhabitants and the authorities.

The suppression of the flow of smugglers, rebels and refugees arriving from the Greek mainland in connection with the anti-Ottoman uprising became one of the priorities of the British authorities for ensuring an adequate protection of public health in the islands. In addition, the mainland was perceived as a place with numerous foci of endemic infectious diseases, so people who arrived clandestinely and without undergoing prior isolation in the lazarettos were considered dangerous for public health. The major disease was plague and a lot of epidemics were recorded at the Greek side in Epirus (1812, 1813, 1814, 1815, 1816, 1817, 1820, 1822, 1823, 1824).[35] A typical case of high alert and the preventive closing of the sea-borders of the Ionian State was the declaration of the High Commissioner Frederick Adam in 1822, in order to protect the islands from a plague epidemic in Epirus on the mainland of Greece.[36] In 1822 and 1831, with regard to the problems posed by rebels and smugglers, the High Commissioner Frederick Adam decided to hire spies on the islands and to place more guards (*quardiani*) to protect the coasts.[37] In addition, the authorities ordered the construction of small watchtowers in remote sites of the islands' coastline, the remains of which are still visible. Today, in the coasts and villages of the Ionian Islands, the toponym '*Βαρδιάνοι*' reminds us of the era of the night guards (*quardiani*, in Greek *vardiani*).

Finally, there was the tension between the Greek population and the authorities. After a few years under British protection, the Greek Ionians realised that the nominal independence embodied by the Assembly and the Parliament was more virtual than real. After experiencing the Venetians, the French and the Russians, the Ionians saw the new foreign rulers as an obstacle in their route towards independence or unification with Greece. The first signs of open tension between the two sides dated back to the beginning of the Greek revolution against the Ottoman Empire in 1821. The British foreign policy of neutrality in this conflict, the tactics of the High Commissioner Lord Maitland against the participation of Ionian volunteers in the revolution (those caught and found guilty were to be exiled from the Ionian State and had their property confiscated) and the diplomatic relations of the British with the Ottoman governor of Epirus, Ali Pasha, who had committed notorious atrocities against the Greeks in war and peacetime, were viewed as unforgivable 'British betrayals' by the Ionian Greeks.[38]

In those circumstances, it is no surprise that the outbreak of epidemics became a source of political tension. The blockades and commercial disruption, the compulsory enrolment of Greeks as grave-diggers, the heavy fines imposed upon those who violated the sanitary laws, the high cost of hospitalisation in the lazarettos and, above all, the appointment of the chief of the Executive Police as head of the sanitary institutions during the epidemic outbreaks were main points of friction.[39] A typical case of social turmoil was the appointment of the chief of the Executive Police, William Fayer, as commander during the crisis of the cholera outbreak in Cephalonia in 1850.[40] For the Greeks, the name William Fayer was synonymous with the execution of the Cephalonian rebels, and the sanitary regulations which he imposed resuscitated angry reactions from the population. Indeed, laws and measures imposed during epidemics were perceived by local inhabitants as intrusive acts against their traditions and their liberty. With the introduction of the reforms based on Thomas Maitland's 1817 Constitution and of the law on the 'Freedom of the Press and Abolition of Censorship' by High Commissioner Lord Seaton (18 May 1848), all Ionian Greek political parties were finally able to speak freely and to publish their own official newspapers. As could be expected, a 'free press' would be the starting point for more political tensions between the two sides and for the emergence of an organised movement of political resistance against British rule.[41]

Against this background of political tension, the Magistrate of Health was always in the eye of the storm. He was attacked for malpractice, especially with regard to the functioning of the lazarettos as well as for issuing orders to perform vaccinations.[42] In all these cases the press played an important role. With every epidemic outbreak, the anti-British papers and parties accused the authorities of bad management of the lazarettos. Paradoxically, although the Ionians called for freedom or union with Greece from their British rulers, they looked back to a golden age of quarantine under their former Venetian rulers, when, they argued, the Magistrate was under the control of the Greeks and more democratic procedures were practised. Besides this, the sanitary authorities had to face the problem of the populations' mistrust towards Western medicine. The case of the mass vaccinations against smallpox is a typical example. According to the physician and traveller, John Hennen, who visited the island in the late 1820s, the Ionians had not yet become accustomed to vaccination. When he visited the civil hospital of Santa Maura, he was happy to see that all the inhabitants of the island were at the hospital. Soon, however, he realised that they had not gone there because they accepted vaccination but rather because they were scared that if they refused, they would be punished with isolation and a harsh period of quarantine in the lazaretto.[43]

Given the increasingly complex political situation in the Protectorate, the maintenance and enforcement of sanitary laws – including isolation in the Lazaretto – was an issue that required special handling. As John Chircop argues, in the British Mediterranean possessions of the Ionian Islands, Malta and Gibraltar, a specific form of colonial state ideology based on the philosophy of charitable paternalism was dominant.[44] The strategy of a well-functioning public sanitary system and a welfare policy (civil hospitals, specific care for the poor, orphanages and foundlings) was essential for the upholding of public order and to garner consent – or in other words to foster a sort of 'eternal gratitude' for the colonisers in the natives. Within this context, the fear of contagion from persons 'outside of the Ionian State' (or similarly 'outside' of Malta or Gibraltar) led to strict 'prophylactic measures' against suspicious cases in order to protect both the colonised populations and the military garrisons on these strategic British possessions. At the same time, during an epidemic outbreak, measures of strict quarantine were utilised by the British authorities to prove their supremacy over, but also paternal concern towards, the local populations, legitimising this as being done for the public health and the protection of the 'healthy part of the society'.[45]

In the case of the Ionian Islands, the followers of 'miasmatic' theories, who came to be considered as enemies of the tranquillity of the colonial order, were to be found mainly in the Greek Assembly (asking for more political power), in anti-British parties (asking for reformations) and more widely within the population – very 'ungrateful' towards British charity (and preferring to ask for freedom). The

British physicians in the Ionian Islands studied the diseases, the environment, the climatic disturbances, the agricultural production, the professions of the inhabitants and their diet and their daily social life, but did not pay enough attention to their mentality of multisecular resistance against foreign rule. Unfortunately for the British, any period of tranquillity between them and the Greeks wasn't a result of their welfare policies. British welfare and charity policies were considered a mere 'trap' but one which was well known to the natives after 600 years of Venetian rule based on 'charity' and social welfare. For the Greeks – a nation with a tradition of seatrade from classic antiquity – peaceful coexistence with the British was based on the feeling of freedom at the religious, economic and political levels. It is interesting to note that during periods of social quiet under British protection – due to flourishing trade and political stability – the Ionians conformed to all sanitary orders and notifications. Not so during political crises, when public health was always the first victim of the violation of all laws. This probably owed to the fact that, in the collective imagination of the Ionian Greeks, the 'lazaretto-prison' represented an outstanding symbol of British rule. Accepting isolation in the lazaretto was equal to an obedient and silent acceptance of British domination. In contrast, the violation of sanitary orders, the refusal of isolation or the escape from a lazaretto, were considered brave acts of resistance against 'foreign oppressors'.

The most important example of such recurrent sanitary–political crises took place in 1852 during an epidemic of smallpox in Corfu. According to statistics, 2,123 people fell ill and 365 died. The newspaper *Filalithis* (lit. 'Friend of Truth') accused the Magistrate of false reports about the real scale of the epidemic, as well as the Committee of Vaccination for 'ineffective' vaccines and the malfunction of the Corfu lazaretto. The anti-British parties criticised the General Resident and the Priore of the lazaretto, for in their opinion this incident was just another example of the failure of public health policies under the British, thus signalling that the time had arrived for political reforms or even independence.[46] In contrast to the calm term of office of the High Commissioner Lord Seaton, the period of his successor, Lord Henry George Ward (1849–55), was actually a turbulent one. A few months before the outbreak of an epidemic in Corfu, Ward tried to revoke the constitutional changes introduced by Lord Seaton and to pass a law that would enable the Commissioner to declare martial law. Moreover, in 1852 political elections were being held in the Ionian Islands. The Commissioner disagreed with the functioning of the newly elected Parliament and in March he decided to adjourn its sessions. This act was a disastrous choice as one of the duties of the new Parliament should have been the appointment of the new sanitary officers of the Islands. As a result, the lazaretto of Corfu and other health institutions remained without any of their directors – an act which led to the malfunctioning of the whole public health system with disastrous effects during the upcoming smallpox epidemic.

Conclusions

For fifty years, the British Union Jack flew upon the fortresses of the Ionian Islands as the symbol of British rule. Yet, as this story has suggested, the nature of this rule was quite complex, at least as it played out in the realms of public health and quarantine. In the first place, while this period coincided with a high point of anticontagionist thought in Britain itself, regional factors meant that the quarantine system that the British inherited from previous occupiers of the islands was not only continued but also enhanced. Such a tendency was common throughout the Britain's Mediterranean territories, as it sought to balance the spread of contagious disease with the practical problem of facilitating commerce and the passage of its own ships in a region where quarantine was extensively practised. Abandoning quarantine measures risked the possibility of others imposing quarantine on British ships or vessels that passed through British controlled ports. In part for this reason a hybrid quarantine system seems to have emerged, which sought to reconcile the sometimes competing imperatives of public health and commerce.

Other factors specific to the Islands also fed into the creation of this hybrid system. One was local commerce, which meant that the practice of quarantine was bent to facilitate trade, leading to variations in the rigour with which it was imposed, and the establishment of meeting rooms in the lazarettos to oil the wheels of commerce. Another factor was the reliance of British rule on its ability to intervene militarily, which meant that at times the army was granted immunity from quarantine with, as we have seen, disastrous results during the revolt in

Cephalonia in 1850. Other pressures also ensured that the quarantine system was less rigorous than the British authorities claimed. There was smuggling from the mainland, which meant that people travelled back and forth between the islands and the rest of Greece under the eyes of the British and their public health officials. Similarly, the arrival of Greek refugees escaping Ottoman rule meant a traffic of people keen to avoid official eyes. Finally, the system was also shaped by growing Ionian discontent with British rule, and frustration with barriers to independence or union with the rest of Greece. Perceived failings in the system provided fodder for discontent not only with the British doings in public health but with British rule itself.

Notes

1 D. Nicol, *Byzantium and Venice: A Study in Diplomatic and Cultural Relations*, Cambridge, Cambridge University Press, 1988, 104–148.
2 H. Jervis and W. Jervis, *History of Corfu and the Republic of the Ionian Islands*, London, Colburn, 1852, 205–280.
3 A.D. Cliff, M.R. Smallma-Raynor and P.M. Stevens, 'Controlling the geographical spread of infectious diseases: plague in Italy, 1347–1851', *Acta Medico-Historica Adriatica* 7, 2, 2009, 197–236.
4 A.D. Cliff and M.R. Smallma-Raynor, *Infectious Diseases Control: A Geographical Analysis from Medieval Quarantine to Global Eradication*, Oxford, Oxford University Press, 2013, 2–10.
5 K. Konstantinidou, E. Mantadakis, E. Falagas, T. Sardi and G. Samonis, 'Venetian rule and control of plague epidemics on the Ionian Islands during 17th and 18th centuries', *Emerging Infection Diseases* 15, 1, 2009, 39–43.
6 P. Selmi, 'Il Magistrato alla Sanità', in *Difesa della Sanità a Venezia. Secoli XIII-XIX*, (Mostra Documentaria), Venezia, 1979, 28–50; R. Palmer, *L' azione della republica di Venezia nel controlo della peste. Lo sviluppo della politica governativa, Venezia e la peste 1348–1797*, Venezia, Marsilio Editori, 1979, 105–107.
7 John Lascaratos, 'The Prevention of Disease and the Establishment of a Social Welfare Policy in the Islands under British Protection (1814–1864)', PhD thesis, Athens University, 1984, 23–26; *Empire Français au nom de Sa Majeste l'Empereur, Rois d'iatle et Protecteur de la Confederation du Ruin, Nous Général de Division Donzelot Gouverneur Général des Isles Ioniennes et Mathieu Lesseps Commissaire Impérial dans Dites Isles. Corfu, 1 June 1810* (Archive of the Historical and Ethnological Society of Greece).

8 Ibid.; T. Gallant, *Experiencing Dominion: Culture, Identity and Power in the British Mediterranean*, Indiana, University of Notre Dame Press, 2002, 4–14.
9 V. Kirkwall, *Four Years in the Ionian Islands: Their Political and Social Condition with a History of the British Protectorate*, London, Chapman & Hall, 1864, 186–208; B. Knox, 'British policy and the Ionian Islands 1847–1864: nationalism and imperial administration', *English Historical Review* 94, 1984, 503–529.
10 S. Xenos, *East and West: A Diplomatic History of the Annexation of the Ionian Islands to the Kingdom of Greece*, London, Trubner, 1865, 290–296.
11 *Le Tre Costituzioni (1800, 1803, 1817) Delle Sette Isole Jonie. Sezione V, Della Sanità*, Corfu, Tipografia Mercurio di G. Nicolaides Filadelfe, 1849.
12 K. Konstantinidou, 'Gli uffici di sanità delle Isole Ionie durante il Seicento e il Settecento', *Studi Veneziani* 49, 2005, 379–391.
13 *Report of the Central Medical Society of Corfu to H. Drummont Wolff, Secretary of H.M. Lord High Commissioner, Corfu 24 March 1861* (Historical Archive of Corfu).
14 Spyropoulos Panagiotis, *Chronicle of the Earthquakes in Greece*, Athens, Dodoni, 1997, 174–194.
15 *Gazzetta Delgi Stati Uniti Delle Isole Jonie, 13 Aug 1838* (Historical Archive of Corfu).
16 J. Poland and D. Dennis, 'Diagnosis and Clinical Manifestations', in D. Dennis, K.L. Cage, J. Poland, N. Gratz and E. Tikhormirov (eds), *Plague Manual: Epidemiology, Distribution, Surveillance and Control*, World Health Organization, Geneva, 1999, 43–45; W. Joklik, H. Willett, B. Amos and C. Wirfeut, *Zinsser's Microbiology*, Norwalk, Appleton Lange, 1999, 569, 950; J. Vainio and F. Cutts, *Yellow Fever*, World Health Organization – Department of Emerging and other Communicable Diseases Surveillance and Control, Geneva, 1998, 9.
17 C. Tsiamis, E. Thalassinou, E. Poulakou-Rebelakou, D. Anoyiatis-Pelé and A. Hatzakis, 'Infectious diseases control in the Ionian Islands during the British Protection (1815–1864)', *Journal of the Royal Army Medical Corps* 159, 3, 2013, 247–254.
18 W. Goodison, *A Historical and Topographical Essay upon the Islands of Corfu, Leucadia, Cephalonia, Ithaca and Zante etc*, London, Thomas & George Underwood, 1822, 230.
19 J. Davy, *Notes and Observations on the Ionian Islands and Malta with some remarks of Constantinople and Turkey, and on the system of a Quarantine, vol. 1*, London, Smith Elds & Co., 1842, 218, 226, 239, 242.
20 *Statistical Report. Parliamentary Papers, LIX (1639), ii*, 1852–1853, 112–145.

21 C. Typaldos-Preténdéris, *Du choléra épidémique observé à Cephalonie en 1850*, Athènes, 1850, p. 38; Newspaper *'Filalithis'*, fol. 26 July, 22 August, 13 September, 30 September, 15 October, 23 October, 31 October, 8 December, 16 December 1852.

22 P. Chiotis, *History of Ionian State (1815–1864), vol II.*, Zante, 1877, 355–364; C. Lavrano, *Sulla meningite cerebro-spinale-miasmatica che la dominato nell'Isola di Corfu nei mesi di Novembre e Decembre 1843, Gennajo e Febbrajo 1844*, Corfu, Nella Tipografia del Governo, 1844.

23 *Ioniki* (Zante), 15 April 1816.

24 Hugh Williams, *Travels in Italy, Greece and the Ionian Isles (Letter XLVI, Corfu)*, Edinburgh, 1820, 150.

25 E. Giffard, *A Short Visit to the Ionian Islands, Athens and the Morea*, London, 1837, 383.

26 Samuel Barrows, *The Isles and Shrines of Greece*, Boston, 1898.

27 E. Poulakou-Rebelakou, C. Tsiamis and N. Tompros, 'Travellers' impressions from the Ionian Islands lazarettos during the British Protection (1815–1864)', *Proceedings of 39th International Congress on the History of Medicine*, Bari, 2004, 38–45.

28 Williams, *Travels in Italy, Greece and the Ionian Isles*, 150.

29 Typaldos-Preténdéris, *Du choléra épidémique*, 38.

30 Ibid.; M. Salomon, *La Statisica Generale Dell'Isola di Cefalonia una delle sette componenti lo stato politico Jonio sotto denominazione di Stati Uniti Delle Isole Jonie*, Corfu, Tipografia Jonia, 1859, 2.

31 Stanley M. Lemon, Margaret A. Hamburg, P. Frederick Sparling, Eileen R. Choffnes and Alison Mack, *Ethical and Legal Considerations in Mitigating Pandemic Disease*, Washington D.C., National Academic Press – Forum on Microbial Threats Board on Global Health Institute of Medicine and National Academies, 2007, 37, 27.

32 Lascaratos, 'The Prevention of Disease', 151–153.

33 Ibid.

34 *Declaration of His Excellency, High Commissioner General Lord Thomas Maitland, Per Ordine de Sua Eccellenza Segretario Pubblico, William Meyer*, Corfu 18 May 1815; Chiotis, *History of Ionian State, vol II.*, 364.

35 Kostas Kostis, *The Time of Plague: Societies of the Greek Peninsula (14th–19th Centuries)*, Heraklion, University Press of Crete, 1995, 406–411.

36 *Proclamazione Dal Palazzo, Per Comando di Sua Eccellenza Fred. Hankey, Raccolta di Tutte le Proclamazioni Pubblicate da Parte di Sua Eccellenza il Lord Alto Commsionario*, Corfu, 23 Luglio 1822.

37 *Declaration of His Excellency*, Corfu, 28 September 1831.

38 *Declaration of His Excellency*, Corfu, 18 May 1815; Chiotis, *History of Ionian State, vol II*, 364.

39 Lascaratos, 'The Prevention of Disease', 145–153.
40 C. Tsiamis, 'Military campaigns and public health: the case of cholera outbreak in Cephalonia (1850)', *Proceedings of the Workshop on the History of Public Health during War in the Mediterranean Region (19th–20th c.)*, Army Navy Hospital of Athens, Athens, 2006, 65–71.
41 Knox, 'British policy and the Ionian Islands', 503–529.
42 *Filalithis*, fol. 13 September 1852.
43 J. Hennen, *Sketches of the Medical Topography of the Mediterranean comprising an account of Gibraltar, the Ionian Islands, and Malta to which is prefixed a sketch of a Plan for Memoirs on medical topography, vol 2*, London, Thomas & George Underwood, 1830, 190–91, 204, 228, 377, 415.
44 John Chircop, 'Public Health and Poor-Relief in the British Mediterranean Colonial Context 1800–1860s', in Laurinda Abreu (ed.), *European Health and Social Welfare Policies*, Lisbon, Blansco, 2014, 297–320.
45 Ibid.
46 *Filalithis*, 26 July; 22 August and 30 September 1852.

11

Inland sanitary cordons and liberal administration in southern Europe: Mallorca (Balearic Islands), 1820–70

Joana Maria Pujadas-Mora and Pere Salas-Vives

Coastal and inland sanitary cordons were often used, as in much of southern Europe, during the nineteenth century, to protect the island of Mallorca against imported epidemics.[1] Esteban Rodríguez Ocaña states that during the eighteenth century in Spain: 'Watch [*resguardo*] was a widely used synonym in public health, a product of a strictly defensive definition of the duty of public health; no wonder it is the same term that described frontier vigilance.'[2] However, isolation in the nineteenth century cannot solely be identified as a refinement of previous practices. It was inseparable from the novel sanitary approach of the new liberal states and the new requirements emerging with the development of commercial capitalism. In order to carry out potentially successful public health policies, use of political power was necessary and, as argued by Norbert Elias,[3] social acceptance (consensus) played an important part in this.[4] In Michel Foucault's terms, the development of medicine in the nineteenth century must be seen as inseparable from policies of public health involving 'the consideration of disease as a political and economic problem'. There is no doubt that liberal governments, under the pretext of healthcare and national defence, had the authority to restrict any constitutional freedom which citizens might have had in order to maintain discipline. Their power of decision extended over life and death, showing how liberal governments could reinforce the use of sanitary cordons.[5]

The fact is that in the pre-bacteriological era quarantine remained an important sanitary practice. The tremendous rise in international commerce during the nineteenth century, especially between Europe and its new African and Asian colonies, involved a reinforcement of quarantines. This was so in spite of the reluctance of the great colonial powers, especially Great Britain. However, in general terms, during the second half of the century, complete isolation – mostly inland – was progressively relaxed in compliance with the requirements of health authorities at those times. This can be seen in the debates and agreements of the International Sanitary Conferences that began in 1851, and the Spanish Health Law of 1855 that adopted many of its recommendations. These developments affected the nature of sanitary cordons in various ways. For example, control was transferred from local to central authorities. Only the central governments had the authority to decide how and when cordons should be imposed, even though these came to be generally confined to the sea borders of the state. The new liberal legislation therefore clearly placed itself against cordons in general and more so against local cordons in particular, while medical experts were divided. Such development can be observed in the Spanish Royal Orders of 24 August 1834 and 31 August 1854, as well as in the Health Law of 1855. The indiscriminate use of cordons was progressively coming to be prohibited by various states and considered by many in the scientific community as ineffective and subject to corrupt activities.[6]

The main aim of this chapter is to study the evolution of these isolationist measures taken in response to a series of epidemic outbreaks in specific inland areas of Mallorca during the nineteenth century. The main outbreaks were: 1. plague in the *Levante* (eastern) area of the island in 1820; 2. an outbreak of yellow fever in Palma in 1821; 3. cholera epidemics in Andratx in 1854 and Palma in 1865; 4. an outbreak of yellow fever again in Palma in 1870. We shall also analyse the relations between these isolationist measures with the scientific paradigms and the new public health laws of the time. Our initial hypothesis is that the relative success of the long tradition of local *cordon sanitaires*, and their observation by the population, in the absence of an accepted effective sanitary alternative, prevailed over the restrictions to their use imposed by the liberal laws. This de facto situation was founded on a tacit consensus between the local authorities and the citizens in one part, and the central government delegates in the province, especially the civil governor, on the other. The main objective would have been to overcome the conflicts created around this issue among the various authorities involved.[7]

For this study we have used various types of provincial and local documentary sources. Among the first one must highlight the collection of orders sent by the provincial authorities to the town councils dealing with epidemic outbreaks and kept in various municipal archives.[8] We have also examined the information related to public health issues contained in the municipal memorandums (*minutas*) – documents which form a continuous series throughout the century – the analysis of which is time consuming. Finally, the information deposited from 1854 onwards in the archives of the *Consell de Mallorca* (Mallorca's Council regional archive), the present-day inheritor of the nineteenth-century Provincial Council,[9] was also of importance. This institution was responsible for the organisation of quarantines and the sanitary cordons, though it counted on the cooperation of the town councils[10] and, in addition, needed the approval and assistance of the army and of course of the Ministry of Interior itself.[11] Finally, news exerpts that appeared in the official bulletins and newspapers at the time have enhanced our understanding of what happened in some detail. The different types of sources used have helped us to overcome the dispersion and fragmentation of the documentation related to the topic, enabling us to compare the perspectives of the different administrations which occasionally expressed conflicting interests.

The 'period of legality' of inland cordons (1817–55)

The period in which sanitary cordons were legally permitted and could therefore be deployed with the full support of the authorities began with the Royal Instruction of 25 August 1817 and ended with the Health General Law of 1855. This period covers the outbreaks of plague in Son Servera, Artà and Capdepera (eastern region) in 1820, and of yellow fever in Palma in 1821. In both these outbreaks similar procedures were implemented. First, as was mandatory, a blockade was put into practice, which affected the full length of Mallorca's littoral. Once the plague broke out in Son Servera, the town was cordoned off by the army to prevent the entry or exit of people. Finally, the rest of the island's towns, including the capital Palma, proceeded to set their own inland cordons, for which they mobilised their respective citizens following the decisions of the government authorities. In this way, a triple isolation affecting the different spatial realities of Mallorca was completed.

As an example of inland *cordon sanitaires*, once an outbreak of 'malignant disease' was declared in Son Servera on 27 May 1820, the provincial authorities isolated the inhabitants of this town from the rest of the island. Neighbouring towns were also included in this directive. The next day, lazarettos installed outside the walls of Palma began to function. All mail sent to the capital was sanitised with vinegar.[12] Everything indicates that before this second day of official epidemic – certainly by 19 May when rumours of infection became persistent – the rest of the island's towns had already begun to isolate themselves in an autonomous and spontaneous manner. Some weeks later, on 14 June, the provincial authorities tried to regulate their operations. They never tried to lift cordons, but they did attempt to prevent abuses and improve communication between the towns and with the capital Palma. These early measures were so successful in preventing the propagation of the epidemic beyond the towns of Son Servera, Artà and Capdepera[13] that the provincial and local authorities, as well as the population as a whole – including the medical profession – agreed to support the same 'contagionist policy'.

The greatest efforts were focused on the cordoning of the three affected localities, with the addition of nearby San Llorenç due to a suspicion of contagion which, however, was unfounded. At first, all citizens of Mallorca were urged to participate in the cordon as part of a 'sacred' and patriotic duty. The dramatic character of the official call is evident in the following text signed by Antonio María Peón, High Commander of the army in the Balearic Islands:

> the love for the Country, your individual and your countrymen's Good demand the sacrifice of yourselves if it were necessary, and of your own interests, by happily going to reinforce the line that cuts communications of those towns with the rest of the Island, and to help those who have the misfortune of being inside it.[14]

But the patriotic zeal demanded from the citizens was not considered enough to preserve the rest of the island from contagion. Direct participation of the army became necessary, although its contribution to the island's blockade and, especially, to the inland sanitary cordon that isolated the affected localities proved insufficient. Precisely 1,000 men were mobilised for the interior cordon, but the army could only gather 400 infantry and forty cavalry civilians.[15] Additionally, artillery pieces were placed on the perimeter of the isolated area and support was sought from Catalonia's Captain-General, with the intention of further increasing the military presence.[16] In parallel, repressive measures were intensified to make the cordon more effective. On 28 June 1820, 'in view of the horrible devastation caused by the infection in Son Servera and Artá', the military authorities announced the following measures:

> Those who break the cordon, or try to, will be executed on the spot. Those who escape, and the fact being proven, will be sentenced to death within 24 hours. Everybody who leaves Son Servera, Artà, San Llorenç and Capdepera after May 19th and does not report to the authorities without justification will be sentenced to death. If any of the guards or watchmen, out of negligence, let anyone pass, they will also be sentenced to death. The troops in the cordon are at war and confront an enemy. They are all subject to the Penal laws promulgated by the General Ordinances of the Army.[17]

Ultimately, the establishment of the inland sanitary cordon and the mobilisation of militarised citizens transformed the whole island into a battlefield in which war was waged for the sake of preserving health. Thus, sick people within the cordoned area were described as 'enemies', and so were those who contravened the orders included in the mandates issued by the civil and military authorities. Such mandates granted them new powers over life and death of the citizens, regardless of the 1812 Constitution restored by the liberal revolution of 1 January 1820. Isolation measures and the associated state of emergency would not be lifted until 1 February 1821.

Paradoxically, once the plague was extinguished, normality lasted only for a short time. During the month of August 1821, news of the influx of yellow fever in the port of Barcelona became increasingly persistent. In early September, rumours spread that the population of Palma had been affected. On the 13th of the same month, Mallorca's capital was blockaded with troops coming from the coastal sanitary cordon that had recently been lifted, just in time for the authorities – and surely the well-off classes – to flee from the city. It is interesting to note that in another order dated the same day, the *Junta Superior de*

Sanidad (Higher Health Board) ordered the local health committees of the rest of the island to adopt isolation measures in each of their respective localities. They were told to prepare lazarettos in order to isolate anyone arriving from the capital and to keep them under observation for ten days.[18] The isolation of Palma was now complete, to the extent that just a few days after the establishment of the local cordons, the capital was running short of food because the rural population refused to keep trade relations. Consequently, the provincial authorities established a series of safe points to restore commerce with the rest of the island. Furthermore, the self-imposed isolation of each municipal community was so effective that communications between them had also been disrupted. The provincial government of Mallorca took action to soften the situation as far as possible.

On 3 October, 1,660 civilians inhabiting *Part Forana*[19] were mobilised with the purpose of widening the perimeter of Palma's sanitary cordon, which also comprised all the healthcare facilities built since the epidemic broke out. All these men, chosen by means of quotas imposed on each locality, had to show up with guns and ammunition. Though no one was excused from being deployed on the basis of class or social station, the possibility of paying for a substitute was allowed, so that day labourers would not lose their wage. Furthermore, to guarantee interior communications, from the 5th of the same month, pedestrians were required to use passports issued by local health authorities that included details of place of origin and health condition of the holder. Individuals travelling undocumented would be arrested immediately, while those coming from Palma were required to undergo ten days of observation in the lazarettos established for local quarantines. In the end, coercive measures based on permanent surveillance and the use of the army were found to be the most effective means to preserve public health on the island.[20] As already discussed, the measures taken by the authorities did not intend to eliminate cordons but to rationalise them, in order to make them more effective and to prevent abuses against the people of Palma. Moreover, the cordon in that city was justified as the only guarantee for the restoration of some form of controlled trade exchange and secure supplies. All the time, support for isolation was total among the citizens and the authorities, as it had been during the preceding plague outbreak in the eastern region. Indeed, as occurred in the latter case, it was again possible to contain the epidemic concentrated within the inland cordon. Preventive measures had been successful.

The experiences of 1820 and 1821 are essential for understanding the favourable attitude of the general public in Mallorca, of the medical community and of the authorities, towards sanitary preservation for the rest of the century. This trend was especially reinforced when coastal blockades succeeded in preventing cholera from entering the island on various occasions until 1854. Andratx was the only place affected in August of that year.[21] In this case, as in the past, a stringent coastal cordon was established around the whole island and maintained until the danger was over. Andratx was also probably cordoned. However, we have no data about other localities[22] nor have we found orders establishing local cordons or spontaneous actions supporting them in any local sources consulted. The reasons for this may include lack of documentation and confirmation that the threat was not considered strong enough to activate local self-isolation. But this may have also been either because the number of cholera cases in Andratx was not high, or because the instructions of the medical community in Mallorca (in line with international opinion) failed to classify cholera as infectious,[23] relying on hygienist measures.

The 'period of illegality' as from 1855

As we have just shown for the case of the 1854 cholera epidemic in Andratx, the law had been progressively restricting the use of inland cordons by local communities. This situation peaked when the Health Law of 1855 declared them illegal. Thus, cordons encouraged by Mallorca's provincial authorities as a measure of sanitary watch in perfect agreement with the island town councils ended up being prohibited by the central government. Ten years after the approval of the aforementioned law, Palma experienced a first outbreak of cholera. This epidemic can be used as a case study to examine sanitary practice under the frame of the new law. The first news about the advance of cholera in the Mediterranean and in the European continent arrived in Mallorca around 21 July 1865. Curiously, the first reaction of the local press was to ask the Provincial Health Board to implement quarantine and isolation measures.[24] Not surprisingly, when the epidemic touched the peninsular coasts, between the 27th and 28th of the same month, the press intensified their demands on the authorities, insisting on the setting up of a military cordon and for stringent observation of the 'sanitary watch' in the port of Palma. Clearly, inland cordons had not lost their popularity.

At the same time, the mayor of Palma, a businessman and member of the Progressive Party, Miquel Estade Sabater, passed an edict to bring public hygiene to the top of the agenda and to make known the appointment of a permanent municipal commission with this in mind.[25] The City Council also published a number of *Health Provisions* on 22 July, based on a report requested eight days before from the local *Real Academia de Medicina y Cirugia*. Their most important contribution was to request the adoption of an eclectic point of view on cholera in relation to the dominant medical trends, which basically meant a shift from the dominant contagionist/isolationist to the miasmatic/hygienist perspective. First, the Academy 'proclaimed that the only safe and infallible means to prevent the entrance of such a frightful disease in a country is isolation of the infected localities [...] Guard the coasts of the Balearic Islands, watch suspicious ships, build lazarettos [...].'[26] In sum, it recommended the adoption of more vigorous and safe isolation measures. Nevertheless, the Academy also recommended that 'the hygienic rules Your Honor issued in the edict of last 29th of July should prevail, deserving as they do the applause and gratitude of the Academy'. Generally, we have found evidence of a special concern for the avoidance of dirt and overcrowding, as well as for the maintenance of 'clean air' in private houses.

In fact, despite the increase in coastal surveillance, a military cordon over the whole perimeter of the island had not yet been established at the beginning of August. The lazaretto in the port of Palma was unable to cope with the arrival of merchant and passenger ships.[27] On 12 August the Provincial Health Board decided that ships carrying letters suspected of contamination (initially only those coming from Marseilles and Valencia) had to move to the lazaretto of Mahon for quarantine.[28] Finally, on 20 August, the government of the province, directed by an interim governor, ordered the establishment of a militarised sanitary cordon along the coastline that, initially, was funded by all the town councils of the island, including, naturally, the capital's council.[29] Some arguments in favour of the cordon expressed by the medical authorities, and even by the press, were its ability to stop smuggling, which had been a causal factor in previous epidemics. It would also prevent potential problems posed by pilgrims returning from Mecca.[30] This last point was not a real concern for the authorities in Mallorca, but it was being widely discussed among the local and international medical profession, as shown by the minutes of the third International Health Conference that took place in Constantinople in 1866.[31]

Last, we must stress that from the arrival of the first news about cholera, during the month of July 1865, and until the end of August, it was the Palma City Council, through its board of health, that led the inland preventive sanitary measures as required by the 1855 law. For this reason, an attempt to rationalise management was made through the creation of a commission subordinated to the board, the Permanent Commission of Health and Welfare. In addition, a loan of 180,000 *escudos* was obtained from the Balearic Bank thanks to the endorsement of ten great contributors: the mayor and nine councilmen.[32] In this climate of increasing uncertainty, on 28 August, the news of the death of three people in suspicious conditions in different areas of the city was made public. It was enough to create panic and, although the authorities did not officially declare a cholera epidemic, or maybe because of this, the exodus of the middle and upper classes was massive. The more modest sectors were left, de facto, within the city.[33] Faced with this situation, the city councils of the *Part Forana* immediately decided to cordon their respective localities at their own risk, clearly contravening the law but following – as we have seen – an effective tradition. However, as a sign of the new times and differently from 1821, the capital city was not cordoned.

Curiously, on the previous day, 27 May, the new civil governor, Adolfo García de León y Pizarro, Marquis of Casa Pizarro, had arrived in Palma. His arrival had been actually delayed more than a week because the paddle steamer *Mallorca* on which he was travelling to the capital of the Balearic Islands was forced to undergo mandatory quarantine in the lazaretto of Mahon, where it remained anchored for ten days. In other words, there were no privileges with regard to quarantine measures. There is no doubt that when the civil governor finally disembarked in Palma, he found a situation that could not be more chaotic. If the escape of a large part of the population wasn't dramatic enough, the paralysis of the administrative and economic activities, combined with the serious threat of shortages of food and other supplies caused by the immediate and illegal self-isolation of the rest of Mallorca, increased the alarm exponentially.[34] In fact, the ideal conditions for a rise in poverty and social misery were being created. Hygienist doctrines had remarked that foci of unhealthiness coupled with social discontent, already under way, could lead to serious public disorder.

The new civil governor tried to develop a different approach to deal with the situation. Almost immediately, he issued a battery of seven new measures that put the focus on building special hospitals, improving medical and pharmaceutical care and securing supplies for the community. At the same time, he declared himself completely opposed to isolationist measures. This resulted in a relaxation of the coastal cordon surrounding the island.[35] The terrestrial cordoning of Palma from the rest of Mallorca was stopped, as demanded by the press and by the majority of the local political elite. Of course, the mayors of the island's towns were ordered to dissolve their defensive cordons. It was an evident hygienist turn. Naturally, right from the start, the position adopted by the civil governor raised mistrust among the municipal authorities at all levels. Let us remember that contagionist measures had always enjoyed a high degree of consensus in Mallorca. Not surprisingly, the first to reject the provisions were the mayors from localities other than Palma who, faced with the rush of emigrants from the capital, refused to lift their own cordons. Such refusal led the civil governor to issue a circular letter reminding the local authorities that their actions were unlawful.[36]

Despite this, the order had little effect. Right from the start, it was rejected in many cases and de facto in almost all. We have evidence to prove that the mayors of the *Audiencia* (judicial district) of Inca agreed that all persons arriving from Palma or any other infected place should undergo six days of quarantine before being allowed to enter their respective localities.[37] Other sources specify that, at least, Inca, Establiments, Sóller, Alaró and Alcudia[38] kept stringent isolation measures. In other localities there were incidents with the public when town councils met to decide whether to follow or not the circular letters coming from the provincial government.[39] As if this was not enough, the press, even progressive newspapers, agreed with the municipalities of the *Part Forana* and supported the reestablishment of the cordons. It is of some interest to note that the main argument raised by the press was not strictly sanitary but social and economic. Contrary to the belief of the civil governor, sanitary cordons emerged as the only real element capable of restoring confidence between the capital and its rural hinterland and, thus, as the only measure that would enable commercial exchanges, the solution for Palma's problems of subsistence. According to the daily newspaper *El Isleño*, the main problem was that food shops and taverns were closed.[40]

The strife between local mayors and the civil governor persisted until some weeks after the epidemic was over. In addition, the press echoed the fact that one of his last circular letters (dated 25 September) – which again prohibited 'categorically' the mayors and the local boards of health to set up cordons – was systematically disobeyed, generating many incidents.[41] It seems that the highest provincial authority finally gave up prohibiting cordons in practice, since everything indicates that, from this moment, his main concern was to prevent abuses rather than to eliminate them.[42] On the other hand, in reference to the coastal blockade, the army did not return to their quarters until 22 October when the danger of disease importation had completely disappeared.[43] If there was opposition from the mayors for the lifting of the cordons, the wish of the Permanent Commission of Public Health formed by individuals of the local and provincial boards of health was also favourable to establish a cordon around the capital. On 18 September, news spread that the aforementioned commission had agreed that 'Palma and villages of Mallorca should set up sanitary cordons around their cities, like the ones established in 1821 [during the yellow fever episode], in line with the wishes of the majority of the inhabitants of the island.' To a large extent opinions published in the press agreed that 'this measure rejected by the Civil Governor allowed many families to find food without incurring extraordinary costs'.[44]

Finally, it was judged unnecessary to cordon off the city of Palma because the epidemic was controlled there/elsewhere.[45] This was a result of the package of charitable and sanitary measures adopted, the creation of hospitals for the diseased and the responsibility for local isolation delegated to the city councils of the *Part Forana*. Nevertheless, the death toll was very high in Palma: some 1,962 people according to the official statistics.[46] As interesting as these figures was the conflict that broke out between the civil governor and most of the political and medical authorities of Palma over the type of sanitary measures to be adopted. Attempts to impose a strictly hygienist point of view, in addition to political circumstances – among which being the relationship between the central and local authorities within the new frame of the liberal state – created a conflict that ended with the resignation of the mayor of the city in the last days of September and the transfer of the Marquis of Casa Pizarro to another province on 4 February 1866.

The events of 1865 had a notable influence on the response to the last epidemic declared in Mallorca during the nineteenth century – the 1870 outbreak of yellow fever in Palma. From the moment that news started spreading that yellow fever was wreaking havoc in the city, most of the other localities proceeded to set up cordons to protect themselves from the capital. Hence, the three localities of the *Levante* region – Artà, Capdepera and Son Servera – decided to isolate themselves in a joint action, as noted in the agreement of the Council of Capdepera dated 30 September 1870.[47] Other towns followed suit like Alaró, on 10 October, and Alcúdia. In this last case, five days of observation for people and three days for goods coming from Palma were declared.[48] As had happened before, with the spread of news – and rumour – on the isolation of each community, travel directions in the interior of the island were established by local arrangements. Thus, the mayor of Manacor informed his counterpart in Alaró that because of the news on the outbreak of yellow fever in Inca, the transit between Alaró and Manacor should only follow the route that passed through the communities of Consell, Sencelles, Sineu and Petra.[49] These arrangements remained in place until the last week of November. It is interesting to observe the change of attitude of the provincial government during this episode and to compare it with the case of cholera in 1865. If on that occasion strict implementation of the 1855 General Law attempted by the civil governor, in evident opposition to the local authorities, triggered a political crisis of major magnitude, there was now a relaxed interpretation which clearly reduced conflicts. In fact, the governor did not forbid local cordons at any time but neither were they encouraged. All actors were just reminded that compliance with the sanitary laws was necessary and, if the communities decided to establish inland sanitary cordons, they should follow the criteria laid down by – and remain under the responsibility of – their respective health boards.[50] Recent experience had demonstrated that both coastal and inland cordons had the consent of the population and of the local medical groups.

Conclusions

During the nineteenth century, the authorities, the medical profession and the population of Mallorca positioned themselves almost unanimously in favour of inland cordons, just as they did with coastal ones, either when the law covered and encouraged this type of measure, or when these were outlawed, mainly after 1855. Medical and public preference for inland isolation had a long historical tradition. The medical profession and the media demanded the establishment of cordons even when the provincial authorities were in doubt. This made sense since the aetiology of infectious diseases was unknown until the 1880s. Additionally, the containment of the plague in the eastern area of the island in 1820, of yellow fever in Palma the next year, the preservation of the island from cholera from 1833 to 1854, and the Andratx outbreak in the latter year through the adoption of isolationist measures, all helped cordons become accepted and demanded by the Mallorcan population.[51] The restructured medical body, which came to include academics, now followed international trends and readily accepted isolation measures.[52] We must add that there was no conflict between contagionist politics and hygienist measures. Even the conflict between commercial interests, strong in the city of Palma, and contagionist politics[53] disappeared. A good sanitary watch policy enabled commerce both within the city and with its rural surroundings. In effect, one of the arguments in favour of the isolation of Palma in 1865 was the reestablishment of its exchanges with the *Part Forana*.

On the other hand, public health issues did not escape the political twists of the time. There was a clear need for negotiations between local elites and central authorities in order to increase the administrative efficiency and control of the sanitary institutions. In this sense, on the occasion of the cholera epidemic of 1865, the crisis provoked by the disputes between a majority of the population and the local authorities, on the one hand, and the civil governor (as state representative) on the other, served to further discredit Queen Isabel II's political system, which came to an end with the *Gloriosa* Revolution three years later. Moreover, let us remember that the 'social question' had appeared during the latter epidemic and transcended the power struggle that was taking place on the island. The irruption of cholera at a moment of consolidation for the new model of a liberal and centralised State produced a disruptive effect, which entailed the need for the negotiation of the Health Law of 1855.

Taking those events from a broader view, the persistence of epidemics, real or 'invisible',[54] in an increasingly globalised world and the potential they demonstrated to penetrate Mallorca's island territory, reinforced the idea that the right way to overcome this problem unavoidably involved increasing outer and inner surveillance, social control – especially of poverty – and the progressive medicalisation of society. This fact had two consequences. First, scientific and technical factors influenced political practice. As Charles E. Rosenberg[55] has argued, administrative rationale and medical advances in Western Europe were sufficient, despite their imperfections and errors, initially to minimise and finally to eradicate the danger of epidemics over less than a century. In fact, all subsequent epidemic outbreaks analysed in Mallorca were contained in their foci of origin. And from 1870 the island was free of epidemics until the influenza pandemic of 1918.

In effect, sanitary control and isolation became more adapted to the emerging culture of liberalism. In parallel with new State legislation, the advances of hygiene in certain areas of medicine, in addition to the legal reservations that might arise in the more liberal sectors of society, explain the gradual relaxation in the use of inland cordons from the second half of the nineteenth century in Mallorca. This was shown when the city of Palma was not cordoned either in 1865 or in 1870, despite the havoc wreaked by cholera and yellow fever and in spite of the calls of the press and the Permanent Commission of Health, something happened that was the exact opposite of what occurred in 1820 and 1821. From then on, one of the three most repressive means of isolation disappeared. Terrestrial containment of infectious foci was no longer used. Protection from the continent by a coastline cordon continued, as did inland defensive cordons in villages considered healthy. This implied the elimination of the most brutal form of coercion practised during epidemics of the plague in the eastern region of the island and yellow fever in Palma in 1820 and 1821, when the army acted with the right of life or death over the population. In subsequent epidemics, the troops were never used to confine the population in infected places: military forces were used only to cordon the coastline. In any case, it was the exclusive job of the local authorities to organise defensive isolations from their neighbours and, obviously, without the repressive presence of the army. These were the early signs of radical changes to come that would involve the consolidation of liberalism and the appearance of bacteriology. Yet, the persistence of coastal cordons until 1899 and of defensive isolation at the time of rupture, indicate that these measures were never completely abandoned, as the sanitary crises of the twenty-first century remind us.

Notes

We would like to express our gratitude to Mr Michael Pietroni FRCS for reviewing the text.

List of abbreviations: AGCM: Arxiu General del Consell de Mallorca (Regional Archive).

AMA: Arxiu Municipal d'Alcúdia (Municipal Archive of Alcúdia, Mallorca).

AMAl: Arxiu Municipal d'Alaró (Municipal Archive of Alaró, Mallorca).

AMAlg: Arxiu Municipal d'Algaida (Municipal Archive of Algaida, Mallorca).

AMAn: Arxiu Municipal d'Andraitx (Municipal Archive of Andraitx, Mallorca).

AMC: Arxiu Municipal de Capdepera (Municipal Archive of Capedepera, Mallorca).

AMP: Arxiu Municipal de Pollença (Municipal Archive of Pollença, Mallorca).

AMPa: Arxiu Municipal de Palma (Municipal Archive of Palma, Mallorca).

AMS: Arxiu Municipal de Sineu (Municipal Archive of Sineu, Mallorca).

BOPB: Boletín Oficial de la Provincia de las Baleares (Official provincial bulletin).

1 Pere Salas Vives, 'Libertad y/o derecho a la vida. El resguardo sanitario durante el primer liberalismo (Mallorca, siglo XIX)', *Historia Social* 68, 2010, 69–85.
2 Esteban Rodríguez Ocaña, 'El resguardo de la salud. Organización sanitaria española en el siglo XVIII', *Dynamis* 7–8, 1987–88, 145–170 (145).
3 Norbert Elias, *El proceso de la civilización. Investigaciones sociogenéticas y psicogenéticas*, Madrid, Fondo de Cultura Económica, 1987.
4 This consideration must be generically related to Max Weber's systemic theory of State growth as a part of a unique process of rationalisation (Joaquín Abellán, *Poder y política en Max Weber*, Madrid, Biblioteca Nueva, 2004). Moreover, we can specify that the new State will adopt a

mixed character, both social and military (see Michael Mann, *The Sources of Social Power, Vol. II: The Rise of Classes and Nation-States, 1760–1914*, Cambridge, Cambridge University Press, 1993; or Abram de Swaan, *In Care of the State. Health Care, Education and Welfare in Europe and the USA in the Modern Era*, Cambridge, Polity Press, 1988).

5 Traditional historiography dealing with state responses to epidemics using the arguments of Erwin H. Ackerknecht (in his article 'Anticontagionism between 1821 and 1867', *Bulletin of Historical Medicine* 81, 1948, 511–532) perpetuated the argument of assimilation, on the one hand, between the contagionist positions and the absolutist state, and on the other hand, anticontagionism and the liberal state. However, Peter Baldwin in his book *Contagion and the State in Europe, 1830–1930* (Cambridge, Cambridge University Press, 1999) revealed how restrictive sanitary politics were related to economic, geographical and administrative factors. For this reason, the importance given to commerce by Mediterranean nations facilitated the use of cordons as prophylactic measures as their costs were lower than epidemics themselves, and commercial activity tended to recover after an epidemic. Another factor that could explain why these preventive measures were used was the *geo-epidemiology of disease* related to the entry routes of epidemics. For this reason, Baldwin pointed out 'the importance of geography is revealed in the basic split between the Mediterranean countries, in close contact with the Oriental sources of cholera, and the Atlantic nations at a further remove. The division between Atlantic and Mediterranean Europe separated nations afraid of epidemics that threatened directly from the Orient from those for whom the disease became a problem mainly once it had invaded Europe itself' (Baldwin, *Contagion and the State in Europe*, 212).

6 Juan José Fernández Sanz, *El año de la vacunación de Ferrán. Trasfondo político, médico, sociodemográfico y económica de una epidemia*, Madrid, Fundación Ramón Aceres, 1990, 47–48.

7 Concepción de Castro, *La Revolución Liberal y los municipios españoles (1812–1868)*, Madrid, Alianza, 1979 and Arturo Cajal Valero, *El Gobernador Civil y el Estado centralizado del siglo XIX*, Madrid, Ministerio de Administraciones Públicas, 1999. For the Spanish context of the time, see Fernando Molina Aparicio and Miguel Cabo Villaverde, 'Historiografia i nacionalització a Espanya. Reflexions finals', *Segle XX. Revista catalana d'història* 4 2011, 161–169; Salvador Calatayud, Jesús Millán and María Cruz Romeo, 'El Estado en la configuración de la España contemporánea. Una revisión de los problemas historiográficos', in S. Calatayud, J. Millán and M. Cruz Romeo (eds), *Estado y periferias en la España del siglo XX. Nuevos enfoques*, València, Publicacions de la Universitat de València,

2009, 9–130 and Fernández Sanz, *El año de la vacunación de Ferrán*, 48–49.

8 We specifically analysed the series entitled '*Health Orders*' – a collection of orders from the superior authorities to the mayors of the towns of the island, from 1784 to 1870, deposited at the Municipal Archive of Pollença.

9 The provincial government was an elected institution presided over by the governor until 1870, and which had its origins in the 1812 Constitution. It had responsibility over all the territory of the province, in this case the Balearic Islands. Basically, it had an administrative character and collaborated or supervised the municipal activity.

10 de Swaan, *In Care of the State*; Mann, *The Sources of Social Power, Vol. II*; Lutz Raphael, *Ley y orden. Dominación mediante la administración en el siglo XIX*, Madrid, Siglo XXI, 2008; Pedro Carasa Soto (ed.), *Ayuntamiento, Estado y Sociedad. Los poderes municipales en la España contemporánea*, Valladolid, Fundación Municipal de Cultura – Instituto de Historia 'Simancas', 2000; or Joaquín del Moral Ruíz, 'Las funciones del Estado y la articulación del territorio nacional: símbolos, administración pública y servicios', in J.d. Moral Ruíz, J. Pro Ruiz and F. Suárez Bilbao (eds), *Estado y territorio en España, 1820–1930. La formación del paisaje nacional*, Madrid, Los libros de la Catarata, 2007, 17–358.

11 Joan Serrallonga Urquidi, 'Epidemias e historia social. Apuntes sobre el cólera en España, 1833–1865', *Historia Social* 24 1996, 7–21.

12 AMP-Health Orders-1681, 27, 28 and 30 May 1820.

13 AMP-Health Orders-1681, 14 June 1820.

14 AMP-Health Orders-1681, 28 June 1820.

15 Joana Sureda Trujillo, *La pesta de 1820 a Son Servera, Artà i Capdepera*, Palma de Mallorca, El Tall editorial, 1993.

16 According to the edict of 18 July that contained the final agreements of the Superior Board of Health, an official had been sent to the General Captain of Catalonia asking for the dispatch of 200 tents for troops and a new battalion of soldiers (AMP, Health Orders-1681).

17 *Antonio Maria Peón*, AMP, Health Orders-1681.

18 AMP, Health Orders–1681: notice from the Balearic Superior Board of Health, 13 September 1821.

19 The historical name of the Island territory excluding the capital city.

20 AMP, Health Orders–1681: notice from the Balearic Superior Board of Health, 3 October 1821 and public announcement from the Balearic Superior Board, 5 October 1821.

21 Unofficially, news of cholera cases in Andratx arrived from at least 8 August (AMAlg-Municipal minutes, 9 August 1854), while the Official Bulletin of the Balearic Province did not offer confirmation until the 25th of the same month (BOPB-3390 25 August 1854).

22 The Municipal Archive of Andratx was destroyed during the 1868 Revolution.
23 Stephen Halliday, 'Death and miasma in Victorian London: an obstinate belief', *BMJ* 323, 2001, 1469–1471; Krista Maglen, '"The first line of defence": British quarantine and the Port Sanitary Authorities in the nineteenth century', *Social History of Medicine* 15, 3, 2002, 413–428 or Valeska Huber, 'The unification of the globe by disease? The international sanitary conferences on cholera, 1851–1894', *The Historical Journal* 49, 2, 2006, 453–476; these among other authors discuss the scientific debates that occurred to determine whether cholera was an infectious disease or not.
24 Juan Llabrés Bernal, *Noticias y relaciones históricas de Mallorca: siglo XIX*, Palma de Mallorca, Imprenta Alcover, 1959, 301.
25 Joana Maria Pujadas-Mora, 'Les epidèmies "invisibles" i "visibles" de còlera a la Ciutat de Palma: gestió municipal (Segle XIX)', Departament de Ciències Històriques i Teoria de les Arts, Palma de Mallorca, Universitat de les Illes Balears, 2005.
26 Alcaldía Constitucional de Palma, *Disposiciones sanitarias*, Palma de Mallorca, Imprenta de Pedro J. Gelabert, 1865, 2.
27 Junta Provincial de Sanidad de las Baleares, *Memoria dirigida por la Junta Provincial de Sanidad de las Baleares al M. I. Señor Gobernador de la provincia sobre la aparición y desarrollo del cólera en estas islas en el año de 1865 y resoluciones acordadas para combatirle, principalmente en la capital, precedida por una comunicación documentada con que dicha autoridad la eleva al Exmo. Sr. Ministro de la Gobernación*, Palma de Mallorca, Imprenta de Pedro J. Gelabert, 1865, 30.
28 Llabrés Bernal, *Noticias y relaciones históricas de Mallorca*, 305.
29 AGCM, Establishment of the sanitary cordon (ECS), S-III-249/33. For more information on this issue, see: Salas Vives, 'Libertad y/o derecho a la vida', 69–85. On the other hand, it should be remembered that the participation of the Captain-General was essential to establish a military cordon (Pujadas-Mora, 'Les epidèmies "invisibles" i "visibles" de cólera').
30 This circumstance is already highlighted in the first page of the book by the Alcaldía Constitucional de Palma, *Disposiciones sanitarias*, or by the Junta Provincial de Sanidad de las Baleares, *Memoria dirigida por la Junta Provincial de Sanidad de las Baleares*.
31 Valeska Huber, 'The unification of the globe by disease?', 462; and Josep Lluis Barona Vilar and Josep Bernabeu-Mestre, *La salud y el Estado. El movimiento sanitario internacional y la administración española (1851–1945)*, València, Publicacions de la Universitat de València, 2008, 39.
32 The loan was finally signed on 28 August (Llabrés Bernal, *Noticias y relaciones históricas de Mallorca*, 308).

33 Ibid. Obviously this was not a unique reaction, since similar actions are to be observed in many other cities struck by epidemics, as argued in Francesc Bonamusa and Joan Serrallonga, *Del roig al groc. Barcelona, 1868–1871. Quintes i epidèmies*, Barcelona, L'Avenç, 1995, 135.

34 To be precise, the Health Law of 1855 specified that: 'As a general rule, the adoption of quarantine systems is prohibited. When special circumstances suggest some interior coercive measures, the Government will advise how they should be put in place' to avoid abuses as in the cases that occurred in Spain during the previous epidemic in 1854–1855 (F. Javier Blanco Segarra, Mariano Galant Torregrosa and Francisco Sala Aniorte, 'La Junta de Sanidad de Torrevieja en el cólera de 1885', in À. Beneito Lloris, F.-X. Blay Meseguer and J. Lloret Pastor (eds), *Beneficència i sanitat en els municipis valencians (1813–1942)*, Alcoi, Seminari d'Estudis Sobre la Ciència – Associació Cultural Alcoià-Comtat – Centre Alcoià d'Estudis Històrics i Arqueològics, 1999, 311–330, 317).

35 Thus, on 5 September the Governor let the General-Captain know that he could remove his troops from the district of Palma and later from the rest of the island (AGCM-Establishment of the sanitary cordonS-III-246/21, 5 September 1865).

36 Notice from the Provincial Government, 29 August 1865 (BOPB, núm. 5129, 30–8–1865).

37 AMA-Municipal minutes, 10 September 1865.

38 J. de Oleza y de España, 'Episodio en la vida de un pueblo. El cólera de 1865 en Palma. La Gente balear durante la epidemia. Lazareto, cuarentenas, cordones sanitarios y disposiciones legales', *Boletín Estadística Municipal de Palma* 59, 1966, 5–9, 5.

39 This was the case in Sineu (AMS-Municipal minute: 1–9–1865), for example. In Alcúdia, however, the cordon was imposed on 3 November, right after the Governor's circular letter (AMA-Municipal minute: 3 September 1865).

40 *El Isleño,* 12 September 1865 and Llabrés Bernal, *Noticias y relaciones históricas de Mallorca,* 313.

41 Ibid., 317.

42 BOPB-5132, 25 September 1865.

43 AMA-Municipal minutes, 22 October 1865.

44 Llabrés Bernal, *Noticias y relaciones históricas de Mallorca,* 316. Nevertheless, we must note that the Mayor of Palma, Miquel Estade, never voted in favour of the land cordoning of his city, although at the end he did not speak publicly against the decision that was adopted by the Health Board of Palma that he chaired (Minute of the Municipal Board of Health and Charity, AMPa, FP, 1514 / VII).

45 For more details about the cholera epidemic that hit Palma in 1865, see Pere Salas and Joana M. Pujadas, 'El Cólera como conflicto y factor de legitimación', *Ayer* 101, 2016, 189–212.
46 Due to the lack of a precise epidemiologic study, this fact has been obtained from the mortuary registry of the deaths in this city and its municipal area from 1 August to 15 December during the cholera epidemic of 1865 (AMPa, Lligall Nou, 2102/2).
47 AMC-Municipal minutes, 30 September 1870.
48 AMA-Municipal minutes, 30 October 1870. We must note that local doctors considered the number of days of quarantine as insufficient.
49 AMAl-Municipal minutes, 30 October 1870.
50 Specifically, the council of Andratx received a circular letter from the Civil Government dated 24 October which stipulated 'Applicable Health laws have to be fulfilled and councils are responsible for this. Such boards must observe the case of establishment of terrestrial sanitary cordons.' Curiously, Andratx was one of the only cases in which its health board recommended not establishing any sanitary cordon (AMAn-Municipal minutes-92/48, 26 October 1870).
51 Similar terms to those proposed in Elias, *El proceso de la civilización.*
52 Eva Canaleta Safont and Isabel Moll Blanes, 'El discurso de los cirujanos como vía de formación científica y de reivindicación, 1847–1868', in I. Porras, B. Gutiérrez, M. Ayarzagüena and J. de las Heras (eds), *Transmisión del conocimiento médico, e internacionalización de las prácticas sanitarias: una reflexión histórica; XVI Congreso de la SEHM celebrado del 15 al 18 de junio de 2011*, Ciudad Real, 2011.
53 For George Davey Smith, 'Commentary: behind the Broad Street pump: aetiology, epidemiology and prevention of cholera in mid-19th century Britain', *International Journal of Epidemiology* 31, 2002, 920–932 (930) following Sylvia Tesch, the most relevant fact about sanitation in the nineteenth century was its proximity to capitalism, searching for a unique or reduced group of causes resposible for cholera that helped to minimise other types of problems arising from the economic and social structure.
54 Pujadas-Mora, 'Les epidèmies "invisibles" i "visibles" de còlera'.
55 Charles E. Rosenberg, 'Cholera in nineteenth-century Europe: a tool for social and economic analysis', *Comparative Studies in Society and History* 8, 4, 1966, 452–463.

Index

EU authorised representative for GPSR:
Easy Access System Europe, Mustamäe tee 50,
10621 Tallinn, Estonia
gpsr.requests@easproject.com

www.ingramcontent.com/pod-product-compliance
Ingram Content Group UK Ltd.
Pitfield, Milton Keynes, MK11 3LW, UK
UKHW021834100926
8556IPUK00004B/335
* 9 7 8 1 5 2 6 1 1 5 5 4 6 *